GOVERNING
GLOBAL
HEALTH

GOVERNING GLOBAL HEALTH

*WHO RUNS THE WORLD
AND WHY?*

CHELSEA CLINTON AND DEVI SRIDHAR

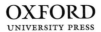

OXFORD
UNIVERSITY PRESS

OXFORD
UNIVERSITY PRESS

Oxford University Press is a department of the University of Oxford.
It furthers the University's objective of excellence in research, scholarship,
and education by publishing worldwide. Oxford is a registered trade mark of
Oxford University Press in the UK and in certain other countries.

Published in the United States of America by Oxford University Press
198 Madison Avenue, New York, NY 10016, United States of America

Names: Clinton, Chelsea, author. | Sridhar, Devi Lalita, author.
Title: Governing global health : who runs the world and why? / Chelsea
Clinton and Devi Sridhar.
Description: New York, NY : Oxford University Press, [2017]
Identifiers: LCCN 2016022370| ISBN 9780190253271 (hardcover : alk. paper) |
ISBN 9780190253295 (e-book) | ISBN 9780190253295 (e-book)
Subjects: | MESH: World Health Organization. | Global Health |
International Cooperation
Classification: LCC RA441 | NLM WA 530.1 | DDC 362.1—dc23
LC record available at https://lccn.loc.gov/2016022370

1 3 5 7 9 8 6 4 2
Printed by Sheridan Books Inc., United States of America

For Charlotte and Aidan, with all my love, Chelsea
For Sadegh, with all my love, Devi

TABLE OF CONTENTS

Preface   viii
Abbreviations   xiii

1. Governing Global Health   1

2. Big Questions and Case Studies   23

3. Shifts in Governance   48

4. Who Funds Global Health?   83

5. Twenty-First-Century Governance   119

6. Disruption and Reform   161

7. Final Reflections   202

Notes   217
Index   267

PREFACE

Throughout our travels across the world, whether to slums in New Delhi, health clinics in Port-au-Prince, or ministries of health in Liberia and Brazil, the health of all people has been at the forefront of our minds. How can we, alongside so many others, make a contribution to global health?

That question is what prompted us to write this book. The same question should be at the top of the agenda set by every government, international development institution, and nongovernment organization (NGO). While health policy debates raise enormously complex issues about institutions, finance, behavior, and the role of markets, no issue has a more profound bearing on the human condition than health. As mothers of young children, we are acutely aware of the role that health systems play during periods of vulnerability. Efficient and equitable health systems save lives and break the link between sickness and poverty. They are an integral part of the social contract.

We are also aware that for millions of women, children, and disadvantaged people around the world, the absence of efficient, effective, and equitable health systems is a source of vulnerability and distress, and part of a vicious cycle of poverty. Our concern in this book is to ask what at a global level can be done to change this picture.

Why now? At first glance, we live in the best of times of public health. People live longer than ever before. Child mortality is falling at an accelerating rate. In the first fifteen years of the twenty-first century, child deaths fell from ten million to just under six million deaths per year. According to UNICEF, roughly forty-eight million lives have been saved through a combination of more skilled birth attendants and higher vaccination rates (along with increased economic development and girls' education, and other factors).[1] Major killers like malaria, pneumonia, measles, and HIV/AIDS are in retreat in the face of improved access to effective prevention, care, and new medicines. In all of these areas, national policy backed by international cooperation has made and continues to make a difference. Untold millions of people are living healthier, more productive, and longer lives than ever before.

Viewed from a different perspective, we are living in the worst of times. Never has the gap between what we are capable of achieving—based on what we already know works—and what we actually achieve been greater. HIV/AIDS rates are not falling for all populations, everywhere. In 2014, tuberculosis, one of the world's oldest diseases, claimed more lives than HIV/AIDS. And, while we live in a world of astonishing technical progress and scientific advance, every year one million children die on the day of their birth and another million die in their first week. If there is one figure that demolishes any cause for complacency over what we have achieved since 2000, it is the sixteen thousand child deaths that occur every single day. The overwhelming majority of these deaths could be prevented through simple, effective, and affordable health interventions or preventative measures we know work. Yet the human toll continues.

For anyone needing a reminder of the destructive potential of ill health it arrived in the form of the 2014/2015 Ebola outbreak. The epidemic was preventable and containable. Yet more than twelve thousand people died and worldwide fear about a global pandemic took hold.

Both the ongoing crisis in child mortality and the Ebola epidemic illustrate in very different ways what happens when health systems fail. Of course, what is achievable in health is influenced by national wealth. Yet we know of all too many cases of relatively wealthy countries that achieve far less than they could, in part because of their failure to combat health inequalities. Equally, there is no shortage of compelling counterexamples of relatively poor countries that "over-perform" because they have put in place the foundations for equitable health systems and received international support to bolster their efforts.

We both have spent much of our academic and professional careers thinking about where we can make a unique contribution to solving major global health challenges and then working toward doing so. What is clear from our experiences—working at different levels from a village to a boardroom—is that all health problems, whether child mortality, infectious diseases, Ebola, or mental health, need institutional support and resources. In addition to our academic work, we are deeply engaged with institutions such as Partners in Health, the Clinton Foundation, the Clinton Health Access Initiative, and Save the Children. This reflects our conviction that far more should be done to join up the best academic research with practical action.

We share a long-standing interest in institutions for the simple reason that institutions matter. It is through institutions that nations have organized and focused efforts to protect and improve the health of their citizens. Today, however, health governance has gone global.

We identify three key drivers of global governance in health. First, there is a growing recognition that health problems go beyond borders and the capacity of national governments alone—and that intergovernmental cooperation is required for an effective response, even within a country. Second, the increasingly important roles that NGOs, the private sector, and philanthropies have played over the past few decades has led to new demands from these groups for a voice—and even votes—in global governance decision-making. Third, it is increasingly evident that global challenges require collective action solutions that need to be efficient and equitable, with fair sharing of the benefits and costs of cooperation.

Global governance is formally conducted by and across national governments through international institutions, underpinned by financing to enable them to fulfill their missions and by rules to structure interaction. Traditionally, studies of international global health institutions look at what exactly they do, exploring questions such as how many lives have they saved, or whether they provide value for money. These are crucial questions. In this book we take a different approach, stepping back to ask why institutions behave the way they do, what decisions are made by whom, and how influence is exercised, whether by governments or nonstate actors.

This book grew out of a series of conversations between the two of us and with our colleagues about recent scholarship on global health in general and the role of the four largest institutions in global health, as measured by annual resources invested—the World Health Organization; the World Bank; the Global Fund to Fight AIDS, Tuberculosis and Malaria; and Gavi, the Vaccine Alliance.

We were struck by what was missing from that vast body of scholarship. For example, international relations scholars have paid scant attention to all four global health behemoths although the World Bank has received scrutiny in areas beyond health. As a consequence, most of the questions we probe here have not been explored in a coherent, comparative manner, including the governance of each institution, their respective financing bases, and how each includes, or does not include, nonstate actors in its governance at the Board or operational level. We believe using tools drawn from international relations provides insight into each question's answers and helps explain the differences across the four large players in global health. We hope our efforts here fill some of the scholarship gaps, for the students we teach in our respective global health governance courses and for anyone else who may be interested in understanding the global health landscape—who runs that world and why.

We are deeply grateful to everyone who helped make this project possible. Professor Ngaire Woods has been a mentor to us, and we are grateful for her guidance and her wisdom, and for making our initial connection to one another. Our respective colleagues at Columbia University's Mailman School of Public Health and the University of Edinburgh have provided support and encouragement throughout every stage of this book. In particular, we are grateful to professors Michael Sparer, Igor Rudan, Harry Campbell, and Sarah Cunningham-Burley.

To Tim Evans of the World Bank (and formerly of WHO), Mark Dybul of the Global Fund, Seth Berkley and Kevin Klock of Gavi, and Marc Van Ameringen of GAIN, thank you for all of the time each of you took with us throughout our work on this book: it is stronger for your input. Additionally, we are grateful to everyone in your respective offices who worked to coordinate our calls and conversations.

This book would not have been finished as quickly, nor would it have been as much fun to work on and write, without the instrumental support of research and editorial assistance from Karolina Puskarczyk, Ishani Premaratne, Anthony Maher, Katharine Heus, Gabrielle Geonnotti, and Marine Kiromera. We are also thankful to Mailman's Health Policy and Management Department's research support program for providing funding at a crucial juncture.

A number of people were generous in taking time to read all or part of the manuscript, including our editor at Oxford University Press (OUP) David McBride, and our copy editor, Mary Sutherland, as well as our reviewers, Eric Goosby, Larry O. Gostin, and several anonymous readers. We are also grateful to Amy Whitmer and Katie Weaver at OUP for their advice and assistance. Additionally, we could not imagine our work without the work and inspiration of Eric, Larry, and so many other colleagues in the fields of global health and international relations, and we want to thank professors Peter Piot, Kevin Watkins, and Julio Frenk in particular.

None of what we do today would be possible without our families, including our grandparents, our parents, our husbands, and our children. We thank all for their support, whether over decades or years, and we could not imagine our lives or our work without all of you. Thank you to Marc, Charlotte, and Aidan, Sadegh, Lea, and Kian for your support, your faith, your joy, and your love.

This book is possible only because of all the people we have thanked and the countless others who over the years have taught us, informed us, worked with us, and inspired us. Any mistakes that remain are our responsibility alone.

ABBREVIATIONS

———⟫•◦•⟪———

AMC	Advance Market Commitment
BMJ	Formerly *British Medical Journal*
CASs	Country Assistance Strategies
CCMs	Country-coordinating mechanisms
CHAI	Clinton Health Access Initiative
CRS	Creditor Reporting System
CSOs	civil society organizations
CVI	Children's Vaccine Initiative
DAC	Development Assistance Committee
DAH	development assistance for health
DALYs	Disability Adjusted Life Years
DFID	Department for International Development
ECOSOC	UN Economic and Social Council
FAO	Food and Agricultural Organization
FIFs	Financial Intermediary Funds
GAIN	Global Alliance for Improved Nutrition
Gates Foundation	Bill & Melinda Gates Foundation
GAO	U.S. Government Accountability Office
Gavi	Global Alliance for Vaccines and Immunization
GHO	Global Health Observatory

GNI	gross national income
GOBI	Growth monitoring, Oral rehydration, Breastfeeding, and Immunization
GPEI	Global Polio Eradication Initiative
GPSA	Global Partnership for Social Accountability
HNP	Health, Nutrition, and Population
HSS	Health Systems Strengthening
HRITF	Health Results Innovation Trust Fund
IAVI	International AIDS Vaccine Initiative
IATI	International Aid Transparency Initiative
IBRD	International Bank for Reconstruction and Development
ICSID	International Centre for Settlement of Investment Disputes
IDA	International Development Association
IEG	Independent Evaluation Group
IFC	International Finance Corporation
IFFIm	International Financing Facility for Innovation Mechanism
IHME	Institute for Health Metrics and Evaluation
IHR	International Health Regulations
ILO	International Labor Organization
IMF	International Monetary Fund
IRC	Independent Review Committee
LFAs	Local Fund Agents
LNHO	League of Nations Health Organization
MAP	Multi-Country HIV/AIDS Program
MDGs	Millennium Development Goals
MERS	Middle East Respiratory Syndrome
MIGA	Multilateral Investment Guarantee Agency
MSF	Médecins sans Frontières/Doctors Without Borders
NCDs	Noncommunicable Diseases
NGO	Nongovernmental Organization
OCHA	UN Office for the Coordination of Humanitarian Affairs
ODA	Official Development Assistance
OECD	Organization for Economic Cooperation and Development
OHCHR	Office of the High Commissioner for Human Rights

OIHP	Office International d'Hygiène Publique
PAHO	Pan American Health Organization
PBF	performance-based funding
PEPFAR	U.S. President's Emergency Plan for AIDS Relief
PHEIC	Public Health Emergency of International Concern
PPP	Public-Private Partnerships
PRs	Principal Recipients
PSI	Population Services International
QAG	Quality Assurance Group
QER	Quality Enhancement Review
RBM	Roll Back Malaria
SDGs	Sustainable Development Goals
SIP	Strategic Investment Plan
SMS	short message service/text message
TRIPS	Trade-Related Aspects of Intellectual Property Rights
TRP	Technical Review Panel
UHC	universal health coverage
UNAIDS	United Nations Programme on HIV and AIDS
UNDP	UN Development Programme
UNESCO	UN Educational, Scientific and Cultural Organization
UNFPA	UN Population Fund
UNHCR	UN Refugee Agency
UNICEF	UN Children's Emergency Fund
UN-IGME	United Nations Interagency Group for Child Mortality Estimation
UNODC	UN Office on Drugs and Crime
WFP	UN Food Programme
WHO	World Health Organization

GOVERNING
GLOBAL
HEALTH

1

Governing Global Health

The 2014/15 outbreak of the highly infectious and often fatal Ebola fever in West Africa and the ongoing challenge of containing Zika virus highlight the need for global cooperation in health. Ebola in particular exposed a global community altogether unprepared to effectively manage a lethal infectious disease outbreak and ensure that the most vulnerable communities did not suffer needlessly and on their own. As of March 2015, Ebola had infected more than twenty-eight thousand people and claimed over eleven thousand lives,[1] brought national health systems to their knees, rolled back hard-won social and economic gains in a region still recovering from civil wars, sparked worldwide panic, and cost billions of dollars in short-term control efforts and economic losses.[2]

Ebola, along with the outbreak of Middle East Respiratory Syndrome (MERS), the resurgence of polio in the Middle East, South Asia, Africa, and Ukraine, and as of early 2016 the newly arrived Zika virus throughout the Americas, with its confirmed terrible effects for pregnant mothers and unborn children, are only the latest examples demonstrating that governments acting in isolation cannot control the spread of infectious diseases. With Zika, this posture may have been understandable had the virus's multidecadal pattern lasted into perpetuity. From when Zika was first identified in Uganda in 1947 until 2007, health officials confirmed a scant fourteen sporadic cases across Africa and Southeast Asia. As we know now, tragically, Zika did not stay confined to that pattern. The first major Zika outbreak occurred on the Micronesian island of Yip in 2007. At the time, no serious illnesses were identified in conjunction with that Zika outbreak; there were no Zika-linked cases of microcephaly, a condition in which a baby's head is significantly smaller than average and which often leads to an underdeveloped brain.[3] Zika's most recent outbreak is much more frightening, particularly because of the now confirmed link to microcephaly as well as other brain and autoimmune diseases.[4]

The current outbreak of Zika began in Brazil in May 2015. Less than a year later, as of early March 2016, local Zika virus transmission is gripping more than two dozen countries and US territories, with travel-related cases showing up around the globe. The Zika virus is expected to soon mimic the geography of where Dengue fever is endemic today, given the two diseases share a vector in the same type of mosquito. Similar to Zika, Dengue remained largely isolated until the mid-twentieth century. Today, Dengue is endemic on every continent save Antarctica, and more than 40 percent of the world's population lives in countries with local Dengue virus transmission.[5] The rapid spread of Zika following so closely on Ebola's heels—in a different part of the world—reveals yet again how vulnerable we are and how collectively unprepared we remain. In fact, in December 2015, Zika virus did not appear on a list published by the World Health Organization (WHO) on the most likely pathogens to cause severe outbreaks without vaccines and drugs (Ebola did appear on the list).[6] A little over a month later during the WHO Executive Board meeting in Geneva, Margaret Chan, the Director-General, announced that Zika virus and its associated conditions, such as microcephaly, constituted a Public Health Emergency of International Concern.

In the book's conclusion, we offer thoughts on how we believe the world can better prepare to combat Zika, the next outbreak of Ebola, and whatever unsuspected infectious threat may (or will) emerge in the future. What is clear is that in the twenty-first century, preparing for a specific, known disease or virus in isolation is not an adequate strategy for protecting public health anywhere.

The AIDS epidemic, now into its fourth decade, is the most obvious example of isolation's failures to protect public health at a national or global level. Recognition of those failures is evident in the global cooperation that led to the creation of the Global Fund to Fight HIV/AIDS, Tuberculosis and Malaria. Yet, it is clear that the world needs periodic reminders that global agreements negotiated among governments are crucial to protecting the health of their individual countries' citizens. The 2015 Lancet–Harvard School of Public Health (HSPH)–London School of Hygiene and Tropical Medicine (LSHTM) Independent Panel on the Global Response to Ebola, which we both were members of, argued that the outbreak was "a stark reminder of the fragility of health security in an interdependent world, and of the importance of building a more robust global system so that all people may be protected from such threats."[7]

While contagion, or fear of contagion, has been the main driver of cooperation between governments over the past few centuries, other health challenges are equally important. For example, in 2015, under-five child mortality was 5.9 million worldwide, a staggeringly high number though considerably lower than the 12.7 million children under five estimated to have died in 1990.[8] What makes these deaths so tragic is that many are vaccine-preventable, and many more could be averted if every expectant mother delivered under the care of a trained birth attendant. In addition, more people in the twenty-first century die of noncommunicable diseases (NCDs), such as heart disease, cancer, and diabetes, than of communicable diseases, such as tuberculosis (TB) and HIV/AIDS, in all but the poorest countries.[9] NCDs now kill thirty-eight million people around the world every year, yet we know how health systems can help effectively prevent and treat many of the most significant NCDs.[10] Road traffic accidents kill 1.3 million people per year and are the single biggest source of fatalities among fifteen- to nineteen-year-olds in developing countries and the second leading cause of death among five- to fourteen-year-olds. For every death in this category, up to fifty people are injured or disabled.[11] We know how to prevent many of these deaths as well, through a combination of better infrastructure, safer and more affordable transportation options, more safety-conscious laws, education, and, yes, stronger health systems. All these challenges require transnational and multisectoral solutions.

Outbreaks such as Ebola are precisely the type of crisis world governments had in mind when they created the WHO in 1948 and placed it at the center of global health governance—the rules and the related formal and informal institutions, norms, and processes that govern or directly influence global health policy. The essential functions of health governance, which historically have been the purview of WHO and its governing board, include convening key stakeholders, defining shared values, establishing standards and regulatory frameworks, setting priorities, mobilizing and aligning resources, and promoting research. All of these are vital to mounting responses to prevent and treat infectious diseases and NCDs alike.

Global governance requires governments to forgo aspects of their individual sovereignty by delegating certain prerogatives and authorities to an international agency like WHO. The clearest delegation comes in rule-setting, as is evident in the International Health Regulations (IHR), which establish how countries must respond to international health risks.[12]

In recent years, new organizations have crowded the global health stage; WHO no longer stands alone in global health governance, nor arguably even at its center. Specific concerns—about HIV/AIDS and child mortality for example—have brought more money into the global health system. But those additional funds are often channeled through new institutions created specifically for such purposes (both to address specific health concerns and to steward funds dedicated to those specific areas). Some new efforts work with WHO, some outside it, and some do both. In contrast to the wide, integrated mandate of WHO, most of these new organizations have a vertical focus, concentrating on relatively narrow goals, such as a particular disease (like HIV/AIDS) or challenge (like child mortality). We now turn briefly to examining how global cooperation for health has evolved over the past century and a half before addressing questions of cooperation today.

HISTORY OF GLOBAL HEALTH COOPERATION

The earliest efforts among states to cooperate focused on the control of infectious disease, specifically cholera.[13] In 1348, the first recorded quarantine laws were introduced in Venice as an effort to control the spread of the bubonic plague, or the Black Death. But it was not until the nineteenth century that governments began to recognize that, in an era of increasing international travel and trade, individual quarantine efforts would not be sufficient to contain cholera. Between 1816 and 1899, there were six global cholera pandemics, all of which are presumed to have originated in Asia and the Middle East. Each time, cholera spread rapidly along established routes of travel and commerce into Russia, Poland, Austria, and eventually the rest of Europe (1816–26, 1829–51, 1852–60, 1863–75, 1881–96, 1899–1923).[14] It was these cholera pandemics, as well as threats of yellow fever, bubonic plague, smallpox, and typhus, that inspired the development of modern international health regulations, echoes of which are still evident today in the most recent IHR edition.[15]

The first International Sanitary Conference convened in Paris in 1851, a few years before John Snow's famous Broad Street map linking cholera transmission to polluted water in England and Filippo Pacini's discovery of the cholera bacteria in Italy.[16] Through eleven successive meetings of the International Sanitary Conference, delegates from across Europe, Latin America, China, Japan, Turkey, Persia (today Iran), Haiti, Liberia, and the United States would at various points join the efforts to establish a set of rules and norms governing how the world would respond to cholera and other serious infectious outbreak threats.[17]

Cooperation was also occurring at regional and local levels, as well as in what today we would refer to as civil society and professional associations. The International Red Cross emerged in part as a response to the needless loss of life due to poor medical care for soldiers during the Second Italian War of 1859 (sometimes referred to as the Franco-Austrian War or the Austro-Sardinian War). The first International Congress of Charities, Corrections, and Philanthropy met in Brussels in 1865 and periodically thereafter until 1914; one of the topics their meetings addressed was that of infant mortality.[18] International professional associations emerged for chemists (pharmacists), ophthalmologists, and surgeons. At the regional level, in 1902, the United States helped found the Pan American Health Organization (PAHO) in response to a yellow fever outbreak that had started in Latin America and spread north; PAHO remains the oldest international public health agency in the world today.

In 1903, twenty countries—the "great powers" in Europe, the United States, Persia, Brazil, and Egypt—gathered in Paris and joined in a consolidated agreement, including guidelines and rules, on how all signatories would deal with future outbreaks of cholera, plague, and yellow fever. The first putatively global health agency came into being four years after that 1903 agreement. In 1907, international cooperation in public health further advanced when governments created the Office International d'hygiène Publique (OIHP), based in Paris. Applying the quickly evolving techniques of epidemiological surveillance, data collecting, disease reporting, and communications technologies, OIHP's member governments intended that this new office would help keep them – as well as the broader international public health community – informed about possible disease outbreaks. They also expected OIHP to provide guidance toward refining quarantine policies that better matched new innovations in rail, automobile, and steamship travel. It is worth nothing that OIHP was entirely dependent on its member states to self-report outbreaks to it, similar to WHO's continued reliance today on self-reporting by its member states of suspected outbreaks or other health concerns.[19]

With the creation of the League of Nations in 1919, following the end of World War I, negotiations coalesced around a proposal for an international health organization that would work in collaboration with OIHP as well as PAHO, the International Red Cross, labor groups, and philanthropies such as the Rockefeller Foundation's International Health Board. The resulting League of Nation's Health Organization (LNHO) was positioned as an advisor to the League of Nations, not independent of it, and as a cooperating partner of the International Labor Organization and the International Red Cross, although those expectations were relaxed over time. Perhaps the most intriguing aspect of the League of Nations' health legacy was the hope among some constituents that it would expand its focus beyond infectious epidemics to include nutrition, parasitic infestations, improved housing and working conditions, safe water supplies, maternal and child health, alcohol and drug abuse, and health systems design. Indeed, the LNHO worked with China throughout the late 1920s and early 1930s on designing a health-care system, including a strong focus on maternal and child health, and with selected Latin American countries on infant mortality in the late 1920s.

Much of the actual work of the short-lived LNHO, however, was devoted to the surveillance and control of epidemic disease. This was arguably the inevitable result of it being a small institution dependent on a small group of powerful member states. It never employed more than thirty people at its headquarters, had a relatively small budget, and relied significantly on preexisting entities like OIHP as well as volunteers or temporary assignments (secondments) from the wealthier member states. By 1927 the LNHO received regular surveillance reports, largely by telegraph, from 140 port cities around the world.[20] From the wealthier states' perspective, infectious diseases posed a significant threat to their trading businesses, particularly for those with colonial empires and territories, and consequently to their citizens living and working around the world.[21] These concerns were similar to what had motivated the Sanitary Conferences—an emphasis on keeping national populations secure, wherever they may reside. Additionally, strategies on how to prevent and control such threats also would have appeared obvious to wealthier member states' representatives. In fact, in the nineteenth and early decades of the twentieth century, advancements in public health (such as separating out sanitation and water), medicine, and surgical care in the wealthier world led to lower burdens of disease in children and fewer maternal deaths.

Still, the LNHO's heavy focus on infectious disease monitoring and reporting did not mean that no attention was paid to noninfectious disease health concerns. In addition to country-specific work, it did provide guidance on what appropriate sanitation entailed and made health systems recommendations, such as suggesting that countries have one doctor for every two thousand people, a ratio many developing countries are still far from reaching today. However, declining donor support throughout the 1930s limited the LNHO's work, particularly on noninfectious diseases. While the Health Committee (the LNHO oversight body) last formally met in Paris in 1939, the League of Nation's Health Section (the working body of the organization) continued working throughout the early 1940s on issues such as how countries could best protect refugees' health.[22] Despite these efforts, international health cooperation was largely stagnant until after World War II.

As was true in international cooperation broadly, World War II and its aftermath reshaped international cooperation in health. In 1948, governments created WHO to direct and coordinate international health work. Its constitution defined health as "a state of complete physical, mental and social well-being and not merely the absence of disease or infirmity." Going even farther, Thomas Parran, the US Surgeon General at the time, noted, "The World Health Organization is a collective instrument which will promote physical and mental vigor, prevent and control disease, expand scientific health knowledge, and contribute to the harmony of human relations. In short, it is a powerful instrument forged for peace."[23] The faith governments had in WHO at inception was clear in its membership. All member states of the United Nations (UN) signed WHO's constitution, the first UN agency to be so broadly sanctioned.[24]

In its early years, WHO built on the work of the LNHO and OIHP.[25] It worked with governments on their efforts to improve hygiene and environmental health; it supported the development and application of new technologies to control major infectious diseases such as malaria, syphilis, tuberculosis, and yaws (a contagious, debilitating bacterial infection). These and other such missions largely went hand in hand with postwar reconstruction efforts. WHO's most cited success from its early years was its initiative to eradicate smallpox.[26] This effort was also notable as it marked a rare moment of US and Soviet Union cooperation in the UN system. The Soviet Union sponsored the first global smallpox eradication resolution in 1958. Yet the effort lacked momentum until 1966; that year, the United States and other countries joined the Soviet Union in a new eradication resolution with a time horizon of eradicating the disease within ten years. Under WHO leadership, the world almost made the ambitious decade goal; in 1979, an expert WHO commission certified the world had indeed defeated smallpox.[27]

Even during this so-called golden era of smallpox eradication, WHO struggled with an internal debate over its fundamental mission.[28] There was ongoing tension between a "vertical" approach, which tackled specific (largely infectious) diseases without addressing general health services and prevention needs, and a "horizontal" approach, which looked to strengthen entire health systems and support basic-care services that would deliver broad-based, integrative, and long-term improvements in public health including, over time, making progress against infectious diseases.[29] Almost from the beginning, bilateral donors favored vertical interventions because measurable results were easier to demonstrate over a shorter time frame, by quantifying, for example, the number of bed nets delivered or vaccines administered. These programs were also easier for donors to monitor and control, given that they typically had separate funding allocation processes, delivery systems, and budgets, even within WHO. However, champions of primary care believed that WHO should dedicate resources and efforts to a horizontal approach, arguing with equal fervor that short-term advances in certain diseases or vaccination coverage risked fragmenting general health services and weakening the role of governments as the main stewards of national health systems.[30]

Like a pendulum, the vertical-versus-horizontal debate has regularly swung over the past fifty years.[31] In 1978, WHO and UNICEF convened the International Conference on Primary Health Care in Alma-Ata, the Soviet Union (in current-day Kazakhstan). Representatives from all WHO member states attended this conference, and for the first time health-care challenges in disadvantaged countries were seriously examined and linked with development opportunities.[32] The resulting Alma-Ata Declaration strongly emphasized health as a basic human right, the role of the state in the universal provision of health care, and community participation as a fundamental prerequisite for effective health care.[33] The declaration acknowledged the importance of community-oriented comprehensive primary health care for all nations, and also recognized the changes needed in economic, social, and political structures at national levels to enable equitable health care access.

Soon after Alma-Ata, the financial crisis in the early 1980s, coupled with a desire for greater donor control over aid budgets (particularly from large donors such as the United States), resulted in declining Official Development Assistance (ODA) for health.[34] Most of the recommended horizontal strategies codified in the Alma-Ata Declaration were criticized as being unattainable, especially in resource-deprived countries, due to vague implementation strategies, immense costs, and the need for a large trained workforce to execute. Vertical strategies that focused on medical interventions, such as vaccinations, were proposed to achieve more immediate results.[35] One consequence of this friction was a move by WHO toward advocating what was known as selective primary care, an approach emphasizing cost-effective interventions such as GOBI (growth monitoring, oral rehydration, breastfeeding, and immunization). The aspiration was that adopting such a strategy would enable a country to successfully attain a short-term, measurable public health goal, an approach seen as reflecting both horizontal and vertical thinking (an early "diagonal" approach).

WHO's *Health for All by 2000* initiative in the late 1980s failed to catalyze comprehensive global primary health care based on the delivery of basic services. This failure further fuelled a paradigm shift from horizontal to vertical funding strategies. In conjunction, greater support for vertical health funding grew from both success and failure: success seen in the focused efforts that achieved smallpox eradication; failure seen in the explosion of HIV/AIDS throughout the 1980s, and the clear verdict that the world's response had been woefully inadequate. As had proven true with previous epidemics, HIV/AIDS would not be confined geographically or demographically.[36] Yet, throughout the late 1980s and early 1990s, new approaches or significant funding streams to combat HIV/AIDS or respond to other "vertical" challenges did not materialize.

Interest in vertical-versus-horizontal health funding rose further with the release of the World Bank's 1993 World Development Report *Investing in Health,* which focused on Disability Adjusted Life Years (DALYs) gained by particular vertical disease interventions. While the concept of DALYs was met with criticism similar to what had been levied against vertical-focused programs historically, it quickly became part of the global health lexicon. With the new millennium approaching, traditional donors, such as the United States and other G7 countries as well as new donors like the Bill & Melinda Gates Foundation (hereafter, Gates Foundation), looked favorably and donated generously to vertical efforts. Two such efforts will be discussed at length later in this book: Gavi, the Vaccine Alliance; and the Global Fund to Fight AIDS, Tuberculosis and Malaria. The United Nations Millennium Development Goals (MDGs) in 2000 articulated eight goals with a set of specific and largely vertical indicators. This further encouraged the development and growth of multiple vertical programs to target certain health interventions, thus reinforcing funding approaches that target particular diseases. Even broader goals, such as improved maternal and child mortality, largely manifested in increased vertical support for issues like more vaccines or more family planning.[37]

While there is near universal consensus that optimal health systems are the key to improving health, vertical strategies continue to receive substantially more funding. In fact, there has been an incredible rise, especially in the past decade, in the number and types of funds allocated through vertical funding mechanisms. Much of the increase in monies for global health has been directed to address HIV/AIDS, malaria, and tuberculosis (TB). A 2008 study of the four major donors in global health noted that in 2005, funding per death varied widely by disease area, from US $1029.10 for HIV/AIDS to $3.21 for NCDs.[38] This finding suggests that donors do not base their decision-making processes on morbidity or mortality data alone. The study also noted the difficulty in discerning the amount of aid money that flows vertically versus horizontally in the health sector given the complicated manner in which donors categorize their aid.

Over the late twentieth century and into the twenty-first, new institutions have emerged that reflect both vertical ambitions and the frustrations of member states with the leadership of WHO. For example, the Joint UN Programme on HIV/AIDS (UNAIDS) was created in 1994 to be the main advocate for global action on HIV/AIDS. It is formally an umbrella organization that brings together eleven cosponsoring UN agencies to lead, strengthen, and support an expanded response to HIV/AIDS.[39] The first independent evaluation of UNAIDS highlighted three reasons to explain why it was created: first, the dissatisfaction among donors with the overall management of WHO, encompassing, in part, criticism that WHO could not manage the role of coordination of rival UN agencies related to HIV/AIDS; second, an interest by donors in having more direct control over the use of their contributed funds plus the recognition that because of the multisectoral nature of HIV/AIDS, agencies with sector-specific mandates were individually poorly positioned to respond; and third, the broader impetus toward UN reform, with UNAIDS seen as an opportunity to demonstrate the potential of the UN as a whole to work more effectively through UNAIDS' joint work plan and shared budget among the cosponsoring agencies.[40]

Scholars too have pointed toward WHO's shortcomings and also to the lack of trust that donors had in WHO's effectiveness to explain the origins of UNAIDS. Michael Merson et al. note, "There was also growing concern about the senior leadership of WHO among donor governments, who reacted to the reelection of Hiroshi Nakajima to a second term as Director-General by decreasing their overall support and voluntary contributions to WHO, calling for organizational reform, and devising new health-related initiatives outside the agency's influence or control."[41]

Arguably the same logic explains at least in part the history of the Global Fund. As mentioned previously, both Gavi and the Global Fund's creations demonstrate a strong belief by donors and others that vertical approaches can attract more resources to greater effect than horizontal approaches alone (though both Gavi and the Global Fund have funded horizontal approaches complementary to their core vertical work through their health systems strengthening programs). The Global Fund and Gavi are just two examples of the rise in prominence and number of public-private partnership models to address major health challenges. One study from 2015 found more than two hundred global health actors of significant scope, including eighteen formal public-private partnerships, many with a strong vertical focus.[42]

THE RISE OF PUBLIC-PRIVATE PARTNERSHIPS

Starting in the late twentieth century, partnership models involving governments, nongovernmental organizations (NGOs), for-profit companies, and other nonstate actors increasingly became viewed as necessary mechanisms to address major challenges in global governance. Global health was arguably the first domain to attempt major "experiments" in this area, particularly in addressing infectious diseases (the Global Fund), childhood vaccinations (Gavi), and food security (GAIN, the Global Alliance for Improved Nutrition). Those experiences contain lessons for how best to address other challenges in health, such as NCDs, including by what are often called "public-private partnerships" (PPPs). We also believe that such lessons offer insight into how traditional institutions, such as WHO, could, and possibly must, adapt to the challenges of the twenty-first century, from preparing for whatever outbreak or pandemic may next emerge to working with developing countries on meaningful health systems strengthening and the adoption of health insurance.

The universe of global health–focused institutions includes organizations that are multilateral, defined as involving two or more governments (e.g., WHO), bilateral, generally defined as one government giving directly to another government (e.g., the UK's Department for International Development [DFID]), regional (e.g., [PAHO]), financing mechanisms (e.g., the Global Fund), coordinating bodies (e.g., UNAIDS), and hybrids that provide both financing mechanisms and direct programmatic support (e.g., Gavi, the Vaccine Alliance, formerly, the Global Alliance for Vaccines and Immunization and colloquially referred to as Gavi). Among the actors listed, whether financing mechanisms or hybrids, PPPs are the newest and arguably most innovative form of governance being attempted.

No single definition of what constitutes a PPP exists. Broadly speaking, such a partnership involves financial and/or in-kind commitments from nonstate actors such as corporations or foundations to enhance public projects. Ideally, the partners share common goals and a shared approach to achieve those goals. For example, Sonja Bartsch defines PPPs as output-oriented cooperation of local, national, transnational, and international actors from the public, the private, and the NGO sector.[43] Wolfgang Reinicke and colleagues use the phrase "Global Public Policy Networks," which refers to bridges built between the public sector and the other two sectors of most societies, the business community and civil society.[44] These so-called trisectoral networks pull diverse groups and resources together and address issues that no one sector can resolve by itself. Instead of PPPs, the Gates Foundation refers to "Global Health Alliances," which are initiatives involving two or more institutions characterized by shared goals and decision-making, coordination or combination of resources, and some shared accountability. Kent Buse and Gill Walt define health global public-private partnerships as collaborative relationships, which transcend national boundaries and bring together at least three types of parties, among them a corporation (and/or industry association) and an inter-governmental organization, so as to achieve a shared goal on the basis of a mutually agreed division of labor. Roy Widdus adds that such partnerships must be achievement-oriented with joint venture attributes such as shared objectives, shared risk-taking, shared decision-making, contributions from each participant, and benefits to each participant.[45] These are only a few of the different conceptualizations of PPPs.

Regardless of definition, it is indisputable that the financing available to support PPPs has exploded over the past two decades. As one notable example, USAID increased its investment in PPPs by almost 40 percent between 2012 and 2013, allowing it to leverage more than $380 million from private sources to support USAID-funded programs. Additionally, the European Union has issued an increasing number of research bids cofinanced by the pharmaceutical industry and philanthropies requiring successful applicants to form a public-private alliance with clear public goals.[46]

EXPLAINING THE GROWTH IN PPPs

One of the significant drivers for PPPs targeting vaccines (Gavi) and HIV/AIDS (the Global Fund) was perceived market failures. In the late 1990s, vaccine prices remained high despite tragically high demand. The same was true for antiretrovirals, the main treatment for human immunodeficiency virus, or HIV, the virus that causes AIDS. In 2000, antiretroviral prices per patient per year ranged from $10,000 to $12,000. In sub-Saharan Africa, fewer than fifty thousand people were receiving the drugs needed to help them stay alive and healthy, even as more than two million people in the region died that year of the disease.[47] The advent of the Global Fund was not the only effort geared toward shifting the antiretroviral market from a high-price–low-volume dynamic to a high-volume–low-price dynamic. Indeed, a partnership set up in 2000 between the UN Children's Emergency Fund (UNICEF), WHO, UNAIDS, the World Bank, the UN Population Fund (UNFPA),[48] and five major pharmaceutical companies with HIV/AIDS medicines worked to make those drugs more affordable to low-and middle-income countries.[49] By 2001, measurable drops in prices were evident. Arguably the advent of the Global Fund's monies to further incentivize additional price decreases in exchange for more volume of drugs purchased only accelerated the preexisting trend line. Partnerships in global health now exist for a variety of reasons beyond compensating for or correcting market failure, including (1) financing, exemplified by the Global Fund to Fight AIDS, TB and Malaria; (2) product delivery and technical assistance, such as Merck's Mectizan Donation Program for the treatment of onchocerciasis or river blindness; (3) issue advocacy such as the Roll Back Malaria partnership that includes WHO, UNICEF, the UN Development Programme (UNDP), and the World Bank; and (4) knowledge mobilization for improved policy as in the Save the Children United Kingdom/GlaxoSmithKline partnership.

Previous work has attributed the rise of these partnerships to a variety of distinct and interrelated factors, including a general ideological shift toward working with, rather than against, the private sector, including to ameliorate market failures; a growing disillusionment among state and nonstate actors with the UN system as a means to achieve ambitious health goals; frustration with chronic funding shortages by the UN for health objectives; unreliable funding over time by traditional bilateral and multilateral aid mechanisms; and a widespread recognition that health challenges, like HIV/AIDS, were beyond the capacity of any individual stakeholder and require collaboration among recipient national governments, the private sector, NGOs, and technical consultants.[50] The rise in PPPs helps explain the explosion of global health-focused efforts mentioned earlier.

Benedict Bull and Desmond McNeill narrow in on four factors driving the emergence and increasing influence of PPPs.[51] The first factor was the rise of transnational corporations with significant market power. The second factor was increased privatization of previously government-owned services such as health care, largely the result of governmental preference (developed world) and for some due to World Bank loan conditionality (developing world). Given the increasing need for the provision of global public goods, as such goods become greater in number and relatively more affordable, the question then becomes *who* was going to provide these. The third factor Bull and McNeill point to was the emergence of new private philanthropic organizations, such as the Gates Foundation, in an environment in which the multilateral system (and the member governments) had fewer resources.

The Gates Foundation has invested significantly in PPPs, including its founding $750 million grant to Gavi to help close the so-called vaccine gap. Additionally, the move to adopt business approaches in global health, including the use of markets, advocated by Gates and others, has been one factor in PPP's emphasizing performance criteria, efficiency, and technology in what they fund. In fact, the Global Fund's Executive Director Mark Dybul believes that PPPs were constructed to both leverage new funding sources and to challenge, and ideally improve, traditional health organizations.[52] The final factor for Bull and McNeill is the concentration of power in a defined set of pharmaceutical companies who wield power in global health largely as a strong voice in global trade negotiations, such as during the negotiations for the Trade-Related Aspects of Intellectual Property Rights (TRIPs) agreement. This concentration of power has been somewhat weakened by the rise of the generic pharmaceutical industry in countries such as India and South Africa. Arguably, PPPs reflect this greater concentration of power and also are intended, at least by some participants, to act as a counter to it.

Thus, given all these factors, multilateral organizations have had no choice but to directly engage with the private sector, what has been described by Kenneth Abbott and Duncan Snidal as inclusion power: "When an actor has inclusion power, it is difficult to create an effective and legitimate institution without it."[53] Multilaterals such as WHO are coming to recognize they must make compromises between their aspirations of being solely the province of governments and their limited power to advance public health goals in the face of globalization and market forces. The recognition of these pressures does not necessarily come with a value judgment. Former UN Secretary-General Kofi Annan succinctly noted in 1999 that "Our post-war institutions were built for an international world, but we now live in a global world."[54] The recognition that more power exists in more places—governments, civil society, the private sector, the public—is arguably even truer today in the twenty-first century than it was at the end of the twentieth.

LEGITIMACY OF PPPs IN HEALTH GOVERNANCE

Legitimacy can be defined either in terms of process, such as inclusiveness and accountability (input legitimacy), or in terms of outcomes, such as lives saved and value for money (output legitimacy). Some allege that there is an inherent trade-off between input and output legitimacy, but this has yet to be rigorously studied, and we remain unconvinced that organizations cannot aspire—and be held accountable—to both standards of legitimacy.[55] In terms of input legitimacy, critics posit that PPPs give private interests a seat at the table—such as with the Board of the Global Fund to Fight HIV/AIDS, Tuberculosis and Malaria, and Gavi—resulting in priorities skewed more toward their interests than those of governments and their citizens. While normative rhetoric is abundant, empirical evidence of such an effect is lacking.[56] The methodological difficulty in such a study is whether it is possible to differentiate the challenges of PPPs from any other targeted effort (public, private, or joint) and from challenges common to all efforts in developing countries which are externally funded. Are there unique aspects to PPPs in these contexts? It is difficult to say. For example, civil society groups have criticized both the US Presidential Emergency Plan For AIDS Relief (PEPFAR) and the multilateral World Bank for being captured by private interests. Even the definition of private is contested—does private mean the private sector, à la a pharmaceutical company or beverage company? Or does private mean any nonstate actor, all of the above listed plus the Gates Foundation and the nongovernmental Save the Children? Disagreement over definitions further complicates such analyses.

In terms of output legitimacy, previous efforts have examined how effective PPPs have been at improving health outcomes and tend to be positive in assessment. Mark Zacher and Tania Keefe have documented three specific successes. These include the Onchocerciasis Control Programme, the Guinea Worm Eradication Partnership, and the Global Polio Eradication Initiative.[57] Aside from these three examples, most of the praise PPPs garner is broad and not tied in any identifiable way to their structure. For example, Kent Buse and Andrew Harmer note that partnerships can get specific health issues onto the national and international agenda, stimulate research and development, mobilize funds, and result in the private sector bringing expertise in product development, marketing, and distribution.[58] In line with those thoughts, Thomas Pogge notes, "we will reach our common and imperative goal of universal access to essential medicines either in collaboration with the pharmaceutical industry or not at all."[59] He makes what we believe to be an important point that "the root of evil lies not in how corporations do business, but in how we regulate and incentivize them," and thus argues that rather than critiquing partnerships, more attention needs to be given to incentivizing companies to behave in a morally responsible manner through either financial or reputational incentives.[60]

REVOLUTIONIZING AID

One driver for the growth in PPPs, particularly seen in the Global Fund and Gavi experiences, was the shared belief by various government officials, activists, and others that these new institutions would revolutionize the very definition and business of development assistance, starting with health, making it more demand-driven (i.e., giving countries with the highest disease burden and the fewest resources a legitimate voice in determining what would be funded) and, over time, providing a disproportionate share of funding to proven, cost-effective interventions (i.e., implementing "pay-for-performance").[61] Arguably, nothing captured this latter motivation more succinctly than the Global Fund's inaugural Executive Director Richard Feachem's oft-repeated mantra: "Raise it, Spend it, Prove it" and his frequently added addendum, "for those who need it most."[62] Private companies bring not only financial resources to the partnership but also business acumen.[63] In theory, the networks and knowledge of the private sector (companies and NGOs) can strengthen the delivery of health-care solutions in remote areas, and perhaps result in the greater availability and delivery of measles vaccines, polio drops, and even bed nets. Yet, there is little empirical evidence that the private sector's involvement alone leads directly to these and other similar effects versus when the private sector works in partnership with developing country governments, multilaterals, NGOs, or all of the above.[64]

From the perch of 2016, it remains an open question whether the Global Fund and the Gavi Alliance will ultimately transform the business of aid, on their own or through their indirect influence on WHO and the World Bank. We just do not yet know. Despite the rapid growth in the number and financing channeled through PPPs, no independent scholarly work—versus self-commissioned independent evaluations—has evaluated the Global Fund holistically (the largest of any PPP in health or any sector), nor has any substantial scholarly work assessed Gavi against their initial founding principles and promises or even another set of metrics beyond programmatic performance. Several descriptive accounts have been published on such partnerships but no academic study has been conducted to assess the performance of partnerships and attempts to explain their strengths and weaknesses. Notably, the Global Environmental Facility, an organization with significantly fewer financial resources than the Global Fund, has received more attention than any global-health-related PPP.[65] This raises questions on the existence of an evidence base to justify the level of investment by the global community in PPPs broadly or in any one area, such as global health.

Part of the explanation for this gap in the literature is that quantifying the impact of PPPs on health using transparent metrics is not straightforward. Every PPP collects data using its own systems, and each organization makes publicly available varying amounts of this data. These constraints also exist when examining WHO and the World Bank. Such data needs to be supplemented with interviews and review of internal and external documents. We provide additional details in chapter 2 of the mixed methods we employed for this research project though we are not looking to fill the scholarly gaps here with a deep dive on any particular PPP.

Interestingly, some of the Global Fund's most strident critics—including those in the US Congress, the European Commission, and policy analysts on both sides of the Atlantic—have acknowledged that it has achieved or helped achieve a great deal.[66] No individual from these institutions or any others that we are aware of has disputed the Global Fund's output legitimacy, nor that of Gavi's, at any juncture in the last fifteen years. There is clear data on the upsurge in vaccine coverage, antiretroviral coverage, insecticide-treated bed-net coverage, and TB-treatment coverage, in which Gavi and the Global Fund clearly played a part. Whether their impact was magnified by the actual or perceived greater legitimacy each derives from their inclusive PPP structures remains an open question.

OUR OBJECTIVES

Put simply, this book is about governing global health with a focus on the role of the "traditional" players in global health, WHO and the World Bank as well as the most significant new health PPPs, the Global Fund and Gavi, the Vaccine Alliance, and the powers that oversee them. Validating the Global Fund's and Gavi's—or WHO's and the World Bank's—assertions about how much they have helped in the fight against specific diseases epidemiologically or for health broadly is not the emphasis of this account. This is partly because our focus lies elsewhere and partly because this is not an epidemiological endeavor. Additionally, just looking at the Global Fund as one example, other organizations occupying a similar space, including PEPFAR, have agreed to share credit for progress in the fights against HIV/AIDS, TB, and malaria given the myriad of efforts on the ground in most countries where Global Fund grantees work alongside PEPFAR-funded efforts and others.[67] For example, in Tanzania, the Global Fund has funded bed-net programs to prevent malaria, rapid-testing programs for TB, and HIV/AIDS drug purchase programs, while simultaneously PEPFAR has supported abstinence education, HIV/AIDS drug purchase programs, and large-scale health literacy campaigns, and the World Bank has provided financing for the clinics in which Global Fund grantees and PEPFAR-funded health workers operate.[68] Disentangling who is responsible for what effects and impacts in that ecosystem is beyond the purview of this book.

Stepping back, our book tackles four interrelated questions: first, how are WHO, the World Bank, the Global Fund, and Gavi governed, and how do their different governance structures influence their role in the global health system? Second, how do the ways in which each is financed influence their agenda and priorities? Third, how inclusive and transparent are our case study organizations? All of these questions go to the institutions' legitimacy and also to how effective they are in achieving their mandates. Finally, we turn to a forward-looking question: What reforms are needed to ensure these structures are able to tackle the major health challenges of the twenty-first century?

We employ principal-agent theory to address our questions. Principal-agent theory concerns the relationship between member states (principals) and an international organization (the agent, often a secretariat).

It emphasizes that while an international organization may often act in ways that are consistent with member states' preferences, at times it may act in ways inconsistent with them, even those of the most powerful members, instead reflecting the agents' interests.[69] This is crucial for our examination of our case studies because each was created at least in part to act with autonomy from its powerful member states, in the best interest of all constituents (at least as perceived by the organizational bureaucracies and professionals themselves). For the newer PPPs, strong secretariats were intended to help safeguard the integrity of the various organizations' grant processes, including implementing countries' ownership of them. Ultimately, principal-agent theory helps us to dissect how the initial aspirations of each were helped (or not) by their governance structures and financing dynamics initially and over time.

BOOK OUTLINE

This book is split into seven chapters that together attempt to provide a robust answer to the questions posed throughout. This introductory chapter outlines how global health governance has evolved over the past century with a focus on the rise of public-private partnership (PPP) models. We provide a short explanation given by scholars and policy makers for the rise in this type of model, including that they are a more accountable form of governance. We conclude the chapter by putting forth our research questions.

In the second chapter, we introduce the case studies that illustrate the shift in governance from traditional UN member-state-led agencies to public-private partnerships. The institutions we examine are WHO and the World Bank ("the old") and the Global Fund to Fight HIV/AIDS, Tuberculosis and Malaria, and the Gavi, the Vaccine Alliance ("the new"). Building on the introduction, we then locate our work in the context of the existing literature on international cooperation, particularly academic work on the shift of power toward nonstate actors. Again, our analysis is guided by principal-agent theory, which concerns the relationship between member states (principals) and an international organization (the agent, often a secretariat). We conclude the chapter by providing a detailed description of our data sources and material.

In the third chapter we take a detailed look at key governance features of the four focal institutions. We identify five key differences between the "old" and "new" institutions and provide an explanation rooted in principal-agent theory for the shift to the newer model. We also take a closer look at the Gates Foundation as an important new type of principal in global governance.

In chapter 4 we take a closer look at financing flows. We first look at how the work of WHO and the World Bank is funded and how their respective financing has changed over time. We then turn to the Global Fund to examine whether it has been able to mobilize more resources from more funders than previous global health efforts (as it initially aspired to do). Similarly, we look at Gavi's funding to assess whether a range of public and private donors provided substantial financial contributions to Gavi and how critical Gavi's multi-stakeholder model and governance has proved to be to its work in lowering vaccine prices.

In chapter 5, we pay particular attention to whether the four institutions are displaying key elements of "good governance" now expected in the twenty-first century, chiefly whether the organizations are inclusive and transparent. We use comparisons between each as well as between the "new" and the "old" to assess whether the "new" agencies are indeed more transparent and accountable than the "old."

In chapter 6 we draw together lessons from the previous chapters on the governance of global health. In the first half of the chapter we assess whether the new models have lived up to the expectations of their founders and provide some granularity on their achievements and disappointments. In the second half we examine the impact of the "new" models on WHO and World Bank and their efforts to reform.

The final chapter summarizes our findings and turns to the consequent implications for major health challenges in the twenty-first century such as the prevention, management, and treatment of NCDs, achieving universal health coverage and strengthening pandemic preparedness.

2

Big Questions and Case Studies

The WHO, the World Bank, Gavi, and the Global Fund all are products of international cooperation. Even Gavi and the Global Fund, which enfranchise nonstate actors, include significant cooperation and resource pooling by their member states, such as the United States (the largest contributor to the Global Fund) and the United Kingdom (the second largest contributor to Gavi after the Gates Foundation). To understand what motivates these institutions, we must first ask what determines when and how states and nonstate actors cooperate in global health.

In international relations, theories of cooperation posit that individual states confront certain dilemmas in which otherwise rational behavior—thus maximizing their individual preferences—would result in suboptimal outcomes for all states concerned. One way states choose to ameliorate such collective action problems is through formalizing their cooperation, often (though not always) in the form of international organizations; this has proven particularly true in global health. A collective action problem is one in which multiple (or even all) individuals would benefit if a certain action were taken. But, given the high costs associated with that particular action, it is unlikely that any one individual would solve—or could afford to solve—the problem alone. Preventing and responding to health concerns, or even threats, are often collective action problems. Indeed, given the painfully apt cliché that diseases do not need passports to cross borders, it is not surprising that in the mid-nineteenth century, health concerns catalyzed some of the first international meetings and agreements, or collective actions, related to issues other than war or peace as discussed in chapter 1. The mid-nineteenth-century discovery that microorganisms—rather than miasma—caused diseases such as cholera arguably only added impetus to these early meetings, the so-called International Sanitary Conferences, and the resulting International Sanitary Conventions.

From the first International Sanitary Conference in Paris in 1851 through to the present, states have chosen to cooperate on health issues in numerous ways. In the twenty-first century, the increased number and density of interactions among states, and between states and nonstate actors, means even the most powerful states are sensitive to events elsewhere and confront their inability to achieve their goals, including as relates to health, alone.[1] This inevitable "interdependence" drives cooperation, even if that cooperation varies dramatically across different health questions and over time.[2] As documented elsewhere, and as we touch on later in this chapter, HIV/AIDS is a good example of such an iterated interdependence, in which states' interests and earlier cooperative efforts shaped their subsequent decisions about when and how to cooperate.[3]

International organizations, at least in theory, help states close the gap between their own interests and those of other states through providing equal access to higher-quality information, lowering transaction costs, enabling economies of scale, spreading systemic risks, and ultimately making it more difficult for any one state to renege on its commitments than to meet its obligations.[4] Over time, international organizations develop their own organizational cultures, norms, and identities that may, in turn, influence the preferences and behavior of their member states, even the most powerful ones.[5] International organizations are the primary way global health law is enacted through either binding agreements, or "hard" law (e.g., treaties), or those that are nonbinding, or "soft" (e.g., codes of practice).[6]

The more independent an organization is from its member states, the more it arguably may be able to facilitate cooperation because its independence theoretically translates into greater legitimacy with each individual member state, and this, in turn, generally leads to greater participation by all states, including the most powerful.[7] In other words, states may design an institution that possesses some autonomy from the governing body composed of member states, and certainly from any one member state, because doing so increases the ability of the newly minted institution to deliver on its mission. This theory, best articulated by Abbott and Snidal, contends that institutions themselves then create the conditions for continued cooperation, including lowered transaction costs in their mandated area, distribution of risk associated with any one action, and increased access to technical expertise and knowledge; the last factor has been a significant driver of cooperation in global health over time. When an institution fails on its core mission or to provide those fundamental elements to its member states, states can either adapt the institution or, failing that, create a new one.[8] Institutions can also at times inhibit or distort cooperation, such as when the self-interests of an institution's bureaucracy run counter to the interests of its member states.[9]

The history of the world's fight against HIV/AIDS over the past thirty-five years illustrates this pattern of adaptation and institution switching or replacement, partly in reaction to beliefs held by powerful member states that extant institutions were failing on their mission and incapable of course-correcting. The early efforts of global cooperation to fight HIV/AIDS global cooperation were first pursued largely within WHO, later through a combination of efforts within WHO as well as with the World Bank's Multi-Country AIDS Program (MAP) and a new institution in UNAIDS, and then most recently through principally the Global Fund, with surveillance and technical expertise still coordinated through WHO and UNAIDS.

More broadly beyond HIV/AIDS, the panoply of global health institutions detailed in chapter 1 evidences a central tension in international organizations (and in the study of them): states often recognize formalized cooperation through international organizations as the means most likely to achieve their individual global health goals, but then are often loathe to invest those same organizations with sufficient authority and resources to successfully discharge their mandates. They instead create new initiatives and institutions to pursue similar or even equivalent objectives; indeed, the creation of both Gavi and the Global Fund are inseparable from this tension.

It cannot be said that the significant challenges in global health result from a paucity of international institutions focused on health. Adding further nuance to the categories of health organizations listed in chapter 1, within the UN system alone, while the WHO may have health most firmly and obviously in its mandate, these UN agencies also have health within their areas of responsibility: the UN Children's Emergency Fund (UNICEF); the UN Population Fund (UNFPA); the UN Development Programme (UNDP); the Food and Agricultural Organization (FAO); the UN Educational, Scientific and Cultural Organization (UNESCO); the UN Refugee Agency (UNHCR); the World Food Programme (WFP); the UN Office on Drugs and Crime (UNODC); the UN Office for the Coordination of Humanitarian Affairs (OCHA); UN Women; and the International Labor Organization (ILO). It is not a short list. When organizations focused on health outside the formal UN system but connected to it in various ways are added, such as UNAIDS; Gavi, the Vaccine Alliance; the Global Fund to Fight AIDS, Tuberculosis and Malaria; and the Global Alliance to Improve Nutrition (GAIN), the list grows even longer. The United States, including through its PEPFAR program, is the single largest global-health funder by far, both directly and indirectly, and is not on this expanded list.

Perhaps the continued preponderance of states as the major funders of global health is not surprising if one understands aid primarily as donors purchasing policy concessions from recipients, as Robert Keohane argued during the Cold War era.[10] If that understanding remains correct in the post–Cold War era, we would then assume that bilateral aid mechanisms would be the dominant paradigm for states to provide official development assistance for health (DAH). While DAH encompasses both financial and in-kind contributions from donors targeted to improving health in developing countries, the vast majority of DAH is financial in nature.

A heavy reliance on bilateral assistance would make sense if development assistance (or foreign aid) were extensions of a donor's overall foreign policy. However, looking at donor financial flows for health reveals that bilateral assistance is not always the dominant paradigm. In 2012, for example, Norway directed more than 60 percent of its DAH through multilateral channels while for the United States, in contrast, that ratio was less than a quarter (much of it through the Global Fund). Over the past twenty-five years, the United States has generally directed somewhere between 60 and 75 percent of its DAH bilaterally, with a preference for trackability of funds and working through US-based organizations as likely an explanation for this ratio as any other. In 1990, France directed more than 90 percent of its DAH through bilateral mechanisms. But in 2012, even as its total DAH had shrunk significantly, more than 80 percent of its DAH that year flowed through multilateral channels.[11] The picture of DAH globally becomes more complex when including multi-bi aid (bilateral contributions to multilateral organizations earmarked for a specific purpose, sector, region, or country as well as trust funds and noncore funding). Countries' DAH channel preferences generally track their overall development assistance preferences, as seen in figure 2.1.

It is not only states that arguably look to influence global health through formalized cooperation or significant direct investments. The Gates Foundation is the largest private, or nonstate, funder of global health concerns; through 2014 it had contributed more than $21 billion to global health programs since its inception less than twenty years ago.[12]

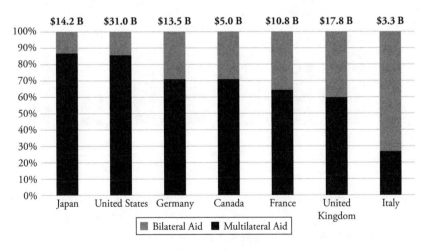

FIGURE 2.1 Bilateral vs. multilateral aid for G7 countries in 2013. Development Co-operation Report 2015: Making Partnerships Effective Coalitions for Action, http://www.oecd.org/dac/development-co-operation-report-20747721.htm.

Yet, even in years in which the Gates Foundation has contributed hundreds of millions of dollars to the Global Fund and Gavi, and millions more to NGOs working in global health, the US government contributed significantly more through its myriad efforts. Indeed, the United States is the single largest funder of global health efforts around the world by any measure. In 2014, it disbursed more than $12 billion in DAH, an amount more than three times as large as that from the United Kingdom, the next largest global health donor, and four times what the Gates Foundation gave that year to global health (fig. 2.2, 2.3).

The emergence of the Gates Foundation as a significant player in global health in the late twentieth and early twenty-first centuries coincided with two phenomena. The first was the greater focus from traditional bilateral donors on global health concerns, including HIV/AIDS. The second was the shared belief among donors that conventional instruments, such as WHO, were not capable of stewarding large inflows of resources intensely focused on solving specific problems, chiefly closing the vaccine gap and HIV/AIDS. Donors' search for more focused, nimble, and efficient solutions (showing more "value-for-money,"

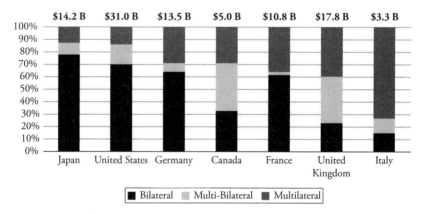

FIGURE 2.2 Bilateral, multi-bi, and multilateral aid for G7 countries in 2013. Some G7 donors direct a majority of their aid through bilateral channels while others rely more on multilateral channels. Development Co-operation Report 2015: Making Partnerships Effective Coalitions for Action, http://www.oecd.org/dac/development-co-operation-report-20747721.htm; 2015 report http://www.oecd.org/dac/multilateral-aid-2015-9789264235212-en.htm.

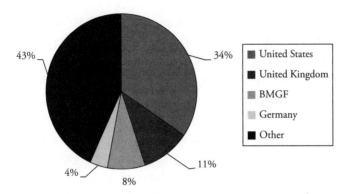

FIGURE 2.3 DAH by source of funding 2014. In 2014, the United States accounted for just over one-third of all DAH. IHME, *Financing Global Health 2014: Shifts in Funding as the MDG Era Closes.*

a concept and term much in vogue with the new millennium) led to new organizations and new pressures on the old ecosystem. While we focus on the largest of these in global health—Gavi and the Global Fund—we recognize their creation reflected a broader shift in donor thinking.

STUDYING THE EVOLUTION OF GLOBAL HEALTH GOVERNANCE: PRINCIPAL-AGENT THEORY

We know personalities are important in the story of global health governance in the twenty-first century, and perhaps none more so than Bill and Melinda Gates. Even though we will touch on the Gates Foundation throughout, our focus in this book is not on personalities and the ways in which specific leaders influence institutions, whether from within or outside. We look instead at our case studies' formal governance structures, financial flows, and their respective policies and practices around the inclusion of civil society, nonstate actors, and the broader public. To help us understand why and how institutions behave, we employ principal-agent theory.

Scholars and officials both have recognized the utility of principal-agent theory to help advance understanding of international organizations. In its *2011 Report on Multilateral Aid*, released in April 2012, the Organization for Economic Cooperation and Development/

Development Assistance Committee (OECD/DAC) suggested that the principal-agent model, "may best explain the decisions involved in choosing multilateral aid" by individual donor countries.[13] Yet, the OECD/DAC report does not employ principal-agent theory to analyze specific global health institutions and in general gives scant attention to key players. As one example, it mentions the Global Fund only twice (and neither time in a principal-agent context).[14]

Several contemporary analyses of international organizations have deployed principal-agent theory to help explain the governance and behavior of the institution. Roland Vaubel gives a useful overview,[15] while others have analyzed the International Monetary Fund (IMF)[16] and the World Bank but never focused specifically on the World Bank's health portfolio.[17] In our view, principal-agent theory provides the most useful framework for engaging with the questions posed in this book.

As mentioned in chapter 1, principal-agent theory casts the relationship between member states—principals—and an international organization—the agent, often a Secretariat. It emphasizes that while an international organization may often act in ways that are consistent with member states' preferences, at other times it may act in ways that instead reflect the agent's interests.[18] This is crucial for our examination of global health as two of our four case studies were created precisely because principals—both extant and new players—were dissatisfied with and unconvinced that existing institutions such as WHO and the World Bank could perform effectively and efficiently in closing the vaccine gap (Gavi) and in managing a scaled-up response to HIV/AIDS. While the historical context is important, we are more interested in applying principal-agent theory to help understand what has happened since the inception of these new institutions, both for Gavi and the Global Fund themselves as well as WHO and the Bank.

Hawkins et al. offer a clear articulation of principal-agent theory applied to international relations. Governments, as principals, have the power to grant and rescind authority. International organizations, as agents, are the recipients of such grants of "conditional authority." International organizations can be classified in one of two ways. First, as a "multiple principal" model, whereby individual member states are independent of one another and each enters into a contract with its agent, retaining the right to commit resources, financial and otherwise, to the agent as each determines appropriate at various points in time.[19]

Alternatively, international organizations can reflect a "collective principal" model in which binding agreements among member states translate in practice to their acting as a unified principal over time toward their agent, even if individual principals continue to strive to influence the agent outside the sanctioned instruments of communication and decision-making and while retaining the right to make individually determined financial contributions to the agent's institution.[20] Most international organizations, and all we address here, reflect the collective principal model. As Hawkins et al. point out, the establishment of a principal-agent relationship, largely defined by the presence of "delegation," the formal grant of authority from principals to an agent, can occur only after states have first decided to cooperate.[21] The criticisms of principal-agent theory largely fault its failures to accurately predict how states and organizations behave over time, with a particularly sharp critique of the relationship between member states and the European Union, arguably the most evaluated principal-agent construct.[22] Pointing out a failure to predict the future, however, is among the most common critiques against any theoretical framework.

A core dimension of principal-agent theory is that over time agents will pursue their own interests within the limits of the constraints the principals impose driven by their own evolving interests. Principal-agent theory suggests that principals try to control their agents, but such control is costly in terms of time and efficiency and, as such, agents possess some autonomy from the beginning. Thus, they often gain more autonomy over time as principals' attention moves elsewhere and as the asymmetry of information between principal and agent increases. This is often even more of a challenge in collective principals because of the sense that someone else is always watching the shop—versus in multiple principals in which each principal has to tend to its own interests constantly.

As a result of divergent interests over time between an agent and its principal, principal-agent analysis leads us to expect that agents can and do pursue policies that the principal may not—or would not—have chosen. This phenomenon is termed "agency slack" and manifests in one of two ways. The first, "shirking," occurs when an agent does not maximize effort, efficiency, or influence on behalf of its principal, potentially explaining any institutional failure to live up to the high expectations of its founders and early supporters. Or, alternatively, such an explanation could too easily obscure other reasons for why the institution has struggled to match its founders' original aspirations.

"Slippage," the second manifestation of agency slack, transpires when an agent intentionally shifts policy toward its preferences or interests, away from those of the principal.[23] Not surprisingly, when collective principals' individual preferences are heterogeneous rather than homogenous, the risk of agency slack increases. Axiomatically then, when principals' preferences are homogenous and strong, the risk of agency slack is small.[24]

An important dimension of any agent's autonomy is its discretion, what Hawkins et al. define as the agent's ability to interpret how it might achieve the specific objectives a principal outlines. Ultimately all member institutions are subject to their membership, particularly those that are dependent upon their members for the plurality or totality of their financial support. Yet, our case studies are different than those that are often examined in books with titles that include phrases like "Who Runs the World." While almost everyone seems to recognize the importance of the work of WHO, the World Bank, Gavi, and the Global Fund, particularly in an era in which viruses and compassion travel with almost equal ferocity around the world, these institutions hold relatively little political power. Unlike the United Nations Security Council or the World Trade Organization, none of our case studies has the power to impose sanctions. Our case studies are not viewed as stewarding "high" political debates or being the mechanisms through which grand bargains are struck; neither do they have the financial heft of certain global non-health-focused peer institutions. Although the funds discussed are significant, and have become even more so in the past fifteen years, the $32.6 billion the world invested in global health in 2014 (bilateral donors plus private philanthropy, including the Gates Foundation), pales when compared to the bailout packages extended in the last few years to Cyprus or Greece from the IMF and others. Another comparison is more illuminating: in its 2014 fiscal year, the World Bank supported $61 billion worth of loans, grants, and guarantees in the developing world—far less than 10 percent of that went to health. Financing related to maternal and early childhood nutrition programs was "only" $600 million.[25] Total loans to health and social services surpassed $3.3 billion.[26] Still, that is a far higher annual amount than the relative comparisons to WHO, which had a two-year budget over 2013/14 of $3.98 billion. Indeed, the World Bank's total support for health (and related social services) is even higher than the more than $2.8 billion the Global Fund disbursed in 2014.[27] Although Gavi's comparable total is smaller, disbursing close to $1.3 billion in 2014, it belongs in this cohort for financial heft and influential innovation in its governance and financing, all of which we explore in later chapters. Indeed, in part for these reasons, Gavi's influence is arguably much greater than the more than $7.1 billion Gavi disbursed from 2000 to 2014 to improve immunization coverage across the world.[28] We discuss the financing of each institution in detail in chapter 4.

CASE STUDIES

For our case studies, we selected the four biggest international organizations in global health, as determined by the financial resources all attract and disburse (fig. 2.4). Three have exclusive global health foci— WHO, Gavi, and the Global Fund—while the other—the World

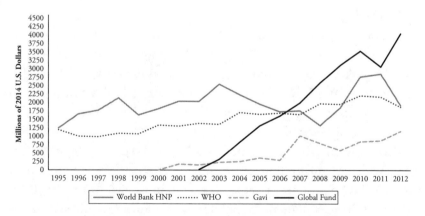

FIGURE 2.4 World Bank HNP, WHO, Gavi, and Global Fund annual disbursements, 1995–2012. Since their inception, Global Fund and Gavi disbursements rose more quickly than those of WHO or the World Bank. IHME, *Financing Global Health 2014: Shifts in Funding as the MDG Era Closes.*

Bank—has become an increasingly significant presence in global health since it made its first grants, or concessionary loans, in health, more than forty years ago.

We examine each institution's governance structures, sources of financing, and their efforts to include actors beyond those who sit on their Boards or provide their funds. The last element includes their respective transparency and partnership policies and practices. This book is not an assessment of their programmatic decision-making nor a technical evaluation as to whether their programmatic investments met with success. For each institution, extensive work has already been done on selected grants, loans, and programs within specific disease areas, programmatic areas, or geographic regions.[29] While we recognize there is a paucity of overall impact evaluations, we do not seek to fill that gap with this work for reasons mentioned earlier. Neither is this a leadership study, though we do acknowledge the impact certain leaders have had on the institutions at various points in their histories. Rather, we hope that our efforts here will help scholars and students alike better understand what influences the behavior and decisions of each institution as relates to the factors we explore.

The "old" actors

The World Health Organization

Arguably the greatest burden WHO bears is its name. Because "health" is in its title, the agency has long borne expectations that it would work to promote and protect all aspects of health, for all people, everywhere. While WHO's constitution defines health broadly as "a complete state of physical, mental, and social well-being, and not merely the absence of disease or infirmity," WHO itself was not intended—nor has it ever claimed—to be an all-encompassing institution with an equally limitless mandate.[30] Rather, from inception in 1948, WHO positioned itself, as it declares in its own words, "to direct and coordinate" international public health efforts.[31] In other words, to help set the world's health agenda, providing technical guidance and support for member states as well as triaging investments (intellectual and capital) based on its assessment of where they would be put to the best use. In its early years, WHO had a relatively more focused mandate and set of goals. Yet, over time, the goals set by the World Health

Assembly, WHO's governing body, have become increasingly diverse and wide-reaching, including the implementation of the International Health Regulations (IHR), the monitoring of the health-related Millennium Development Goals (MDGs) and now those of the Sustainable Development Goals (SDGs), as well as strategies to reduce the harmful use of alcohol, tobacco, and counterfeit medical products, in addition to its continuing work, since inception, on malaria and maternal health, among other areas.

It is not only the scope of priorities that has shifted over time, it is also the specific priorities the World Health Assembly has articulated that have evolved. In the 1960s and 1970s, it charged WHO to work on smallpox eradication (which it succeeded in doing) and to eliminate malaria (which it failed to do). Also in the 1970s, WHO, prompted by the World Health Assembly, pushed for better diagnosis and treatment of mental health and began championing health as a human right, codified in the 1978 Alma-Ata Declaration.[32] In the 1980s, it came belatedly and sluggishly to HIV/AIDS. In the 1990s, smoking cessation and preventing young people around the world from ever picking up a cigarette consumed much of WHO's energy. This prioritization was largely due to WHO's Director-General from 1998 to 2003, Dr. Gro Harlem Brundtland, more than the Health Assembly itself. In the early 2000s, in reaction to SARS and again attributable in part to Dr. Brundtland, WHO supported—and brokered—a strengthened IHR, intended both to help prevent outbreaks from spreading across borders (the IHR's original intent) and to strengthen health systems in low-income countries (which was viewed as an important goal in and of itself and crucial to preventing epidemics). In the later 2000s and into the second decade of the new century, for some in WHO, a more robust IHR and pandemic response remained paramount, while for others, more technical support on areas ranging from tuberculosis control to maternal health held center stage. The result was an ever-fragmented WHO budget and splintered organizational attention.

Some critics point to this lack of focus over time as making WHO inevitably vulnerable to the weaknesses that the 2014/15 Ebola epidemic revealed. Whether this is fair is almost beside the point given the perception of failure. It is also possible to view the growth of the World Bank as a major global health actor and the entrance of Gavi and the Global Fund onto the global health scene as indictments of

WHO's inability to provide the technical and programmatic support governments need to provide improved public health and health care for their populations, regardless of health priority or fashion. One could make a similar argument as well about the institutions that track the global burden of disease through morbidity and mortality data, including the Institute for Health Metrics and Evaluation (IHME); arguably, IHME's creation revealed the Gates Foundation's lack of confidence in WHO to produce such data.

Additionally, WHO does not put forward a consistent message about its mission and work. Unlike the other three institutions we discuss in which there are very clear achievements heralded for any given year and over time, it is difficult to find an analogous articulation on WHO's website. The organization does not even publish an annual report beyond its audited financial data. What are WHO's greatest achievements, according to WHO? We don't know. It is also not clear what WHO believes its successes to be after examining various issue- and programmatic-specific reports that WHO issues or from looking at Executive Board and World Health Assembly documents. Annually, WHO provides aggregated health statistics from its member states but often other sources, such as the IHME mentioned earlier, are viewed as having higher-quality health data. Additionally, WHO provides reports against certain priority health areas, such as its June 2015 universal health coverage report, but not others. The last World Health Report issued by WHO in 2013 focused on the same topic of universal health coverage.[33] In September 2015, a series of searches on Google and Google Scholar for "World Health Organization Annual Report" and "WHO Annual Report" yielded first a report on WHO's Programme to Eliminate Lymphatic Filariasis; a few results down was the link to the World Cancer Report 2014.[34] Indeed, similar to WHO overall, most WHO programs do not appear to share their greatest achievements on an annual or even regular cadence. Notably, unlike the World Bank, Gavi, and the Global Fund, as we will see, the only eligibility criteria for WHO attention and resources are disease burden (e.g., for TB) and public health preparedness and response or lack thereof (e.g., IHR monitoring), not country income level or WHO's own competitive advantage to make a distinctly positive difference in those areas.

While the Executive Board of WHO makes public its resolutions and certain resolutions relate to specific WHO priorities, it is generally not clear what WHO's role has been in the progress made against those priorities thus far or what responsibility it is claiming for making progress in the future. For example, during the 136th Executive Board meeting in early 2015, the Board passed a resolution recommending the World Health Assembly adopt the proposed new technical strategy on malaria. The resolution (and subsequent adoption by the World Health Assembly) clearly articulates what is expected of member states, WHO partners, and WHO itself to reach a 90 percent reduction in malaria incidence and mortality by 2030. It does not say, however, what WHO had already helped achieve.[35] A search of documents on the Roll Back Malaria Partnership website, until recently hosted at WHO, does not yield greater insight into WHO's view of its own malaria work.[36] Perhaps the approach of consistently not claiming credit on its website, in its governance forums, and in partners' documents reflects WHO's ethos of helping set the stage and mustering partners to advance a sundry agenda. Perhaps it is the result of not dedicating time and resources to "making its case." Perhaps its work is too embedded in that of member states, UN partner agencies, NGO partners, and others, and disaggregating who was responsible for what technical advice or programming would be impossible to do on the ground or consistently across member states and programs in malaria or any area of work. Whatever the reason, it is impossible to share the same level of specificity of results that the Global Fund and Gavi certainly assert across their scope of work and which the World Bank asserts across certain aspects of its global health portfolio.

In this book, we describe how WHO is governed and financed and how the composition of its donors in particular has changed over the years. Of note are the different ways in which the institution's leadership has positioned it as being more technical or member state–driven over time, particularly given it, like traditional international organizations, depends on member support from dues and, even more significantly, discretionary donations. It is important not to confuse those two funding streams even if the source (i.e., the donor) is the same. Additionally, we examine how transparent WHO is in the areas it is most often looked to for leadership, for example around pandemic response, and how it engages, or does not engage, civil society and the public in those areas as well as more broadly in WHO governance.

The World Bank

One thing that always surprises the students we teach on both sides of the Atlantic is that the World Bank is one of the largest players in global health. Established in 1944 to help finance post–World War II European reconstruction and recovery, that legacy remains evident in the official name of its largest constituent institution, the International Bank for Reconstruction and Development (IBRD). Today, the IBRD provides loans and advice to middle-income and low-income countries deemed credit-worthy (at times the loans are contingent on taking the advice offered). The IBRD is only part of the World Bank. Indeed, the Bank is not a monolith but an umbrella enterprise including two institutions: the IBRD and the International Development Association (IDA). Formed in 1960, IDA provides loans and grants to the poorest countries; income level is the only criterion for countries to be eligible to apply for IDA funds.

Furthermore, the World Bank Group encompasses three additional institutions: the International Finance Corporation (IFC), which focuses on helping countries access private-sector capital directly and through the IFC; the Multilateral Investment Guarantee Agency (MIGA), which offers risk insurance to investors and lenders to remove that barrier to foreign direct investment in developing countries; and the International Centre for Settlement of Investment Disputes (ICSID), which provides services in line with its name. (We will not be discussing these three entities in this book.)

Unlike its companion UN institutions, the World Bank, from its inception, has raised funds on global capital markets as well as received funds from its member states. Most of IBRD's funds come from the world's capital markets while most of IDA's funds come from donor countries through a replenishment mechanism. In chapter 4 we examine how similar and distinct the funding approaches and streams are for the World Bank compared to our other case studies.

The World Bank's growing engagement in health coincided with a larger movement within the Bank and broader development community that recognized economic growth, while necessary for development, was by itself insufficient to guarantee development, particularly in places with endemic health challenges such as malnutrition and stunting or water-borne diseases like rotavirus or cholera. In the Bank's language, supporting countries' work in such health areas were investments in "human capital" and "human development." Since the Bank made its first loans in family planning in the early 1970s, it has invested significantly in programs to address malnutrition, onchocerciasis (river blindness), maternal health, primary/basic health services, HIV/AIDS, and more. At times, it has also launched new programs to oversee those investments, notably the Multi-Country HIV/AIDS Program (MAP), started in 2000. We probe the Bank in similar ways to that of WHO, examining both its governance and financing, as well as disbursement of resources to global health projects broadly. We also look at the Bank's inclusion of civil society organizations in various consultative capacities as well as its broader transparency policies and practices.

While its health portfolio has grown significantly in the last forty years, most of the Bank's lending and grants remain outside of the formal health sector. Yet, it is more readily apparent from the World Bank's website, versus WHO's website, what some of its investments in health have yielded, at least according to the Bank itself. For example, the World Bank asserts that from 2013 to 2015, programs funded through IDA provided close to 29 million women with antenatal care, immunized 142.8 million children, and provided basic nutrition services to more than 177 million children, adolescent girls, and pregnant or lactating mothers.[37] The Bank's MAP provided $2 billion for HIV/AIDS programs in thirty-five sub-Saharan African countries from 2000 to 2010, translating into counseling and testing sites and education initiatives across the continent. In total, from 2000 to 2013, IDA-funded efforts, including MAP, tested more than six million people and educated more than 170 million.[38] It is difficult not to be drawn to specific numbers like those, particularly when juxtaposed to WHO's challenges in pointing to equally specific results from its efforts. The desire to match specific results to specific investments—and be able to track the trajectories of each and the relationships between the two—is a major reason why the donor community and others began looking for "new" and more vertically focused health actors at the end of the twentieth century.

The "new" actors

Ensuring that Gavi and the Global Fund were both part of, and separate from, the existing global health governance landscape was essential to the creation of each. Their founders envisioned that they would have the legitimacy of intergovernmental partnerships while also the efficiency of the private sector (and a greater claim then to financial support beyond the conventional donor countries, including from the private sector). Enfranchising both state and nonstate actors on the various Boards was groundbreaking in global health. However, they were not the first international organizations to formally include nonstate actors. From its inception in 1919, the International Labor Organization (ILO) has formally included in its governance member-state governments as well as both employers and employee representatives.

In the 1990s, donor countries largely did not trust preexisting institutions, particularly WHO, to steward amplified efforts to close the vaccine gap or defeat HIV/AIDS, TB, or malaria. This was true even though the donor countries then (even more so than today) heavily influenced, if not actually controlled, the agendas of WHO and the World Bank.[39] Unsurprisingly, such donor dissatisfaction found expression in the emergence and institutional shape of Gavi and the Global Fund, and there are many distinctive features of both Gavi and the Global Fund that reflect frustration with the UN system. As one such example, neither has an in-country nor even a regional presence, meaning they do not have offices in the countries or regions to which they provide grant funding. This was a design decision made by their founders, as we will discuss later, intended to keep both entities operationally focused and lean (preventing the inefficient bureaucracy often pointed to, fairly or not, as a symptom and cause of UN dysfunction). An added benefit of such an operational approach was that it provided donors a more narrow span of monitoring and control. It is much easier to monitor an institution with one office than an institution with 150 offices around the globe as is true of WHO. Today, both Gavi and the Global Fund Secretariats in Geneva employ far more people than their founders likely envisioned. Yet, both employ far fewer people than WHO (despite claims to the contrary.)[40] Still, it is their lack of country or regional presence that arguably is most distinctive from an operational perspective.

Gavi, the Vaccine Alliance

Of all our case studies, Gavi has the most focused mission: to use its market-shaping power to help close the "vaccine gap" to help ensure that children in developing countries receive a full complement of crucial immunizations. Created in 2000 through an initial grant by the Gates Foundation, Gavi has leveraged its financial heft to shift the market around vaccines to a higher-volume, lower-cost dynamic, and also to incentivize future vaccine research and development. From 2000 to 2014, Gavi helped acquire more than $5.3 billion worth of vaccines and disbursed more than $1.7 billion to seventy-seven countries to support the distribution of those vaccines.[41] Given the significant financial resources Gavi has spent, it is not surprising that the number of vaccines provided is also significant. In 2014 alone, Gavi funds acquired 169 million doses of the pentavalent vaccine which includes DPT3, or a three-dose combination vaccine targeting diphtheria, pertussis, and tetanus (hence the DPT3 moniker) plus the vaccines against Hemophilus influenza type B and hepatitis B.[42] Country eligibility for Gavi funds is determined purely by per capita income level, similar to World Bank IDA eligibility.

Arguably, Gavi grew out of both a WHO success and a failure. In 1974, WHO launched the Expanded Program on Immunization to tackle the same vaccine gap Gavi was charged with twenty-five years later, albeit a much smaller one because of WHO's and UNICEF's preceding efforts. In 1974, 5 percent of children in the developing world had received a full complement of basic vaccines, at the time—diphtheria, measles, pertussis, polio, tetanus, and tuberculosis. In 1990, the percentage had risen to 80 percent. Yet, in Gavi's own telling of its origins, donor attention shifted away from WHO's immunization program in the 1990s, either because of its significant progress or because of a lack of confidence in the leadership, or possibly both.[43] Regardless of the reasons, upward progress halted and vaccination rates started to decline. In 2000, worldwide DPT3 (diphtheria, pertussis, and tetanus) rates were 73 percent, down three points from 76 percent in 1990. Throughout the 1990s, DPT3 coverage rates flatlined in low-income countries at even lower levels.[44]

At inception in 2000, Gavi comprised two separate entities with two distinct Boards, one focused on organizing the work of Gavi (the Global Alliance for Vaccines and Immunization), and the other on serving as a fiduciary agent for the funds Gavi raised (the Gavi Fund). The two merged in 2008 bringing all Gavi-related functions under one aegis (we examine this merger and commensurate governance reforms in chapter 6). Gavi's governance today includes donor governments, developing country governments (an equal number of each), the Gates Foundation, the vaccine industry from both donor and developing countries (again, in equal number), WHO, UNICEF, the World Bank, a civil society organization, a research health institute with work relevant to Gavi's mission, and nine "independent" individuals.[45] Only UNICEF, WHO, the World Bank, and the Gates Foundation hold permanent Gavi Board seats. Other Board members are time-limited in their Board service. This is an important principal-agent difference from how the other Boards are constituted and often work in practice, where multiple powerful donors effectively, even if not constitutionally, hold permanent Board seats.

Both UNICEF and WHO have close relationships with Gavi and its work beyond the boardroom. Gavi's impact is assessed by WHO, the organization it arguably displaced. WHO estimates that Gavi support from 2000 to 2008 prevented 3.4 million deaths and protected 50.8 million additional children with basic pentavalent vaccines; DPT3 coverage rose to 81 percent in low-income countries in 2014, up from 60 percent in 2000 (a percentage equal to that of 1990, again indicating the absence of progress made in the late twentieth century on vaccination coverage rates).[46] Gavi's funds are used to purchase vaccines solely through UNICEF; this arrangement is not without its critics, as some argue that more competition for Gavi purchasing would further drive down prices across the system. According to WHO, through 2014 Gavi funds enabled UNICEF and others to vaccinate 213 million additional children with new and underutilized vaccines, including the pentavalent vaccine, Japanese encephalitis, meningitis A, measles-rubella, pneumococcal, rotavirus, and yellow fever.[47] Starting in 2013, Gavi began funding the HPV (Human papillomavirus) vaccine and in 2014, the inactivated poliovirus vaccine. Still, recent research has indicated that 40 percent of Gavi's funds have gone to buying pentavalent vaccines.[48]

The 18 percent rate of return on vaccines investments—in other words, for every $1 invested in vaccination efforts in a given country, that country later realizes $1.18 in economic benefits—is often what Gavi points to as justifying its singular focus.[49] In Gavi's articulation, fewer vaccinated kids get sick than unvaccinated kids, yielding future medical cost savings. Those same vaccinated kids are more likely to develop healthy brains and bodies, and are therefore able later on to contribute to their country's economies and overall well-being.[50] Yet, part of this rate of return is the relatively low cost of vaccines compared to other public health interventions. Hence, Gavi's assertion that vaccines are "Public Health's Best Buy."[51] Using market power to buy a higher volume of vaccines at a lower per-unit purchase price has been part of Gavi's business model, even its raison d'être, from the beginning. While Gavi is careful not to claim exclusive credit for falling vaccine prices throughout the early 2000s, it does note that the price of the Hepatitis B monovalent vaccine dropped from $.56, when Gavi launched, to $.16 in 2010. Similarly, the pentavalent vaccine price declined from $3.50 in 2001 to $2.58 in 2011.[52] Given the significant upsurge of vaccine-dedicated resources that Gavi's creation catalyzed, it would be hard to dispute its market-shaping effects (even if the market results were not the sole product of Gavi's available resources and rather the result of multiple actors working on multiple fronts to lower vaccine prices as well as their underlying costs).[53]

A financial focus is a core part of Gavi's identity. Indeed, as mentioned earlier, unlike WHO or the World Bank, Gavi has no on-the-ground presence in the developing countries where the vaccines it helps fund are delivered. UNICEF, not Gavi, procures all of the vaccines that Gavi's funds buy. Distributing those vaccines safely and effectively immunizing children around the world also is the work of UNICEF, in conjunction with other partners from national governments and NGOs. It makes sense that WHO would track Gavi's progress against its goal of closing the vaccine gap as WHO's Department of Immunization, Vaccines, and Biologicals provides technical guidance to Gavi, including on the quality and safety of which vaccines to purchase. Gavi reimburses WHO and UNICEF for their technical support (WHO) and on-the-ground distribution support (UNICEF). According to Gavi's 2013/14 business plan, it was set to provide $51 million to WHO and $30 million to UNICEF.[54] Gavi raises money to fund these efforts and the vaccine purchases through a replenishment mechanism, similar to that of IDA. A replenishment process is one in which an organization solicits multiyear commitments from donors on a regular schedule, for example every three years, rather than looking for specific contributions every year. We further discuss Gavi's fundraising in chapter 4.

The Global Fund to Fight AIDS, Tuberculosis and Malaria

Like Gavi, the Global Fund to Fight AIDS, Tuberculosis and Malaria, as its name makes clear, also has a focused mission. It too is a financial entity, not an on-the-ground programmatic one. Unlike Gavi, it does not work primarily through multilateral partners like UNICEF, but rather through multi-party grant agreements. In its most recent funding model iteration (late 2013), the Global Fund allocates funds to eligible countries. And unlike Gavi, Global Fund eligibility is determined through a matrix inclusive of both income level and disease burden. It is possible for countries to be eligible to apply for funds in one area (e.g., HIV/AIDS) based on disease burden and not another (e.g., malaria). Country-coordinating mechanisms (CCMs) composed of government and nongovernmental partners then apply for grants within their allocation, specifying whether the requested funds will be used for HIV/AIDS, TB and/or malaria prevention and treatment, or broader health-systems strengthening.[55] While CCMs apply for grants and oversee grant implementation, what are known as Principal Recipients (PRs) are charged with delivering on the grant's program. Many Global Fund grants have both government and nongovernmental PRs working together in conjunction with various subcontractors. In addition, technical assistance for CCMs and PRs comes from other multilateral agencies like WHO as well as donors, like the United States. While principal-agent theory also would help elucidate the dynamics inherent in these relationships (from the Global Fund to the CCMs to the PRs to the subcontractors to technical assistance providers), such explorations fall beyond the scope of this book.

What is relevant to this work is that the Global Fund, like Gavi, has no in-country presence. All Global Fund Secretariat staff work from the Geneva headquarters. This decision was made toward not only keeping the Global Fund lean from a cost perspective but also as a deliberate decision to bolster "country-ownership" of Global Fund grants. Not having Global Fund staff in-country, the reasoning goes, provides more space for CCMs and PRs to make decisions they believe are best for their grants in their country context, not as determined by foreigners or technocrats (or both). This is a major distinction from WHO or Gavi's partner UNICEF, both of which have offices in 150 countries and 190 countries, respectively.[56]

Similar to Gavi, the Global Fund has a multi-stakeholder Board, which comprises an equal number of donor and implementing constituencies.[57] The donor constituency includes eight donor governments, a representative from the private sector, and a private foundation. The implementing constituency includes seven implementing countries, a nongovernmental organization from a donor country, a nongovernmental organization from an implementing country, and a representative of communities affected by HIV/AIDS, TB, or malaria. The World Bank, WHO, UNAIDS, and other technical partners are observers at Board meetings but do not have a Board vote. Additional unique aspects of the Global Fund's Board will be discussed more fully in chapter 3.

Like Gavi, the Global Fund from the beginning has defined itself as solely a financing entity (a claim further bolstered, like Gavi, by its lack of in-country presence). From its creation in 2002 through early 2016, the Global Fund had raised $33 billion and disbursed $27 billion in funding to support grants targeting HIV/AIDS, tuberculosis, and malaria in more than 140 countries.[58] Aside from the US government, more money has flowed to global health through the Global Fund to Fight AIDS, Tuberculosis and Malaria than any other institution in the early twenty-first century. In chapter 4, we discuss the distinction between channels and origins of funding (for example, most years, one-third of the Global Fund's money has originated from the United States through funding from the US PEPFAR program).

According to the Global Fund, through early 2015, the monies it has disbursed have put 8.1 million people on antiretroviral treatment, provided 423 million people with HIV counseling and testing, and prevented 3.1 million children from getting HIV from their mothers during pregnancy. Global Fund grants have also been used to detect and treat 13.2 million cases of tuberculosis, distribute 548 million bed nets, and deliver more than 515 million malaria drug treatments.[59] While these statistics come from the Global Fund's own tracking, the

Fund has worked closely with the US government's PEPFAR program and others to, where possible, distinguish (and assign) responsibility for who is on HIV medication or who has received an insecticide-treated bed net. However, where it is not possible, PEPFAR, the Global Fund, and others have decided to share credit under the understandable rationale that if someone is receiving diagnosis and treatment in a clinic receiving funds from multiple sources, *all* of those sources should share in the credit of saving lives.[60] In 2010 alone, the Fund accounted for 25 percent of all international public funding (multilateral and bilateral) disbursements to fight HIV/AIDS, 60 percent of international public funding for TB control, 65 percent of all funds allocated to TB in the twenty-two most-affected countries, and 70 percent of all funds allocated to malaria around the world.[61] That year, the Global Fund disbursed more than $3 billion.[62] PEPFAR disbursed more than twice as much, investing more than 15 percent of its funds in the Global Fund and many billions more alongside Global Fund around the world.[63]

METHODS

We analyze whether our case study institutions are viewed as effective by their principals through examining their governance, financial flows, and various reform pressures. Are the institutions we focus on governed, organized, and financed in ways that support their stated missions and position them for success against their own declared agenda? How do their principals' views on those questions influence their behavior as well as their funding and governance? Here are only a few such questions we aim to answer in subsequent chapters. For WHO, have its principals and the public perceived it as helping make the world healthier in an effective and efficient manner, as judged by principals' investments in the institution? Indeed, was WHO rewarded by its principals in terms of greater funding for the work it did or only for work that principals wanted it to do? For the World Bank, how central is global health to its work? Was its move into global health a comment on its strengths or on others' failures? For Gavi and the Global Fund, did they each enfranchise developing countries, the private sector, and nonstate actors in their governance in a meaningful and durable way? Or do donors continue to play an outsized role in setting and driving their respective agenda? Were Gavi and the Global Fund rewarded with additional responsibilities and funds for perceived successes and greater legitimacy due to their inclusive structures or merely for meeting donors' expectations?

The data sources we use to answer these questions focus largely on financial flows and various governance policies, particularly on how the principals relate to one another, how they relate to their agent institutions, and how the institutions, in turn, as well as the principals, relate to the public.[64] As noted previously, surprisingly little scholarship has focused on the Global Fund or Gavi, and none that we are aware of examines these questions in a comparative way across these four institutions. We complement the queries with targeted interviews from people leading and working within our case study organizations and hope our mixed-methods approach helps us ultimately answer our book's central question—who indeed runs the world of global health?

3

Shifts in Governance

IN THIS CHAPTER WE take a detailed look at key governance features of WHO, the World Bank, the Global Fund, and Gavi. We identify five key differences between the "old" and "new" institutions and provide an explanation rooted in principal-agent theory for the shift to the "newer" governance models. We then turn to examine the role of the Gates Foundation in this evolution.

KEY DIFFERENCES BETWEEN THE NEWER AND OLD MULTILATERALS

As described in chapters 1 and 2, alongside increases in funding for global health, a major change in international cooperation has been the emergence of new multi-stakeholder institutions for global funding, including the Global Fund and Gavi. The Global Fund is fast becoming the largest multi-stakeholder donor in health with pledges rising from $852 million in 2001 (its creation) to $3.2 billion in 2014. Gavi is also picking up pace from its initial start of $164.7 million in 1999 to $1.4 billion in 2014. These swells in funding will be further discussed and analyzed in chapter 4.

In addition to commanding significant resources that may once have flowed through WHO or even the World Bank, the relatively newer initiatives are marked by a structure of governance that differs in important ways from traditional multilateral institutions. First, a wider set of principals participate in the governance of the new initiatives. Traditional multilateral institutions are governed by boards encompassing only their member states. The World Health Assembly, WHO's governing body, comprises governments each of which have one vote; some of its decisions require a simple majority, others a two-thirds majority of those present and voting. The main functions of the World Health Assembly are to determine WHO's policies, to make recommendations to member states, to approve a general program of work, and to give instructions and directives to WHO's Executive Board and the Director-General.

The World Health Assembly also has ultimate financial authority over WHO and as such reviews and approves the budget and other financial recommendations made by the WHO Secretariat. Significantly, it also elects WHO's Director-General and decides on his or her renewal. The goals set by the World Health Assembly include negotiating and approving normative instruments such as treaties, formalizing public health recommendations (e.g., International Code of Marketing of Breast-Milk Substitutes), and approving global strategies for WHO and, at least aspirationally, public health more broadly (e.g., Global Strategy on HIV/AIDS 2011–2015).[1] Given the solely intergovernmental nature of WHO and the World Health Assembly's one-state, one-vote governing paradigm, it is clear why it remains the most important institution for negotiating international health agreements—both binding treaties and soft instruments such as recommendations—that apply to states within and/or across their borders.

Similar to WHO, the World Bank is governed, as well as owned, by its member states. To join the World Bank, a country must first become a member of the International Monetary Fund (IMF). Then, countries can apply to join the IBRD and subsequently IDA and other parts of the World Bank Group. The Bank's equivalent of the World Health Assembly is its Board of Governors; each member state appoints one World Bank Governor. The Bank's Governors' powers include determining whether to admit new members, to increase or decrease the expected capital allocations of member states, and when and how to cooperate with other international organizations, among other authorities. It also chooses the World Bank's president. Day-to-day, a Board of Directors oversees the Bank's administration. The Board includes a group of twenty-five Executive Directors elected solely by member states and chaired by the president of the World Bank Group. This is the body that approves IBRD loans and IDA grants and credits, as well as the Bank's budget.

In contrast, the Global Fund and Gavi are governed by Boards that include representatives of civil society, the private sector, and philanthropic organizations. At the Global Fund, the Board is responsible for its governance, selecting the Fund's Executive Director, the approval of new policies, and the approval of grants (though the process of grant approval, and what exactly the Board is approving, has changed over the duration of the Fund's existence, as we discuss in chapter 6). As of 2015, the Board itself is made up of a total of twenty-eight members: the twenty voting members include seven representatives from developing countries (one from each of the six WHO regions and an additional representative from Africa), eight from donor countries, three from civil society, one from the private sector, and one from the Gates Foundation. In addition, there are eight nonvoting members which include key partners such as WHO, UNAIDS, the World Bank, a Swiss citizen (as the Fund is legally a Swiss foundation and this is a requirement of Swiss law) and the Global Fund Board's chair and vice-chair (the latter two originally were voting Board members). Enfranchising implementing countries meaningfully on the Board was important to the Fund's founders as evidenced in the balanced constituencies across donors and implementers (albeit with one more donor than implementing country having a voting Board seat).[2] However, implementing constituencies, or countries alone, do not have a blocking majority on the Fund's Board, despite some initial suggestion they might be given such authority.[3] From the beginning, from donors' perspective, "country-ownership" has had clear boundaries.

Civil-society Global Fund Board seats are reserved for one donor country NGO representative, one implementing country NGO representative, and one person who represents the communities afflicted by one of the Fund's three constituent diseases (table 3.1). The chair and vice-chair of the Board each serve two-year terms with their positions alternating between representatives from the donor constituency and from the recipient or implementing constituency.

TABLE 3.1 Global Fund board composition as of January 2016

Implementer constituencies	Donor constituencies	Nonvoting members
Eastern Europe and Central Asia	Canada, Switzerland, and Australia	Chair
Eastern Mediterranean	European Commission (Belgium, Italy, Portugal, Spain)	Vice-Chair
Eastern and Southern Africa	France	Executive Director
Latin America and Caribbean	Germany	Host Country (Switzerland)
South East Asia	Japan	WHO
West and Central Africa	Point Seven (Denmark, Ireland, Luxembourg, Netherlands, Norway, Sweden)	UNAIDS
Western Pacific Region	United Kingdom	Partners (Roll Back Malaria, Stop TB, UNITAID)
Communities (NGOs representing Communities Living with Diseases)	United States	Trustee (World Bank)
Developed Country NGO	Private Foundation (Bill & Melinda Gates Foundation)	
Developing Country NGO	Private Sector	

Source: "Board" Global Fund, accessed 26 June 2016, http://www.theglobalfund.org/en/board/members/

At Gavi, the Board establishes all policies, oversees operations, and monitors program implementation. The Gavi Board consists of four permanent seats for representatives from the Gates Foundation, UNICEF, WHO, and the World Bank; unlike at the Global Fund, Gavi's multilateral partners have voting seats on the Board (table 3.2). In addition, there are eighteen rotating Board members who represent various constituency groups: developing country governments (five seats), donor governments (five seats), research and technical institutes (one seat), industrialized country vaccine industry (one seat), developing country vaccine industry (one seat), and civil society organizations (one seat). The Board also includes unaffiliated Board members (nine seats) with no professional connection to Gavi's work under the rationale that they bring independent and balanced scrutiny to the Board's deliberations.[4]

Since the millennium, the Gates Foundation has become an important new principal in global health. As of the end of 2013, it held the position as the largest philanthropic foundation in the world with an endowment of approximately $41 billion, with many more billions pledged by Warren Buffett to augment its work.[5] It holds seats on the Global Fund and Gavi Boards, reflecting the importance of its contributions to each over time, and is the largest or second largest contributor of voluntary funds to WHO, depending on the year. We discuss the Gates Foundation in more detail in the final section of this chapter and again in chapters 4 and 6.

A second distinguishing feature of how new initiatives are governed concerns their mandates. Narrower mandates characterize the new initiatives—indeed, the narrow (or more vertical) mandates were arguably the catalysts for their creation. Unlike the broad mandates of WHO ("the attainment by all people of the highest possible level of

TABLE 3.2 Gavi, the Vaccine Alliance board composition

Rotating seats	Permanent seats
Independent/Unaffiliated Individuals (9)	Gates Foundation (1)
Governments Donor Countries (5)	WHO (1)
Governments Developing Countries (5)	UNICEF (1)
Gavi CEO (1)	World Bank (1)
Research and Technical Health Institutes (1)	
Vaccine Industry Developing Countries (1)	
Vaccine Industry Industrialized Countries (1)	
Civil Society Organizations (1)	

Source: "Board Composition," Gavi, accessed 26 June 2016, http://www.gavi.org/about/governance/gavi-board/composition/.

health") and the World Bank ("to alleviate poverty and improve quality of life"), both the Global Fund and Gavi have narrowly defined mandates that are problem-focused. The Global Fund's mandate is to attract and disburse additional resources to prevent and treat HIV/AIDS, tuberculosis, and malaria. Gavi's mandate is to save children's lives and protect people's health by increasing access to immunization in poor countries, thus closing the vaccine gap between richer and poorer countries.

A third attribute of the new initiatives is that they are funded solely by voluntary contributions from governments and other donors as well as through innovative financing mechanisms, such as the so-called Gavi bonds and (RED) for the Global Fund. While WHO and the World Bank have moved toward voluntary contributions from donors (with funds to be used at those donors' discretion, not the institutions'), they both still have financial models at least partially based on assessed contributions. The new multilaterals not only rely entirely on voluntary contributions, they have never seriously considered moving to an assessed contribution model. Through the mechanism of replenishment, the Global Fund receives voluntary contributions from governments (the largest contributors), individuals, businesses, and private foundations. These are usually not for specific projects but to replenish the core fund. There are exceptions though. For example, in 2010, Chevron committed $30 million to the Global Fund over three years specifically for programs in Nigeria, Indonesia, Angola, Thailand, and South Africa.[6] Gavi also relies on donor contributions through replenishment, long-term pledges, and pledges to support the development and manufacture of vaccines. Private foundations (largely the Gates Foundation) have donated about a third of Gavi's budget, with the remaining contributions drawn from government. We discuss the financing of the four organizations, and the implications of their financing for their governance, in greater detail in chapter 4.

A fourth difference between new initiatives and more traditional multilateral approaches concerns the way relationships with recipients of funds are structured. Unlike WHO and the World Bank, which work predominately with and through government agencies and have offices and personnel in recipient countries, neither the Global Fund nor Gavi works directly in-country. The Global Fund relies on Country

Coordinating Mechanisms (CCMs) to develop and submit grant pro-posals based on priority needs at the national level. After grant ap-proval, CCMs oversee progress during implementation. CCMs usually consist of representatives from governments, NGOs, donors, people living with diseases, faith-based organizations, the private sector, and the academic community. For each grant, the CCM nominates one or two organizations to serve as Principal Recipient (PR). Since the CCM is a committee and not an implementing agency, while it technically has responsibility for grant oversight, it allocates responsibility for grant implementation to the PR. About two-thirds of all PRs are government institutions, but most recently the Global Fund first allowed and then began strongly encouraging, where possible, "dual track financing" where grants have both government and nongovernmental PRs. In fragile states, UNDP tends to play the PR role in Global Fund grants.

The Global Fund Board sets the parameters to determine which countries are eligible to apply for Global Fund funding. As of early 2016, eligibility is largely determined through a matrix of income threshold (data drawn from the World Bank) and disease burden (data drawn from WHO and UNAIDS). Low-income countries are eligible to apply for all types of Global Fund grants: HIV/AIDS, TB, Malaria, and Health Systems Strengthening. Middle-income countries' eligibil-ity is determined by their overall disease burden of HIV/AIDS, TB, and malaria. Additionally, countries with high disease burdens in vul-nerable populations, even if they have lower disease burdens in the overall population, are eligible to apply for Global Fund grants in those areas; for example, to treat high HIV/AIDS rates in commercial sex workers or injectable drug users.[7] Every eligible country is allocated a maximum amount of funding for each disease, based on income level, disease burden, risk, and whether their infection rates are expected to increase or decrease, among other criteria.[8] As of 2015, 125 countries are eligible to receive or currently are receiving Global Fund monies; the latter category includes countries graduating from Global Fund eligi-bility, with NGOs in those countries often receiving funds through specific transitional arrangements.[9]

Gavi provides funding directly to national governments based on country income. Again, as of 2015, countries with gross national income (GNI) per capita below $1,580 were eligible to apply for Gavi support; until 2010, the income threshold for Gavi applications was a GNI of $1,000. Both levels were determined by Gavi's board. Historically, there was no complementary (or from the countries' perspective, perhaps complicating) additional variable of disease burden or vaccine coverage levels to determine eligibility. More recently, Gavi's board decided that only countries with at least 70 percent DPT3 vaccine coverage, as determined by WHO/UNICEF, could apply for new DPT3 vaccine support (although Gavi has waived this requirement for certain countries).[10] Gavi placed no such thresholds on countries looking to apply for inactive poliovirus, meningitis A, yellow fever, HPV, rotavirus, Japanese encephalitis, or measles-rubella vaccine support. As of 2015, fifty-two countries are currently eligible to apply for at least one type of Gavi support.[11] In contrast to the new organizations, WHO works with virtually every country in the world on different issues while the World Bank engages with countries that meet the various income and credit-worthiness criteria set forth by the IBRD and IDA respectively on a project-by-project basis.

The fifth major difference between the "old" and "new" institutions is that the legitimacy of the new initiatives differs from the state-centric

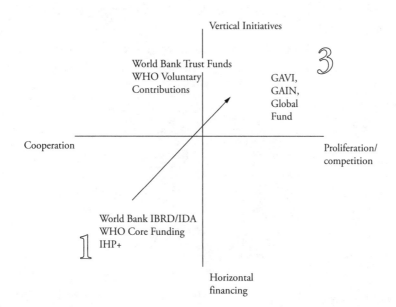

FIGURE 3.1 The new diversity of cooperation. Authors' calculations.

model of representation and interaction in traditional multilateral organizations. Both the Global Fund and Gavi derive their legitimacy from their effectiveness in improving very specifically defined health outputs and outcomes (output legitimacy), which we outlined in chapter 2. As a source of legitimacy, and arguably a proof of legitimacy, the Global Fund and Gavi also claim to better represent those affected by the particular diseases or disease threats they are working to overcome (process legitimacy). We talk more about legitimacy in chapter 5.

The move toward partnerships like the Global Fund and Gavi illustrates three major trends in global health governance more broadly.[12] The first is a trend toward more discretionary funding and away from core or longer-term committed funding. The second is a trend toward multi-stakeholder governance and away from traditional government-centered representation and decision-making. The third is a trend toward narrower mandates or problem-focused "vertical" initiatives and away from broader goals sought through multilateral cooperation. In figure 3.1 we depict these trends across two axes, from box 1 to box 3. The horizontal axis runs from traditional multilateral cooperation on the left, to the proliferation of new initiatives and agencies on the right. The vertical axis runs from horizontal approaches (such as a "health systems" approach) to vertical approaches (some would say "disease-specific").

Figures 3.2 through 3.8 show board composition of each institution and together provide a comparison of Board membership across WHO,

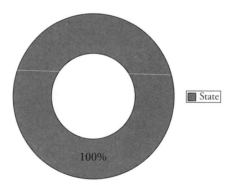

FIGURE 3.2 WHO—World Health assembly composition. "Media Centre: World Health Assembly," WHO, accessed 27 June 2016, http://www.who.int/mediacentre/events/governance/wha/en/.

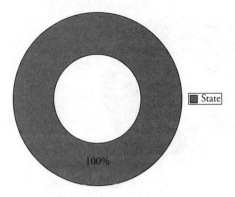

FIGURE 3.3 WHO—Executive Board composition. "Governance: Executive Board members," WHO, accessed 27 June 2016, http://www .who.int/governance/eb/eb_members/en/.

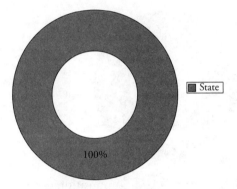

FIGURE 3.4 World Bank—Board of Governors composition. World Bank, accessed 27 June 2016, http://www.worldbank.org/en/about/ leadership/directors.

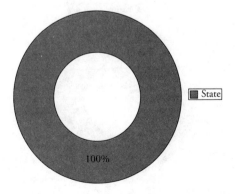

FIGURE 3.5 World Bank—Board of Directors composition. World Bank, accessed 27 June 2016, http://www.worldbank.org/en/about/ leadership/governors.

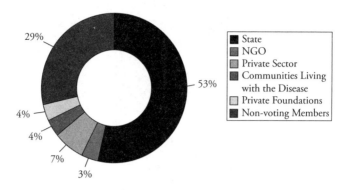

FIGURE 3.6 Global Fund Board composition. Global Fund, accessed 26 June 2016, http://www.theglobalfund.org/en/board/members/.

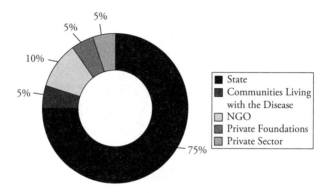

FIGURE 3.7 Global Fund Board composition—voting members only. Global Fund, accessed 26 June 2016, http://www.theglobalfund.org/en/board/members/.

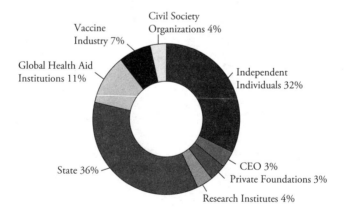

FIGURE 3.8 Gavi Board composition. Gavi, the Vaccine Alliance, accessed 26 June 2016, http://www.gavi.org/about/governance/gavi-board/composition/.

the World Bank, the Global Fund, and Gavi. Please note we use "state" to represent governments in the charts rather than "member state" given the Global Fund and Gavi do not have member states.

WHAT IS DRIVING THE NEW PATTERNS OF GLOBAL HEALTH FUNDING AND GOVERNANCE?

What explains these "new" patterns of cooperation in global health? Why are governments (and other actors) choosing to contribute in the ways described above? And what impact are they having on the "old" institutions such as WHO and the World Bank? In this section, we examine whether new patterns of global health funding and governance reflect a desire by participating governments and other actors to control multilateral agents more tightly. From the principal-agent literature, one of us (Devi Sridhar) and Ngaire Woods propose that governments as well as foundations and other actors could enhance their control over a multilateral agent in four ways:[13]

(1) Through the alignment of the objective interests of the agency with their own

(2) Through the use of material incentives to reward actions and behavior they approve and to punish those which they don't

(3) By reducing the asymmetry of information between them and the agency (such as by contracting out expertise or information gathering activities)

(4) By tightening their monitoring over the agency's work and outcomes, such as through the governance and decision-making rules of the agency.

In the following section we further develop these propositions and apply them to explain emerging forms of cooperation in global health.

Realigning objectives

Classic agency theory assumes that agents and principals do not have perfectly aligned objectives. For this reason, a principal will reduce the autonomy of his or her agent in order to better align its actions with the principal's objectives. Are governments or member states, and donors specifically, reducing the autonomy of international organizations in order to better align global health work with their own preferences?

In global health, differences have emerged between the substantive policy objectives and priorities of multilateral organizations and those (particularly shorter term priorities) of some of their member states. Traditional multilateral organizations have broad objectives such as WHO's objective to improve health; for example, the agency advocates that all countries should meet the International Health Regulations requirements, which would increase countries' capacities to detect and treat outbreaks while also improving their overall health systems (given what is required to adequately detect and respond to outbreaks). Meanwhile, member states in recent years have pushed more specific interests such as to concentrate on funding the treatment of a particular disease, or on specific, nationally defined priorities. For example, as we discuss extensively in the introduction, much of the new funding in global health has targeted specific diseases and in particular HIV/AIDS, TB, and malaria. The new patterns of cooperation exemplified in the Global Fund and Gavi can be seen as a way donor governments (and new actors such as the Gates Foundation) are attempting to better align cooperation with specific interests and goals, including by using trust funds and voluntary contributions (see chapter 4), as well as through creating new institutions and increasing their power in these new initiatives by limiting the size of their boards.

The case of multilateral cooperation on HIV/AIDS illustrates this dynamic process of realigning objectives. In the early 1980s when HIV/AIDS first appeared as a major public health emergency, donor governments were reluctant to invest heavily in WHO's core budget: instead they attempted to ring-fence their contribution. In 1986, the US government gave $2 million to WHO with the condition that half the money must be used for global AIDS control and half that money used to fight HIV/AIDS in Africa. In 1987, donors supported the Global AIDS Programme launched by Jonathan Mann within WHO, but with a governance structure somewhat separate from that entity. Unlike other programs, it did not require approval from WHO's regional offices for policy guidelines it promoted within their respective jurisdictions and its funding was extrabudgetary. Despite this tight grip on funds, donors became rapidly dissatisfied that they were unable to control where additional HIV/AIDS money was being spent.[14] In response to this frustration, WHO created several ways to channel bilateral aid through a new medium-term plan, so that donor governments could give money for the multilateral AIDS program while earmarking for country-specific projects. Yet, in 1990, the US Congress began to question publicly where the extra funds it had given over the last few years to WHO for HIV/AIDS had been used, amid fear that the extra money had led to corruption, not progress, in combating the disease.

In 1992, donors conducted an external review of the WHO response to HIV/AIDS, which called for a new effort that could address HIV/AIDS as a development issue. The external review concluded that "no single agency is capable of responding to the totality of the problems posed by AIDS; and as never before, a cooperative effort, which is broadly based but guided by a shared sense of purpose, is essential."[15] In 1994, major donors and US and European HIV/AIDS activists alike agreed that a joint and cosponsored initiative would be established and one hopefully that would be more accountable to donors and activists alike. The initiative would not be an agency in itself but instead leverage the resources of its cosponsoring UN agencies. The result was UNAIDS—a new initiative launched in 1996—whose creation was the product of weaknesses within WHO, interagency conflict, and donor pressures for more control over a multisectoral approach.[16] In 2015, the UNAIDS Program Coordinating Board included twenty-two member states, eleven cosponsoring entities (including WHO and the World Bank), and four regional NGOs working on the epidemic or representing people living with HIV/AIDS.[17] Despite this broad-based engagement, soon after its creation UNAIDS donors began to view it as being unable to mobilize and spend large amounts of funding to fight the explosion of AIDS in Africa, in part because of its legal status as a UN entity.[18] In other words, donors still remained reluctant to trust the UN system with the substantial funds that were increasingly recognized as being needed to combat the exploding HIV/AIDS pandemic.

As HIV/AIDS shifted to the top of the global agenda, the World Bank increased its HIV/AIDS efforts. In December 2000, the World

Bank launched its Multi-Country HIV/AIDS Program for Africa, better known as MAP, which committed more Bank resources to HIV/AIDS in Africa in 2001—$2 billion over fifteen years—than all previous years combined. Yet, donors worried that the Bank's efforts would similarly result in slow, inflexible, and top-down programs that would take too long to respond to countries' needs. There were also worries that the Bank's procurement rules would hinder developing country-ownership of their own HIV/AIDS agenda.[19] Additionally, by 2000, donors such as the United States and United Kingdom, supported by their fellow G7 members (the largest seven economies in the world), felt that the World Bank supported top-down public sector spending at the cost of supporting more effective NGOs, community groups, or local or international private-sector providers.[20] While the Bank may have hoped its financial commitment to MAP would gain donors' trust, it quickly became clear those hopes were not to materialize in substantial donor commitments. Throughout 2000 and 2001, it was evident that UN Secretary-General Kofi Annan clearly believed a new entity was needed to signal a new level of commitment by the world to combat HIV/AIDS, TB, and malaria—which he referred to as the diseases of the poor.[21] Pressures mounted for another new agency, and the Global Fund took shape.

It is difficult to imagine a stronger donor endorsement for the Global Fund than the US government's persistent levels of high funding, in most years accounting for one-third of the Fund's budget. Most of the US contributions come from the President's Emergency Plan For AIDS Relief program (PEPFAR). Created in 2003 by President George W. Bush, with a strong budget from Congress and reauthorized every five years since, PEPFAR is now the largest source of funds to combat HIV/AIDS, both bilaterally and through the Global Fund. By 2003, early results from Global Fund grants hinted that more money could make a real difference (even while acknowledging growing pains for the Fund and grantees alike).[22] One could argue that at least in the Global Fund's early years, its greatest achievement was in being a catalyst for PEPFAR. Or, one could argue the other way around, that PEPFAR catalyzed more giving by other donors to the Global Fund. It also could be argued that PEPFAR enabled the United

States greater leverage over the Global Fund given its financial importance to the Fund. We will discuss these possible dynamics further in chapter 4.

In 2011, the UK government's Department for International Development (DFID) reviewed the most significant forty-three multilateral organizations, based on amounts of donated funds from the United Kingdom.[23] The alignment of an organization's objectives with those of the UK government was the first key element tested in the review, which rated fifteen of the forty-three organizations as strong in working toward UK development and humanitarian objectives. The Global Fund and Gavi were both heralded in this context, as well recognized for providing good value for money. WHO and the World Bank (both IBRD and IDA) were viewed as more in the middle of the pack on both measures.[24]

In their follow-up to the review in 2013, DFID explicitly discussed how financing and conditionality (no funding "without strings attached") can be used to align the objectives of multilateral agencies with the specific development objectives of the UK government.[25] The UK DFID also expressed its desire to apply "special measures" to four organizations offering poor value for money to ensure, among other things, that they do a better job in delivering on UK objectives.[26] None of the agencies we examine in our book fell into this bottom category.

The evidence highlights that the new governance mechanisms supported by new funding permit governments to realign the objectives of multilateral initiatives with their own. Individual governments (or small groups of governments and like-minded others) are using new funding mechanisms, agencies, or initiatives as a way to articulate a separate, well-defined mandate and to pursue it.

Sharpening incentives

Classic agency literature also draws attention to incentives and, more specifically, to how incentives might be better structured to induce an agent to carry out the principal's interests faithfully. "High-powered incentives," for example, are those that tie an agent's payoffs tightly to realized outcomes, delivering a large reward to the agent when the principal's desired outcome is realized. These are not personal incentives for the management of an agency or secretariat but incentives that reward the agency or institution itself.

We argue that in respect to international institutions, governments can (and do) use membership (on which institutions in part rely on for legitimacy) and budget as rewards and punishments in their attempts to induce international institutions to achieve particular outcomes. However, it is worth noting that incentives are difficult in respect to international organizations because these agencies have multiple principals.[27] If any one principal (i.e., government) were seen to be able unilaterally to manipulate incentives, the continued participation of others would be difficult to assure. For this reason, multilateral institutions such as WHO and the World Bank are structured deliberately to limit the power of any one or group of individual governments to set incentives for the management and staff. The result is a structure designed to ensure a degree of autonomy, which permits the agencies to act as genuinely "multilateral" organizations. For example, in institutions, such as WHO, where assessed member contributions are an obligation of membership, countries have a duty to provide the budget regardless of agency priorities or performance.

Caveats aside, governments or groups of governments do use rewards or punishments to influence the actions of an international organization. Exit, or threatening exit, is one option. For example, the UK government in 2011 announced, as a result of that year's Multilateral Aid Review that it was withdrawing its membership of the UN Industrial Development Organization (UNIDO) given the report found it offered poor value for money and its work overlapped with other, more effective institutions.[28] UNIDO has been particularly criticized for its limited transparency, weak results reporting, weak financial reporting, and most notably, its inability to define its purpose and function. The United States withdrew at the end of 1996.[29]

A much more common incentive that governments use to influence international organizations is financial, wherein they threaten or promise changes to the budget of an organization. For example, in the 2013 UK government follow-up to their initial review, they declared their intention to stop all extrabudgetary funding to the UN International Strategy for Disaster Risk Reduction (UNISDR) and the UN Human

Settlements Programme (UN-HABITAT), and for the UK's Department for International Development (DFID) to stop contributing core funding to the ILO (leaving the UK's core contributions to be made by the Department of Work and Pensions).

Constraining governments from using financial leverage is their obligation to meet mandatory contribution levels and pay into core budgets. For example, as noted (with some implicit frustration) in the 2013 UK DFID aid review follow-up report cited earlier, the United Kingdom has a treaty obligation to the European Commission to contribute to its development assistance budget, regardless of the UK's view on how such contributed monies are being spent. Likewise the United Kingdom—as do all member countries—has a membership duty to WHO to contribute a proportion of the core budget reflecting the UK's wealth and population size. The World Health Assembly determines how that budget is apportioned, and it must unanimously approve every biennial budget. If a country does not pay its assessed contribution, WHO is authorized to suspend voting privileges and services to which a member is entitled, although no provision is made for expulsion. Suspension of voting privileges, while not common, has occurred when the World Health Assembly has concluded that a country has an ability to pay but is unwilling to do so. Governments do not have similar core budget obligations to the Global Fund or Gavi (or the World Bank's IDA).

Tighter incentives are made possible when governments, or others, provide extrabudgetary resources. In WHO this is significant. We discuss in detail in chapter 4 that a majority of WHO's voluntary contributions are earmarked, or designated, for specific purposes. In 2015, such voluntary contributions comprised 80 percent of WHO's overall budget. This requires WHO to work more in the interests of a few states and principals rather than its wider membership.[30] If the specific purposes that funds are given for are judged as being delivered, then funding is likely to be renewed. Thus, through providing funding tied to specific health priorities, donors can ensure that their funding is used to influence the activities and direction of the organization. It is not only newer institutions that are funded entirely through voluntary models. Even some traditional UN agencies, such as UNICEF, rely completely on voluntary contributions. In 2012, 69 percent of UNICEF's contributions were earmarked; the comparable figure for WHO that year was 61 percent.[31]

In the World Bank a similar structure of core capital and discretionary contributions exists. The World Bank's main lending agency is the IBRD, which is funded from three sources. It raises money from private capital markets by selling bonds which are underwritten by its full membership (through required capital contributions, similar to membership fees); it earns money on its interest-bearing loans to members; and it earns income from its investment portfolio (since it invests part of the money it earns from its lending). These sources are independent of members' control.

Discretionary contributions to the World Bank became significant, starting in 1960, when the members of the Bank created the International Development Association (IDA) to make concessional loans to the poorest countries. The funding for IDA is negotiated every few years through a replenishment mechanism during which individual governments determine how much they will contribute. A result of this process has been to open up a new channel through which the Bank can be directly influenced by its wealthier government members, and in particular the United States and the United Kingdom. The resulting relationships between the United States, the United Kingdom, IDA, and the World Bank are worth examining, and we hope other scholars will do so.

The United States has always been an important contributor to IDA. For example, the United States provided more than 20 percent of the total IDA contributions in the thirteenth replenishment, concluded in 2002, and more than 12 percent to IDA's sixteenth replenishment, completed in 2010.[32] The United Kingdom is also a significant IDA donor. In two of the three most recent replenishments, the fifteenth (completed in 2007) and the seventeenth (completed in 2013), the United Kingdom was IDA's largest donor, with the United States just behind it. Even though the IDA itself accounts for only about 25 percent of IBRD/IDA total lending, given the importance of the United States as an IDA donor, one would expect some degree of US leverage within the IDA itself. Historically, the United States has used threats to reduce or withhold contributions to IDA in order to demand changes in policy, not just in IDA but in the World Bank as a whole. For instance, during the late 1970s, the Bank was forced to promise not to lend to Vietnam in order to prevent the defeat of IDA sixth replenishment, and in 1993, under pressure from Congress, the United States linked the creation of an Independent Inspection Panel in the World Bank to IDA's tenth replenishment. This would serve two purposes, from the United States' and other donors' perspectives: first, to give donors more visibility into how their contributions were being used; and second, reports from an independent panel would mean donors would be less reliant on the Bank itself for its own monitoring and reporting. From the US perspective, such conditions were perceived as more than fair, with the reasoning being that the United States should exert greater influence than other donors over an organization—in this instance, the Bank—given it provides a greater share of the total funds. As one scholar frames the US engagement with the Bank over its first fifty years: "with the Congress standing behind or reaching around it, the American administration was disposed to make its catalogue of demands not only insistent but comprehensive on replenishment occasions."[33]

New cooperative initiatives such as the Global Fund and Gavi take financial incentives to another level. They reflect higher powered and more precise incentives on agencies to achieve outcomes explicitly specified by a defined group of principals, given their dependence on voluntary contributions and the absence of assessed membership dues. Additionally, from inception, the Global Fund has linked past grant performance to both future grant funding from the Global Fund and the expectation of future donor support. Gavi, too, has long promised results as part of its legitimacy and as proof of concept to its donors. Confident in its mission and its track record, Gavi first relied on ongoing donations, not the formal mechanism of replenishment, to galvanize and secure donor funds. Gavi launched its first replenishment process in New York in October 2010, more than a decade after its founding. Gavi donors met to agree on how to fund programs to avert an estimated 4.2 million future deaths through immunization. The meeting set the stage for a pledging conference in 2011 where Gavi raised $4.3 billion, significantly exceeding its initial goal of $3.7 billion.[34] United States co-chair Dr. Ezekiel J. Emanuel said, "As a founder of the Gavi Alliance, and by co-chairing this action meeting, the US is pleased to strengthen our continued commitment to the Gavi Alliance and to its ambitious goals. We're all here because Gavi's track record of 5.4 million lives saved makes it both a good investment for the world, and a source of hope."[35]

In contrast to Gavi, resource mobilization within the Global Fund has always been based on a periodic replenishment model on a voluntary basis for donors, complemented by additional ad hoc contributions from any donor and through the (RED) program, discussed in chapter 4. For the Global Fund, replenishment provides a forum for the Global Fund to discuss its achievements, for donors to exchange views on the operations and effectiveness of the Global Fund, and then for donors to consider its funding needs and make financing pledges for the next few years, reflecting their confidence (or lack thereof) in the organization. At the most recent replenishment conference held in December 2013, donors pledged $12 billion to support the Fund's work over the subsequent three years.[36]

Principals express confidence, or make clear the expectations of what is required to maintain or regain confidence (and to maintain or regain funding) in a variety of ways. As one example, the United States was the driver behind the Global Fund Board introducing its Office of Inspector General. At the April 2005 Global Fund Board meeting, the United States shared with the Board that the US Congress had made 25 percent of its contribution contingent on the creation of an Office of Inspector General, which was immediately proposed. Global Fund's Executive Director Feachem opposed the US position, but the Board voted in favor of the US proposal—it is hard to imagine how it could have done otherwise given that US contributions already represented one-third of the Fund's purse. This event is not recorded in the Board Report, although Aidspan, the Global Fund "watchdog" and an observer at the Board meeting, reported that the Board agreed to create an Inspector General because of pressure from the United States.[37] Additionally in 2011, Germany, the third biggest donor to the Fund, withheld 200 million Euros until concerns were answered about identified and alleged fraud and misuse of Global Fund money in Mauritania, Mali, Zambia, and Djibouti.[38]

Thus this "new" cooperation in global health—for both "old" and "new" multilaterals—is characterized by a tightening of the incentives used to shape the behavior of multilateral agents. This has taken two forms: an increase in discretionary contributions to conventional multilateral organizations, and the establishment of new organizations, both of which embody a structure of specific incentives, bolstered by 100 percent voluntary funding models, and a more limited set of principals.

Reducing asymmetries of information

According to classic agency theory, agents derive autonomy from their principals in part because they have greater information or expertise.[39] If principals sought to increase their control over agents, one way would be by reducing the information asymmetry (as between the management and staff of international agencies, and their government principals) inherent in many multilateral organizations. But is this possible in respect to global health institutions? And is it happening?

In this section we explore how information is distributed in the Global Fund and Gavi. Do the management and staff control most of the information on which decisions are made, in the same way that they do in WHO or the World Bank? Or is there a new and different model at work, which puts information directly into the hands of Board members (or principals), rather than into the hands of their agents (the management and staff of the organization)?

Our first observation is that both the old and new institutions look outside for information and technical advice on programs; this is true for staff and member states alike. WHO, for example, while possessing considerable in-house technical expertise, relies on expert advisory panels and committees to support its broad scope of work.[40] Most often these are established for the purpose of reviewing and making technical recommendations on a specific subject of interest to the organization, such as food safety, response to the H1N1 pandemic, or counterfeit medicines.

Crucial to our analysis of the principal-agent relationship is that WHO's Director-General appoints members of a panel based on technical ability and experience, although consideration is also given to the broadest possible international representation in terms of diversity of knowledge, experience, and approaches in the fields for which the panels are established. Such a panel then reports to the Director-General, and thus WHO's management, which in turn submits a report to the Executive Board on meetings of expert committees. The report contains observations on the implications of the expert committee reports and recommendations on follow-up actions to be taken. The texts of the recommendations of the expert committees are additionally provided in annexes. Two points are worth underscoring here: first, the outside experts are putting information initially into the hands of management and staff, not the Board, meaning that a potential asymmetry of information persists; second, the information provided by outside experts is not being used directly in decisions about what to fund and on what conditions.

Both the Global Fund and Gavi rely on out-of-house experts that report directly to the Board, most crucially on grant-making decisions, the main modus operandi of both organizations. In both organizations, external advisers aid the Board's decision-making in terms of which proposals and programs to fund. For this purpose, the Global Fund has a Technical Review Panel (TRP). The panel reviews proposals based on certain technical criteria and makes recommendations to the Board. Affirmative recommendations have been made for approximately 40 percent of proposals submitted through 2014, and the Board has approved almost 100 percent of recommended proposals, both under its Rounds-based and New Funding Model approaches.[41] The TRP consists of a chair and two vice-chairs and a maximum of forty experts who are appointed by the Board for a defined period of time (under the rounds-based model, panel members could serve for up to four rounds). Vacancies on the TRP arise annually, and members are selected from a pool of approximately 100 experts called the Technical Review Panel Support Group. Recruitment for this larger group typically occurs every two years and is managed by the Board's Portfolio and Implementation Committee using an open, transparent, and criteria-based process through a public call for applications. Criteria include broad expertise, both scientific and programmatic, in HIV/AIDS, tuberculosis, and malaria prevention, care, and treatment as well as broader health systems. Unlike in WHO, the Board appoints members of the TRP from a potential pool that a Board committee, not the Secretariat, selects. Importantly, the panel itself has never been accused of favoritism or partiality in early or later years,[42] and although there were more experts from high-income countries in the early years of the Global Fund, efforts have been made to recruit implementing country experts as well. As of 2015, both vice-chairs of the TRP come from implementing countries.[43]

Similarly, Gavi relies on an Independent Review Committee (IRC) composed of experts drawn from a broad geographic and experiential base to make recommendations on countries' proposals for Gavi support. The committee is independent, meaning no member can have a tie to Gavi or any of the entities serving on Gavi's Board. The IRC is divided into three teams to reflect Gavi's core areas: new proposals team, health systems team, and the monitoring team. Each team has a membership varying from eight to eighteen, with members serving for a term of three years. To ensure consistency in methodology and approach, some members serve on two or three teams. When new members are required, Gavi issues a call for nominations to its partners specifying the skills needed. IRC members are selected (primarily from low- and middle-income countries) for their expertise in public health, epidemiology, development, and economics, and specific knowledge of vaccines and immunization. Once nominations are received, the final decision whether to appoint a new IRC member is made by the Gavi Chief Executive, not its Board as is the case at the Global Fund. Grant applications may undergo multiple rounds of revision between Gavi and recipient countries before grant approval, which, like at the Global Fund, fully resides in the Gavi Board's domain. Similar to the Global Fund experience, the Gavi Board approves most of the IRC's recommendations.[44]

The newer institutions in global health are characterized by governance structures that reduce the asymmetry of information between the principals (countries represented on the governing body of an organization) and their agent (the management and staff of the agency). In WHO and the World Bank, the senior management of the organization presents proposals to the various boards, thus ensuring that the management and staff of the organization retain considerable influence and agenda-setting power. By contrast, the decision-making boards of the Global Fund and Gavi have decided instead to take advice from panels composed of independent experts that make recommendations to them directly (at Gavi the IRC recommendations go first to the Chief Executive but are then passed along to the Board). This reduces the potential agency slack afforded to senior management and staff of the agencies concerned, again increasing the authority of the organizations' principals.

Tightening monitoring

A fundamental problem of all principal-agent relationships lies in how to monitor the agent.[45] Typically, agency models assume that the principal cannot directly observe an agent's actions.[46] Instead, all the principal can expect to observe are outcomes, which correlate with an agent's effort but not perfectly so. Reward and punishment schemes are thus constructed around outcomes (such as share prices in the business world or further investments in the global health arena) rather than actions taken. If outcomes are only weakly linked to agent effort, such incentive schemes may have minimal effects. A general problem is that effective monitoring might demand an investment of resources so large that it overwhelms the rationale for delegation.

When governments and foundations cooperate on global health by delegating authority and actions to a global fund or agency, how can they know precisely what their agent is doing on their behalf? The desire to know understandably has become a major preoccupation of donors reflected in priority being given to demonstrating results, typically through results-based management systems, comprehensive results frameworks, an increased use of evaluations (both independent and in-house), and a tightening and deepening of reporting requirements and transparency. This focus can be seen in the UK DFID's review of multilateral aid, in which there is a specific focus on (a) measuring strategic and performance management in multilateral agencies and (b) improving transparency and accountability. The review asked whether organizations make comprehensive information about their policies and projects readily available to outsiders, and whether they are accountable to their stakeholders, including donors, development country governments, civil society organizations, and direct beneficiaries.[47] Similarly, the series of US Government Accountability Office (GAO) reviews of the Global Fund in its early years particularly focused on the Secretariat and grantees' documentation, and how accessible and usable they were to the United States and other constituents. Indeed, the United States would use these reviews to push the Fund for better documentation—and better direct visibility into its processes from Geneva down to the CCMs and PRs.[48] These demands carve out a new direction in principal-agent relations to that envisaged in the more traditional governance structure of multilaterals.

Traditional multilateral organizations have established structures for their member states to monitor their activities. For WHO, the World Health Assembly is the main vehicle by which member states monitor the activities of the organization, albeit at a high level, through various reports the secretariat provides, particularly as relates to proposed shifts in budgets year to year. Member states can also monitor WHO through the Executive Board, which is composed of thirty-four technically qualified individuals in the field of health and from a diversity of member states (although in most years the United States has held a seat), each elected for three-year terms.[49] The Board meets at least twice a year where it works to realize the decisions and policies of the health assembly, to advise it, and to generally facilitate its work.

Despite the World Health Assembly and the Executive Board, one of the main challenges in monitoring WHO relates to its regional structure.[50] WHO is composed of the main Secretariat, in Geneva, and six regional organizations, which are unique in the UN system for their independence and decision-making power. Each member state is allocated to a regional office, which is governed by a Regional Committee—a plenary body largely composed of Ministers of Health. Each office is headed by a Regional Director who serves as WHO's chief technical and administrative officer in that region. Regional Directors are elected by their constituent countries and then formally appointed by the Executive Board. They have full power over personnel in their region including the appointments of country representatives. Regional Committees meet annually to formulate policies, review the regional program budget, and monitor WHO's collaborative activities for health. The World Health Assembly and WHO's Executive Board formally approve these decisions, but in practice, tight policy and budgetary control is not possible. This creates challenges in monitoring the organization. As former WHO Director-General Dr. Gro Brundtland stated, "WHO is one. Not two—meaning one financed by the regular budget and one financed by extrabudgetary funds. Not seven—meaning Geneva and the six regional offices."[51] This telling quote indicates two major challenges facing WHO leadership—the first is where the money comes from and for what purpose (core, mandatory funding versus extrabudgetary, voluntary funding), and the second is managing six semiautonomous regional offices over which the Director-General has limited authority. Despite Brundtland's assertion, not many would have agreed with her then, or agree with her today, given the unchanged regional structure and continued rise of extrabudgetary funds as a percentage of WHO's budget.

In the World Bank, the Board of Governors on which all member countries are represented (some in groups) sits permanently in Washington, DC.[52] Members of the Board have access to large amounts of information about what the Bank is doing, enabling them (in theory) to closely monitor the activities of the staff and management of the organization. In reality, the Directors who sit on the Board (sometimes for only a short period of time) drown in the information to which they have access and strive to little effect to monitor closely the activities of the staff and management of the organization, and to report activities back to their own home governments. The Board has sometimes sought to more actively monitor the activities of the management and staff.[53] For example, as mentioned earlier, in 1993 the Board, driven by the United States, created the Independent Inspection Panel: an institution investigating Bank decisions and actions and reporting directly to the Board.[54] This is similar to what the United States pushed for, and achieved, fifteen years later with the introduction of the Inspector General at the Global Fund.

When contrasted to the new multilateral initiatives such as the Global Fund and Gavi, the World Bank and WHO look particularly difficult to monitor: for starters, their activities are broader and more diffuse, and their budgets are more complex. By contrast (as we discuss in detail in chapter 5), the Global Fund provides detailed financial information about Global Fund grant commitments and disbursements, donor pledges and contributions, and, importantly, grant progress reports, which over time have gotten more specific to their programs rather than the funds received and disbursed. It also discloses the TRP recommendations and subsequent Board funding decisions. An electronic library provides internal and external evaluations of the Fund. The *Global Fund Observer* (produced by NGO Aidspan) reports on the financing of the Global Fund, monitors its progress, comments on the approval, disbursement, and implementation of grants, provides guidance for stakeholders within application countries, and reports and comments on board meetings. Additionally, many donor member states have people from their bilateral aid agencies on the ground in countries receiving funds from the Global Fund who at times are members of the CCMs charged with overseeing the grants. Given the absence of a country presence by the Global Fund, this in-country presence translates into more real-time monitoring for certain donors than even the Global Fund Secretariat could claim. Gavi has a transparency and accountability policy that governs the management of all cash-based support to Gavi eligible countries (see chapter 5) and similarly discloses all IRC recommendations and Board decisions related to Gavi applications and approved grants.

The review of multilateral organizations conducted by UK DFID rated only two of forty-three organizations as "strong" on transparency and accountability, and both were global funds (Gavi and the Global Fund); an additional three were rated as satisfactory.[55] Gavi is praised for "strong financial oversight including a proactive Finance and Audit Committee, and internal Auditor appointments and a robust Transparency and Accountability Policy."[56] The Global Fund is praised because its decision "to publish/require recipients to publish procurement data has been a major driver for a range of innovations in transparency."[57] By contrast the report notes, "the WHO has no formal disclosure policy and does not publish enough specific program or policy details," even though "partners are well represented in governance mechanisms."[58] We talk more about the differences in disclosure policies and practices, and WHO's unique lack of disclosure policies and practices compared to our other case study institutions, in chapter 5.

In sum, the move toward the partnership model in global health is permitting donors to finance and deliver assistance in ways that they can more closely control and monitor at every stage, and for the Global Fund, at every level. This is one of the ways in which new practices of global health cooperation are altering the relationship between principals (governments) and their agents (the management and staff of international agencies). Donors are reducing potential agency slack by using financing and governance mechanisms, as well as the creation of new agencies, to (a) more closely align the objectives of global agencies with their own objectives, (b) more robustly create and enforce incentives for performance, (c) more directly reduce the information asymmetry between them and the agents they empower to deliver health coopera-tion, and (d) more closely monitor what global agencies are doing.

THE GATES FOUNDATION

Even the definition of what kind of actor is a principal in global health has shifted. Most notably, the Gates Foundation has become an impor-tant new principal in WHO, the Global Fund, and Gavi, as well as in a more limited way in the World Bank. This influence comes directly through Board membership and/or financing voluntary contributions. The Gates Foundation, the largest private grant-making foundation in the world, annually gives around $3 billion in grants, and in 2013, gave $1.08 billion for global health.[59] It also holds significant policy leverage and is part of what is known as the H8, along with WHO, the World Bank, Gavi, the Global Fund, UNICEF, UNFPA, and UNAIDS. The H8 was created in 2007 to bring renewed attention to the health-related MDGs and focus on ways of speeding up progress; its fate in the post-MDG era remains, as of early 2016, unclear.[60] In addition, the influence of the Gates Foundation is not only about the money itself, but also about the time and attention Bill and Melinda Gates give to particular health issues that signal their importance to other wealthy individuals, including potential supporters of global health concerns, and also, arguably, the broader world.[61]

In 1997, Bill Gates established The William H. Gates Foundation so that he could pursue charitable endeavors. Over the next three years, Gates's interest in global health grew—perhaps seen nowhere more prominently than in the Foundation's grant establishing Gavi in 1999. A year later, in 2000, the Foundation was restructured into The Bill and Melinda Gates Foundation.[62] In 2006, the Gates Foundation fur-ther refined its mission, including a clear articulation of its three main priorities as global health, global development, and work in the United States, clearly reinforcing its previously made commitments and goals. Additionally, Warren Buffett pledged to give $37 billion to the Foun-dation, doubling its endowment.[63] The Gates Foundation currently has an endowment of $42.9 billion, and, as of summer 2015, has paid out $33.5 billion in grants since its inception.[64] The Gateses and Warren Buffett have pledged to give a majority of their fortunes to charitable causes, largely through the Gates Foundation.

Because of the enormous amount of money at its disposal, the Gates Foundation is able to play a role in setting the research agenda for several public health priorities and to strongly influence policy decisions.[65] The Foundation co-chairs are involved with approving grant-making strategies in advance, and their level of involvement depends on the size of the grant—they do not authorize every one but certainly are involved in decisions of personal priority or involving significant sums.[66] As with all US registered foundations, it is required to report affirmative financing decisions transparently to the United States Internal Revenue Service. It is clear that the Gates Foundation has played a vital role in global health and can aptly claim credit for saving untold lives, including through its strong support of Gavi. Yet, despite its large budget and significant influence in shaping global health policy and financing, or perhaps because of it, there has been surprisingly little examination of the Foundation's health grants or funding policies.[67]

Although private philanthropic foundations such as the Rockefeller Foundation and Ford Foundation have long contributed to global health efforts, the scale and influence of the Gates Foundation is unprecedented. Not only does its annual budget surpass that of WHO, with its annual global health investments totaling more than 50 percent of WHO's yearly spend, but "the Gates approach" of funding almost exclusively disease-specific programs has deeply shaped the global health policy landscape.[68] It is also important to recognize that, as discussed earlier, preferences and pressures for vertical or disease-specific programs pre-date the Gates Foundation's earliest incarnation.

As we discussed in chapter 1, the rise of the partnership model coincided with a surge in global health funding focused on disease-specific or selective interventions.[69] What has been the role of the Gates Foundation in driving the "vertical" model to global health governance and delivery forward?[70] In some areas, the answer might be assumed to be fairly minimal, as we see in the experience of the increasingly vertical focus on HIV/AIDS over time, driven by the United States and other bilateral donors. At the Gates Foundation, the question of the balance between vertical and horizontal health funding is arguably most evident when looking specifically at child health research, a major priority of the Foundation. The issue of child health received renewed global attention following the Millennium Development Summit of the UN in 2000, which drafted eight development targets; MDG 4 specifically highlighted the importance of child health with the aim to reduce child mortality rates by two-thirds by 2015 from the base year of 1990.

Rooted in the Gates Foundation's philosophy that "every life has equal value," Bill Gates has stated his aim to cut in half child mortality over the next twenty years.[71] In line with this, the Foundation has made billion-dollar investments into various different aspects of child health, including funding relevant research. Looking at the period from 2005 to 2014 provides a window into how the Foundation's research priorities have changed over time, including as relates to the attention paid to more vertical interventions.[72]

In order to facilitate analyses, grant data relating to child health research for this period was categorized into five nonoverlapping categories. The five categories are:

- *Cause-Specific funding*: This includes all child health grants that were specifically targeting one or more diseases. Vaccines were not included in this category.
- *Nutrition and Breastfeeding*: This includes all child health grants for nutrition, malnutrition, breastfeeding, food fortification, food supplementation, and improving food systems.
- *Growth and Missed Potential*: This includes all child health grants addressing cognitive and neurodevelopment, and physical healthy growth.
- *Vaccines*: This included all grants for vaccine research. This category was comprised of grants for development of vaccines for specific diseases and grants for general vaccine implementation research.
- *Other*: This included all grants for improving child health data, metrics, and evidence. For example, grants to fund studies on global estimates of child mortality. This category also included

child health grants that did not fit under any of the other categories. Typically, these were grants looking at child mortality overall as opposed to any specific disease or issue.

All child health–related research grants were placed into one of these five categories. Because these categories do not overlap, no one grant appeared in more than one category. Grants were allocated into categories based on the primary goals stated in the grant description. Categorization allowed for analysis of trends in terms of vertical versus horizontal funding. For example, "vaccines" and "cause-specific" grants fall under vertical funding. In contrast, "nutrition and breastfeeding" and "growth and missed potential" fall under horizontal funding as grants in those areas focus on risk factors that affect a wide array of diseases in different ways. Thus, funding into these two categories arguably has a crosscutting effect on numerous diseases and health outcomes, making it horizontal funding.

From 2005 through 2009, 64 percent of all child health research grants by the Gates Foundation went into vaccines (fig. 3.9). Vaccines also accounted for the largest number of grants with 104 of the total 171 grants. "Nutrition and Breastfeeding" and "Other" each received around 13 percent of total grants followed by "Cause-Specific" research which accounted for 9 percent. "Growth and Missed Potential" received the least amount of money during this period with only 1 percent of all funding and one grant.

From 2010 to 2014, "Vaccines" accounted for 74 percent of all child health research grants awarded by the Foundation (fig. 3.10). "Cause-Specific" research received the second largest amount of grants with around 14 percent of all grants going into this category, followed by "Other" which made up 6 percent of all grants. Finally, "Nutrition and Breastfeeding" and "Growth and Missed Potential" accounted for the least amount of total grants with 4 percent and 2 percent respectively.

The Gates Foundation's commitment to supporting research into vaccination development and program implementation is well known and documented. Previous research found that 97 percent of all Gates Foundation grants for global health were allocated to developing new technologies between 2000 and 2004.[73] Given Bill Gates's career, it is

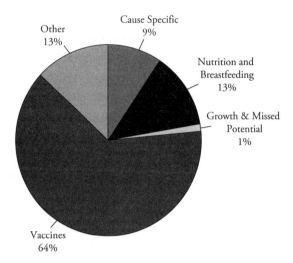

FIGURE 3.9 Distribution of Gates Foundation funding for child health research by category for 2005–2009. Marine Kiromera, "Investigating the Bill & Melinda Gates Foundation's Funding Policies for Child Health Research from 2005–2014"; Gabrielle Geonnotti, "Investigating How the Bill and Melinda Gates Foundation Has Invested in Global Child Health Research from 2005–2014" (MPH diss., University of Edinburgh, 2015).

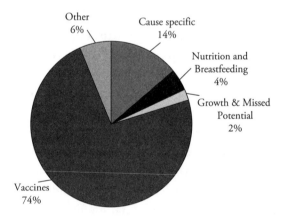

FIGURE 3.10 Distribution of Gates Foundation funding for child health research by category for 2010–2014. Marine Kiromera, "Investigating the Bill & Melinda Gates Foundation's Funding Policies for Child Health Research from 2005–2014"; Gabrielle Geonnotti, "Investigating How the Bill and Melinda Gates Foundation Has Invested in Global Child Health Research from 2005–2014."

not surprising that the Foundation's global health agenda tends to focus on the research and development of new technologies, most notably pharmaceutical innovations. In fact, less than 23 percent of grants made by the Gates Foundation from 2000 to 2004 went to research pertinent to delivery and utilization.[74] While this analysis was not restricted to child health research alone, it highlights the priority technological advancement has within the organization. Therefore, it is unsurprising that in this analysis, vaccine funding was shown to be five times greater than the next most well-funded category in both time periods. This occurred despite a 29 percent reduction in the funding between the periods, a decrease from $1.2 billion to $868 million.

Even with growing consensus throughout the early twenty-first century among major global health actors and institutions about the importance of horizontal funding, particularly with regard to meeting MDG 4 by the end of 2015, the Gates Foundation did not appear to have made any major shifts in their funding policies or programmatic priorities.[75] Overall, despite public statements recognizing the limitations of their preferred vertical funding strategy, there has yet to be any significant shift toward horizontal programs in terms of what the Gates Foundation actually funds.[76] To be fair, much the same could be said of most major bilateral donors as well.

One of the legacies from the MDG era is the role the Gates Foundation has played in creating public private partnerships, most notably Gavi, supporting other vertical initiatives such as the Global Fund, and investing funds in WHO through major voluntary contributions and in the World Bank partnerships at more modest levels.[77] As an important new principal in global health, the Foundation has used financing to create and advance forums where it can, understandably, at least somewhat control and monitor the use of its funds more tightly.

The irony that this chapter brings to the fore is that states historically form and join global institutions such as WHO in recognition of the need for collective action that does not always mesh with their own national interests. Yet, as the shifts in global governance over the past two decades demonstrate, they are loath to provide the support and investment to these institutions, either for lack of trust, sovereignty concerns, or simply because they cannot control and monitor their activities as closely as they would like. As we discuss in chapter 4, the desire for tighter control is reflected in donors moving global health financing toward a discretionary model (in terms of amount and timing of payment) to fund a specific priority (as opposed to the general purposes of the organization), over which donors will be able to exercise closer monitoring and, at least in theory, greater control.

4

Who Funds Global Health?

DEPENDING ON WHERE YOU are sitting, the answer to this chapter's question is either straightforward or rather convoluted. If we take global health to mean the promotion and protection of health in the developing world, the answer to the question is unquestionably developing country governments themselves. In 2012, low- and middle-income country government health expenditures reached above $711 billion, more than double the aggregate levels a decade before and far above the $33 billion in Development Assistance for Health (DAH) provided by donor countries in that same year (fig. 4.1).[1] DAH encompasses both financial and in-kind contributions from donors targeted to improving health in developing countries.

From 1991 to 2001, cumulative Official Development Assistance (ODA) contracted by approximately 30 percent, in real dollar terms. In a stunning reversal, ODA grew 11.4 percent per year on average from 2001 to 2005, again in real dollar terms; excluding debt relief, which grew 63 percent between 2001 and 2005, traditional ODA still grew on average 4.6 percent per year.[2] Looking at the twenty-first century's first decade from 2001 to 2011 tells a similar story to its first few years. Over those ten years, ODA grew in real dollar terms from $82.8 billion in 2001 to $132.4 billion in 2011, an annualized increase of 4.8 percent (fig. 4.2).[3]

Narrowing in on health specifically, DAH experienced an average annual growth rate of 5.4 percent from 1990 to 2000, outperforming

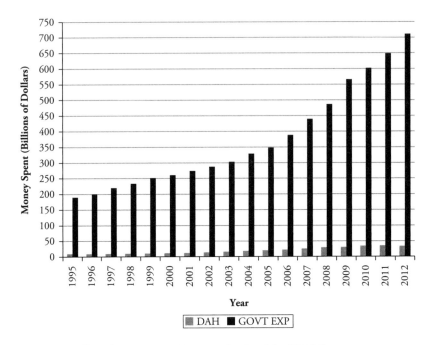

FIGURE 4.1 Development assistance for health (DAH) vs. government health expenditures. IHME, "Financing Global Health 2014: Shifts in Funding as the MDG Era Closes/B2 and B14," accessed 13 January 2016, http://www.healthdata.org/policy-report/financing-global-health -2014-shifts-funding-mdg-era-closes.

significantly the overall ODA (shrinking) trajectory over a similar time period. From 2000 to 2010, DAH increased on average 11.3 percent per year. Since 2010, as the most recent IHME report noted, DAH "has plateaued," staying consistently around $35–36 billion (in 2014, DAH was an estimated $35.9 billion, 1.6 percent lower than in 2013).[4] These overall numbers help provide important context to the financing commitments central to the creation of two of our four focal institutions. It is hard to disaggregate whether those institutions drove funding or their funding was the foregone conclusion of their creation given a greater intensity of conventional bilateral donors' focus on health, specifically on vertical intervention-focused instruments, and the emergence of the Gates Foundation as a significant new donor in health. Indeed, the US government, the UK government, and the Gates Foundation accounted for more than 61 percent of the DAH increase

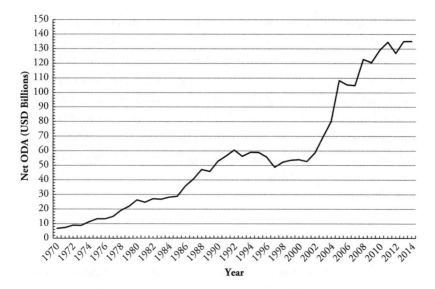

FIGURE 4.2 Official development assistance (ODA) growth from 1970–2014. OECD, 2015, http://www.oecd.org/dac/stats/.

from 2000 to 2014.[5] Still, it bears repeating that if we were focused only on the straightforward answer to this chapter's core question of who funds global health—it is not primarily DAH or even ODA more broadly, it is developing country governments themselves.

If we take this chapter's question to focus on DAH alone (as we do), then the answer is more nuanced, in part because the focus of donors has shifted over recent years in reaction to shifting disease burdens, new knowledge around how best to prevent and treat diseases, as well as donors' priorities themselves. Those nuances include both the ultimate target of those monies as well as the mechanisms that donors rely on to steward those resources. To be clear, DAH only includes efforts (the majority of which are financial in nature, not in-kind) focused primarily on health. This means that DAH does not include other efforts that are focused on water and sanitation, food aid, or humanitarian assistance following a natural disaster or outbreak of violence, although all of those are intimately connected to the maintenance and attainment of health for the people affected. The same could be argued for education efforts—given the well-established correlation between a mother's education and her child's health—or efforts combating climate change—given the causal relationship between rising temperatures and the incidence of certain diseases. The possibility of "health" to include all things—and then to mean in practical, trackable terms, nothing—helps illuminate why DAH is so tightly defined. In this chapter, we first discuss different ways to classify DAH as well as lay out the general ways in which donors contribute to DAH before moving on to discuss the ways in which WHO, the World Bank, the Global Fund, and Gavi are financed—and who is ultimately holding their purse strings and to what effect. It builds on and provides greater context to the observations made in chapter 3.

SOURCE VS. CHANNEL OF FUNDING

"Source" refers to the true origins of DAH, generally donor governments, private philanthropic foundations, and private individuals. From a technical perspective, sources include government treasuries, corporate treasuries, philanthropic capital designated for health or a portion of a philanthropic foundation's endowment, as well as contributions from private individuals or their family foundations (fig. 4.3). We do not believe such qualifications add to our descriptions or analyses and as such will refer only to the main institution itself. For example, the largest source of DAH, by far, is the US Treasury; we will refer to this as the US government or the United States. Similarly, the largest source of private support for global health, again by far, is the Gates Foundation. The "channels" through which the United States and the Gates Foundation, as well as other donors, direct their contributions vary from donor to donor and from year to year. All four of our focal institutions are examples of channels, although arguably the World Bank is also a source of funds given the substantial amounts it raises through its own bond issuances.

Bilateral aid agencies and multilateral organizations not discussed here (such as UNICEF), as well as NGOs and public-private partnerships, are also examples of channels of assistance given their general reliance on bilateral donors, philanthropic foundations, and private individuals (fig. 4.4). Channels differ from implementing institutions, or those actors that do the work on the ground to achieve broad and specific health goals with the funding received from various channels and sources. Sometimes the same institution is both the channel and

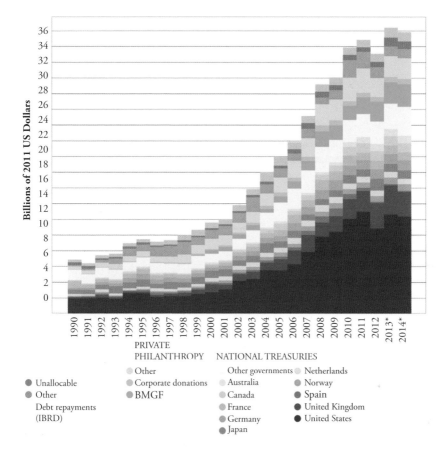

FIGURE 4.3 DAH by source of funding, 1990–2014. IHME 2014, 18.

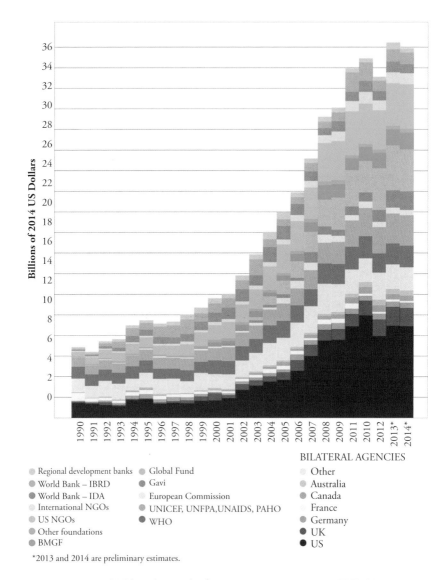

FIGURE 4.4 DAH by channel of assistance, 1990–2014. IHME 2014, 17.

implementing institution, although in global health, more often than not, the two are not synonymous. For example, the United Kingdom makes contributions to Gavi (channel), which would then provide funds for the purchase and distribution of vaccines to UNICEF (implementing institution). Or, the United States donates to the Global Fund (channel) to support financing grants tackling HIV/AIDS in South Africa, in which the South African Health Ministry and various NGOs (implementing institutions) jointly receive funds and work together toward a grant's ambitions.

MEMBERSHIP DUES VS. VOLUNTARY CONTRIBUTIONS

Conventionally, funds move from source institutions to channels through two mechanisms, although increasingly these are complemented by what are often referred to as new or innovative financing approaches. Traditionally, international organizations raise funds through assessed contributions or what are known, more colloquially, as membership dues. Of our focal institutions, Gavi and the Global Fund have no funding stream resembling assessed, or even expected, levels of contributions. The UN itself and many of its agencies, including WHO, levy assessed contributions or fees on its member states. Until Ebola shined a light on the relatively low level that assessed contributions to WHO count toward its overall budget, much of the debate, at least in the United States, around membership fees focused on the UN itself and only periodically on its agencies. This UN system-myopia resulted at least in part because the US Congress, generally more skeptical of international organizations than the executive branch, has to approve budget appropriations for the United States' financial obligations and voluntary contributions to international organizations in which it holds membership. In contrast to the UN system, the World Bank's IBRD is owned by its member states through a system of contributed capital that corresponds to voting rights (though these too could be thought of as expected contribution levels given they are necessary to maintaining preexisting voting rights). Yet, as referenced earlier, most of the monies the Bank ultimately lends are raised on global capital markets through bond issues, making it unique among the institutions discussed here.

Gavi, the Global Fund, and the World Bank's IDA rely entirely on voluntary contributions to fund their work. Over the past thirty-five years, WHO has increasingly relied on voluntary contributions to support its work (and arguably to determine its future work as we discuss later). Since the 1980–81 budget term, at least half of WHO's total budget has come from voluntary contributions. For WHO, voluntary donor commitments, many from WHO's member states, are generally made during WHO's budget cycle.[6] In contrast, the voluntary contributions that fund IDA's, Gavi's, and the Global Fund's work are raised predominantly through replenishment conferences, or meetings convened periodically, generally every three to four years,[7] to discuss the organizations' individual funding needs and to determine, in hard commitments, donors' willingness to meet those needs. We discuss replenishment mechanism more in-depth in the context of each institution as relevant.

THE "GOLDEN AGE" RISING TIDE

Financing is an intimate and inevitable part of the story of these institutions, as too is the overall trajectory and composition of DAH. Indeed, IHME has termed the past fifteen years "the Golden Age" of DAH given the "largess" donors contributed to global health.[8] Both Gavi and the Global Fund were created (at least in part) because of a shared belief across bilateral donors, the Gates Foundation, and even the technical community that if efforts to close the vaccine gap (Gavi) and scale up treatment for AIDS (the Global Fund) were unburdened by the history and bureaucracy of WHO, with an injection of significant start-up capital, more funding would flow over time to each.[9] The corollary expectation was that not just more money would be marshaled for these causes but that the resources would be additional to global health and not redirected from preexisting donor commitments to programs targeting childhood immunizations, HIV/AIDS, TB, malaria, or other health priorities. Advocates for the creation of Gavi and the Global Fund alike were also emphatic that significant levels of new resources would be driven by a coalition of public and private donors. Such tenets were believed so strongly that they appear as aspirations in the Global Fund's 2002 Framework Document.[10]

The Millennium Development Goals (MDGs) articulated in 2000 buttressed that early twenty-first-century optimism. Three of the eight goals focused on health: MDG 4 Reduce Child Mortality, MDG 5 Improve Maternal Health, and MDG 6 Combat HIV/AIDS, Malaria, and other diseases. Indeed, MDG 4 relates directly to Gavi's work and MDG 6 to that of the Global Fund. Whether the MDGs catalyzed additional development funding and more importantly development progress—including as relates to health—remains open to debate; some analyses contend that both funding flows and development progress were already accelerating before the MDGs were codified.[11] What is certainly true is that the concentration of focus on specific health concerns in the late twentieth and early twenty-first century was unprecedented in terms of resource intensity.

One example of this was the advent of the Gates Foundation (see chapter 3). From its inception in the late 1990s, the Gates Foundation, along with its founders, Bill and Melinda Gates, has played a significant role in global health, both in setting the agenda and in what gets funded within that agenda, including as relates to research priorities (which influence the agenda in the future).[12] In 1999, the Gates Foundation provided the initial funding that enabled Gavi to transition from an idea to an institution. The Gates Foundation has been a major funder almost every year to the Global Fund as well. It is not engaged only with "new institutions": through 31 August 2015, for the 2014/15 work plan, the Gates Foundation was the second largest contributor of earmarked voluntary contributions to WHO at almost $516 million.[13] The first was the United States at more than $573 million, a figure that does not include its biennial assessed contributions of more than $230 million.[14] Given that WHO remains the institution most associated with health, we first turn to who funds it, at what levels, and for what purposes.

The World Health Organization

From a funding perspective, WHO is the most conventional of our case study institutions since it receives funding from two tranches: assessed contributions from its 194 member states and voluntary contributions from its member states, philanthropic foundations, corporations, NGOs, and private individuals.[15] The former were known as regular budget funds until 2015, and they are the monies that WHO has full discretion to use as its leadership determines and the World Health Assembly, a body composed of all its member states, approves. In practice, assessed contributions are used to support the administrative costs of running WHO and programs that may not have significant support among member states (or at least donors) given that member states fund their prerogatives through their voluntary contributions to the organization. Individual states' membership dues are calculated in conjunction with WHO's biennial budget process based on the UN's standard scale of ability to pay as determined by a country's gross national product (size of economy) and population.

In 1980, the WHA voted to freeze its membership assessments in real dollar terms; in other words, only inflation and exchange rates (if one currency rose or fell significantly against the US dollar, the currency WHO historically has used to assess membership dues) would influence membership assessment adjustments.[16] This took effect with the 1982–83 budget. To be fair, real budget freezes in the early 1980s were not confined to WHO. Under pressure from donors, led by the United States, such mechanisms were introduced through the UN system and to the UN itself. With regards to the UN, the United States went even farther in the mid-1980s.[17] In 1985, the US Congress voted to withhold funding to the UN's regular budget funds unless UN member states agreed that all budgets must be passed by consensus (giving the United States and any member state an effective veto). In 1986, UN member states passed such a resolution and in 1987 moved to freeze the UN's regular budget funds at then current levels.[18]

Budget pressures did not ameliorate as the 1980s waned. In fact, in 1993, the World Health Assembly voted on an even more stringent budgetary policy for WHO, moving the organization from zero real growth to zero nominal growth for regular budget funds, meaning no inflation or currency adjustments in assessed membership contributions. The UN General Assembly voted on a similar policy for the 1996–97 UN budget.[19] But although the United States relaxed its opposition to real growth for the UN regular budget funds in the early 2000s, WHO received no such amnesty from its governing body. Yet, there was still space for the World Health Assembly to consider raising membership dues. Particularly throughout the early 2000s—when the UN General Assembly voted to increase UN membership dues—the

World Health Assembly repeatedly voted to not raise their own membership dues. It effectively made a similar decision again at its 2015 meeting by not voting on this question. To put this in perspective, such a cascade of failures to increase member states' assessed contributions means that on a per capita basis, member states have paid the same assessments to WHO throughout the history of the HIV/AIDS pandemic.[20]

Throughout the 1980s and 1990s, the failure of member states to pay even their frozen levels of contributions presented a significant challenge for WHO. The United States in particular withheld funds, a move largely interpreted as expressing dissatisfaction with WHO's list of essential medicines (its international guide for governments of the minimum medicine needs for a basic health-care system listing the most efficacious, safe, and cost-effective medicines for priority conditions),[21] in line with public opposition from US pharmaceutical companies.[22] Then WHO's Director-General Halfdan Mahler called the withholding of assessed contribution payments "financial hostage."[23] In 1989, WHO collected just above 70 percent of its assessed contributions.[24] WHO was not alone in facing significant arrears. By the late 1990s, donor and developing countries alike were billions of dollars in arrears to the UN and its agencies.[25] That includes the more than $100 million that went unpaid to WHO in many years; in 1996 alone, member states were more than $169 million in arrears to WHO, or just under 10 percent of its total 1996–97 biennial budget.[26] Although an outlier, in 1995, WHO collected only 56 percent of assessed contributions; in other years in the 1990s, before Dr. Gro Brundtland assumed leadership of WHO in 1998, collection rates were largely in the high 70 percents.[27] As one example, in 1998, close to 80 percent of assessed contributions were collected, yet eighty-eight member states had not paid their dues in full. Of those, WHO suspended voting rights of twenty-five countries (those judged to be able to make some payment, at least sufficient to warrant the reinstatement of voting rights were they to do so).[28]

In the late 1990s and into the 2000s, arrears rates dropped significantly, in part because in 2001, WHO agreed to reduce the US contribution obligation to 22 percent of regular budget funds from 25 percent and also in part because of Dr. Gro Brundtland's success in restoring some measure of member states' faith in WHO over her tenure (although it was coincident with the creation of both Gavi and the Global Fund, both arguably negative comments on WHO's global health leadership).[29] In 2003, WHO's collection rate for membership dues stood at 90 percent.[30] For the 2008/9 budget cycle, the collection rate exceeded 97 percent over the two years. More typically in the early 2010s, collection rates hovered in the high 80 percents and low 90 percents; in 2014, the collection rate was 86 percent.[31] Yet regular budget funds are only part of WHO's financial picture, and over time they have diminished in importance to WHO's financial whole, while remaining vital to WHO's core work. Looking for ways to complement its frozen membership assessments, WHO actively sought out more donors to make voluntary contributions. In 1998, in her first speech to the World Health Assembly as WHO's Executive Director, Dr. Brundtland asserted a set of "basic requirements" for WHO to be the lead agency in global health. Her second speech highlighted that WHO "must reach out to others" for greater support of its work.[32]

WHO is hardly alone in relying heavily on extrabudgetary funds or voluntary contributions. Some UN agencies are entirely dependent on voluntary contributions; there are no assessed dues for member states. The United Nations Children's Fund (UNICEF), the United Nations Population Fund (UNFPA), and the World Food Programme (WFP) all rely entirely on voluntary contributions to fund their core operations and their programmatic work. From inception, WHO has accepted, even depended on, extrabudgetary funds to support a portion of its work. Throughout WHO's history, voluntary contributions have supported some of its most marquee efforts—successes and failures alike. They fueled the work of both the Intensified Smallpox Eradication Programme launched in 1967 (a success) and the Intensified Malaria Eradication Programme launched in 1955 (a failure insofar as malaria is still with us). Yet it wasn't until the 1970s that extrabudgetary funds became increasingly important to WHO's total budget, soaring from 18 percent in 1970–71 to 53 percent of the total budget in 1980–81.[33] Beyond a slight dip—to 48 percent and 49 percent—in the 1984–85 and 1986–87 biennial budgets respectively, they marched through the 50 percents in the 1980s and 1990s and rose to the 60 percents and then 70 percents in the 2000s.[34] In 2014, voluntary contributions accounted for 80.3 percent of received funds,[35] noticeably higher than the 77 percent projected in WHO's biennial budget for 2014/15 (see fig. 4.5).

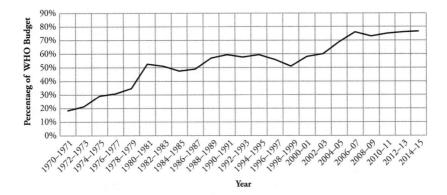

FIGURE 4.5 Extrabudgetary funding as a percentage of the WHO budget. Kelley Lee, *The World Health Organization*, 40 (yrs. 1970–97); WHO, "Financing of the World Health Organization," provisional agenda item, Executive Board Special Session on WHO reform, 25 October 2011, 2, http://apps.who.int/gb/ebwha/pdf_files/EBSS/EBSS2_ID2-en.pdf.; WHO, "Programme Budget 2014–2015," Geneva, Switzerland, October 2014, http://www.who.int/about/resources_planning/PB14-15_en.pdf.

Extrabudgetary funds rose in importance across the UN system over the same period. For example, from 1996 to 2003, more than 65 percent of UNDP's resources, on average, came through extrabudgetary channels.[36] Extrabudgetary funds first breached 50 percent of WHO's total budget in the same budget cycle that the World Health Assembly made the decision to freeze the nominal assessed membership dues. Recent aggregate budget pressures have only further increased the prominence of extrabudgetary funds in WHO's budget. The World Health Assembly slashed WHO's budget by more than 20 percent from 2009/10 to 2014/15, from almost $5 billion to less than $4 billion. These cuts received particular scrutiny during the Ebola crisis given WHO's pandemic and emergency response team, as a result of the organization's shrinking budget, declined from ninety-four to thirty-four staff members over the same time period.[37]

Analyses of WHO have long pointed to member states, and particularly major donors, looking to exert influence over the institution through money given and money withheld. In 1994, Fiona Godlee and others published a series of articles in the *British Medical Journal* elucidating the factors beyond poor leadership (in their view) that constrained WHO's ability to lead. The first on their list was "financial constraints and donor countries' demands."[38] More than twenty years later, Laurie Garrett, writing in *Foreign Affairs*, noted that member states' delegates attending the 68th World Health Assembly in 2015 "declined to raise revenues in order to address a massive budget crisis, accelerating the WHO's decline as a player on the global health stage relative to better-funded, more effective, and less politicized institutions, such as the Global Fund; Gavi, the Vaccine Alliance; the US President's Emergency Plan for AIDS Relief; and the Bill and Melinda Gates Foundation. And they dramatically rearranged the WHO's priorities, shifting resources away from combating infectious diseases."[39]

The rearrangement of priorities, using Garrett's phrasing, to align with extrabudgetary funds was inevitable. The core funding of WHO is used for the purposes decided by member states at the World Health Assembly, often in line with recommendations from the WHO Secretariat. The use of voluntary funding, however, is almost entirely predetermined by the specific donor (which donors could argue is their way of compensating for a perceived lack of WHO attention in certain areas). In fact, WHO's priorities and donors' priorities often do not align. In 2012/13, of WHO's regular budget, 12.9 percent[40] of funds were allocated to infectious disease and 4.8 percent to noncommunicable diseases and injuries.[41] By contrast, 57 percent of the 2012/13 extrabudgetary funding of WHO was used for infectious diseases,[42] while only 2.3 percent was allocated to noncommunicable diseases and injuries. Women's health and maternal health specifically are areas repeatedly pointed to as being underrepresented in donors' extrabudgetary priorities and therefore in WHO's scope of work.[43]

In the 2014/15 budget, donors earmarked 93 percent of extrabudgetary funds. In 2010/11, the top ten donors accounted for more than 70 percent of the total voluntary payments.[44] There is no reason to believe the most recent budget cycle was any different based on 2015 midyear data available. What has changed budget cycle to budget cycle is which entity is WHO's most significant extrabudgetary donor. While the United States remains WHO's most significant donor inclusive of assessed contributions and voluntary contributions (or regular budget funds plus extrabudgetary funds), the Gates Foundation in some years has contributed more through extrabudgetary funds than any other donor, including the United States. It also earmarks 100 percent of such donations (as does the United States).[45] The decision whether to accept these earmarked donations lies with the Director-General. As Peter Piot demonstrated while he served as Executive-Director of UNAIDS, it is challenging, but possible, to reject unflexible monies and to negotiate with donors to increase their share of unearmarked contributions (which is why Piot rejected all hard earmarked contributions, a decision not without controversy).[46]

Figure 4.6 shows WHO's top ten member-state contributors based on assessed contributions or regular budget funds plus voluntary contributions in 2014.[47] If we were to look only at the top ten member-state contributors based on regular budget funds, the list would include four donors—Canada, China, Spain, and Mexico—that contribute less than $15 million per annum to WHO. Only two countries on that list—the United States and Japan—contribute more than $50 million per annum. While not insignificant sums per se, when compared to the monies directed toward global health in recent years and particularly since 2000, these are notably low figures. Additionally, when voluntary contributions are included, the list includes countries like Australia,

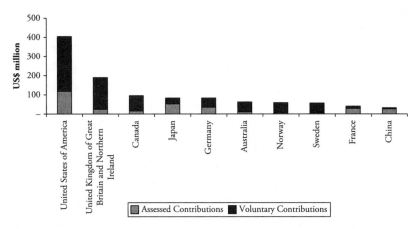

FIGURE 4.6 Top 10 member-state contributors for 2014, combining assessed and voluntary contributions (US$ million). WHO, "Financial Report and Audited Financial Statements for the Year Ended 31 December 2014," provisional agenda item, 68th World Health Assembly, 24 April 2015.

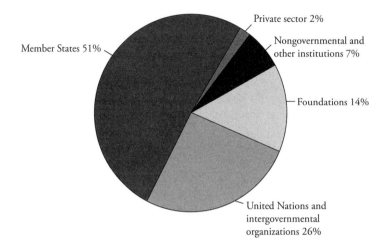

FIGURE 4.7 Revenue from voluntary contributions for 2014, by source. World Health Organization, "Financial Report and Audited Financial Statements for the Year Ended 31 December 2014," provisional agenda item, 68th World Health Assembly, 24 April 2015.

Norway, and Sweden, which are not on the top ten assessed-only list, and excludes countries that are, including Italy, Mexico, and Spain. Yet, member states account for barely half of all voluntary contributions as is evident in figure 4.7.

Looking at a top donor list of member states alone clearly presents a misleading picture of who is funding WHO, particularly given the Gates Foundation's importance to WHO's budget through extrabudgetary funds. Looking only at an extrabudgetary top ten donors list also presents an incomplete, if interesting, picture. On the extrabudgetary list, five of the top ten are not bilateral donors (although one, the European Commission, is composed solely of member states similar to WHO). In 2012/13, the Gates Foundation was the largest extrabudgetary donor to WHO; Gavi was the fourth largest, reflecting Gavi's reliance on WHO at the country and regional level for its support to countries applying for Gavi funds and implementing Gavi-supported immunization programs as well as on WHO headquarters for monitoring countries' immunization levels, among other areas.[48] If we expanded the top donor list in 2012/13 to include the top twenty extrabudgetary donors, only nine would be bilateral donors.[49]

The regular budget fund list will not change unless an appetite develops within the World Health Assembly to change the formulary and the levels of assessed contributions. There is no sign of that occurring in the foreseeable future; in fact, the opposite has proven true, even after the Ebola crisis. In 2015, the World Health Assembly again refused to increase assessed contributions, even the 5 percent annual growth rate that the Director-General had proposed. Even at 5 percent, if extrabudgetary funds stayed frozen, in nominal dollar terms it would take more than twenty-six years for regular budget funds to reach a commensurate level with the 2014/15 extrabudgetary funds.[50] In contrast, in 2012 the UN General Assembly passed updated membership assessments to support the UN Secretariat's work, as well as that of international tribunals and peacekeeping efforts. That decision covers assessments through 2015, with the expectation that the issue will be addressed again in 2016.[51]

Donor preference for voluntary contributions is a clear example of how principals look to exert control over their agents. It is a classic example of supply-driven control. Given the democratic nature of the World Health Assembly—one state, one vote—unlike weighted voting at the World Bank or a more limited Board membership at the Global Fund or Gavi, it is not surprising that donors rely on resources as a principal means of exerting control as, or when, other options are limited.

The World Bank

Alongside the turn toward voluntary contributions as a mechanism of control over WHO activities, donors also turned to other institutions, first the World Bank and then later Gavi and the Global Fund, to further exert influence over their use of funds, and possibly also further limit the ability of WHO to lead in the global health arena.

From 1990 through 2011, the World Bank, according to its own data, disbursed close to $20 billion in grants and loans throughout its health, nutrition, and population (HNP) portfolio. When a broader definition of health aligned with the IHME methodology is used (inclusive of the Bank's HIV/AIDS programming for example), the World Bank disbursed more than $33.8 billion over the same time period in loans and grants, and more than an additional $2.8 billion in-kind—an

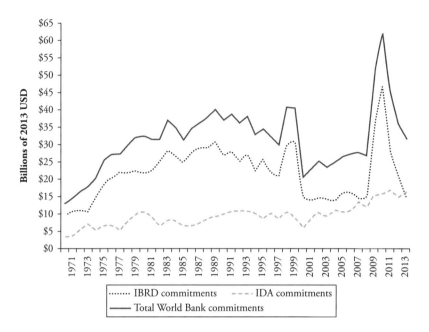

FIGURE 4.8 Real IBRD, IDA, and total World Bank commitments by year (billion 2013 USD). Kevin Currey, "Some Evolving Trends at the World Bank: Lending, Funding, Staffing" (briefing note, Ford Foundation, May 2014), 6.

impressive cumulative amount and an amount higher than the aggregated WHO budgets over the same time period.[52] Still, health represented a relatively small slice of the commitments the Bank has made since 1990. Indeed, as is evident from figure 4.8, $20 billion roughly equals the World Bank's total commitments in 1975, a time when the Bank's involvement in health was only just beginning.

As discussed earlier, the World Bank Group (fig. 4.9) comprises five different constituent agencies. While all are governed as one entity, each agency is financed in distinct ways.

The IBRD is funded by capital contributions from its members and is effectively "owned" by its 188 member states (as of 31 December 2013). As votes are allocated based on capital subscription (or expectation of annual investment), there is clearly an incentive for member states to meet—and even seek to increase—their capital commitments. This pressure is evident in the recent intransigence of the United States (driven by Congress, not the White House) to cede a portion of its

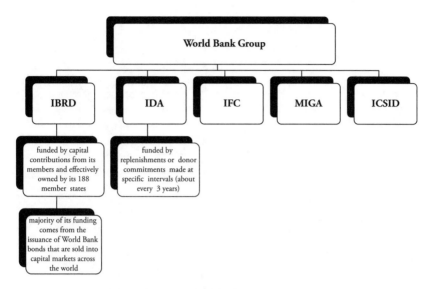

FIGURE 4.9 World Bank group. Authors' calculations based on working knowledge; http://www.worldbank.org/en/about?.

current 16.1 percent voting share (which allows it to effectively block any decision it does not agree with since most of the Bank's key decisions require 85 percent of all votes outstanding to approve) and in China's efforts to invest more into the Bank to gain a commensurate rise in voting power.[53] Similar to WHO, only member states can make contributions to the IBRD. Unlike WHO, there are no voluntary contributions to IBRD. But, similar to WHO, a majority of IBRD funding does not come from its member states' capital assessments. In IBRD's case, a majority of its funding comes from the issuance of World Bank bonds that are sold on capital markets across the world. In 2013, IBRD raised $22.1 billion dollars from bonds issued in twenty-one currencies; only a small portion of those funds would eventually find their way to health (however defined).[54] In its more than seventy-year history, through 2014 the IBRD had provided more than $500 billion in loans predominately to middle-income countries.[55]

In contrast, IDA is funded by replenishments, or donor commitments, made at specific intervals, generally every three years (fig. 4.10). Since its launch in 1960, IDA has convened seventeen replenishment meetings, securing increasing IDA commitments from World Bank members almost every round (as of October 2015). Generally, replenishments are

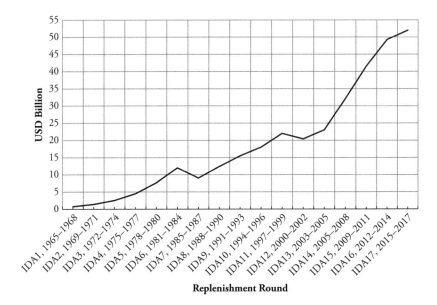

FIGURE 4.10 Funds pledged at IDA 1–17 replenishment meetings. For IDA 1–11, see http://www.worldbank.org/en/about; for IDA 12–17, see http://www.worldbank.org/en/news/all?displayconttype_exact=Press+Release.

held a year or more before the funds will actually be called upon to support IDA's work. Through 2014, IDA had provided more than $312 billion in loans, credits, and grants to the world's least developed countries.[56]

IDA's first replenishment, in 1960, raised $750 million, with the United States accounting for more than 40 percent of total funds pledged, as is shown in figure 4.11. In 1984, in advance of IDA's seventh replenishment, the United States committed $750 million (the total amount of the first replenishment almost twenty years earlier) and said it would not account for more than 25 percent of IDA at any point in time, in line with similar arguments expressed throughout the UN system, including at WHO.[57] IDA's most recent replenishment occurred in 2013 and attracted more than $51.9 billion in commitments. While the World Bank convenes the replenishments, in practice they are actually overseen by donors, not the Bank nor IDA recipients. Looking at the sixteenth replenishment (which covered work through 2014) provides a more complete picture of IDA donors given that

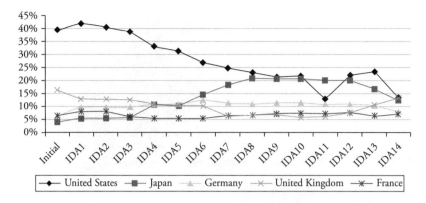

FIGURE 4.11 Donor contributions to IDA. Martin Weiss, "CRS Report for Congress: The World Bank's International Development Association (IDA)," 1 April 2008, http://fpc.state.gov/documents/organization/104719.pdf.

funds for the seventeenth replenishment are still being collected at the time of this writing (see fig. 4.12). It is clear a finite number of donors account for the majority of IDA's coffers, and it is a similar list to those most prominent in the Global Fund or Gavi's top roster, as we will see subsequently in this chapter.

The majority of projects under the Bank's HNP umbrella are funded predominately through IDA, even though IDA- and IBRD-funded projects are informed and approved through the same internal Bank channels. For example, in 2012, of forty-one newly approved HNP projects, IDA provided a significant majority of the funding across the new projects.[58] Even though most countries only qualify for health-related funding under IBRD or IDA (and not both), the Bank's Board and staff work to coordinate loans and technical assistance under the "health, nutrition, and population" aegis across IBRD and IDA funding streams. Similarly, in both the World Bank's annual reports and the Bank's open data and resource tracking, the Bank groups IBRD and IDA health loans and grants under "health and other social services."

In 2014, as has generally been true in recent years, the World Bank was the second largest multilateral funder of global health concerns following the Global Fund; however, within the World Bank, health itself claims a relatively small share of attention. For its 2014 fiscal year, loans in the "health and other social services" space stood at less than

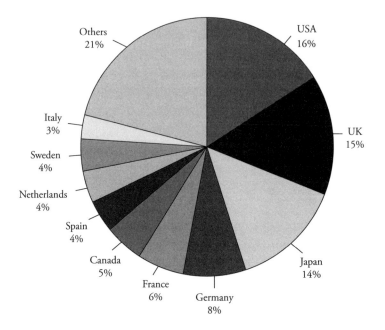

FIGURE 4.12 IDA 16 replenishment donors, covering FY2012–FY2014 (July 1, 2011–June 30, 2014). World Bank, IDA 16 Report, "Report from the Executive Directors of the International Development Association to the Board of Governors, Additions to IDA Resources: Sixteenth Replenishment," 18 March 2011, http://www-wds.worldbank.org/external/default/WDSContentServer/WDSP/IB/2011/03/30/000356161_20110330003335/Rendered/PDF/605750BR0IDA1R1031281110BOX358324B.pdf.

$3.4 billion, out of a total loan pool of more than $40.8 billion.[59] Health loans accounted for less than 10 percent of the Bank's portfolio that year, barely edging above 8 percent of total loan volume. In some years, health loans have accounted for close to twice as much—close to 16 percent (2011). It is fair to say that the World Bank is more important to global health than health is to the Bank, although this is changing as we discuss in chapter 6.[60] From a principal-agent standpoint, such incongruity likely favors the agent's discretion in health given that in 2014, multiple other sectors received significantly more Bank funds than health did. Other sectors—such as public administration, law, and justice, as well as energy, mining, and transportation—have received greater attention from the Bank and the Bank's donors, as well as received more funds. In most recent years, those latter three sectors have received billions more in funding than health and other social services have.[61]

By the early 1990s, the World Bank had become the largest single channel of funding for health. That is a remarkable transformation over a relatively short period of time. In 1980, the Bank granted no loans with a specific health focus.[62] From 1981 to 1990 the World Bank's disbursements for health (not inclusive of population and nutrition loans and grants) grew from $33 million to $263 million.[63] Disbursements for health (inclusive of population and nutrition) topped $1 billion throughout the 1990s, reaching close to $2 billion in 1998.[64] By 2012, disbursements across health, population, and nutrition loans and grants soared past $2.5 billion.[65] Commitments increased even more dramatically. In 2000, commitments were at $1 billion (actually slightly below disbursements that year), and by 2010, commitments had quadrupled to approximately $4 billion across various health, nutrition, and population projects (see figs. 4.13 and 4.14).[66]

This increase in commitments and disbursements across the 1980s and 1990s, and then the largely steady levels of disbursements into the

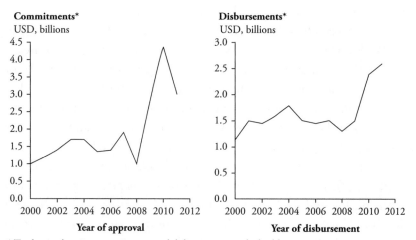

* Total annual project commitments and disbursements to the health sector

FIGURE 4.13 Total annual project commitments and disbursements to the health sector. Cristian Baeza, Director, Health, Nutrition and Population, The World Bank, "The World Bank in Health 2012: Challenges, Priorities, and Role in the Global Health Aid Architecture," 31 January 2012.

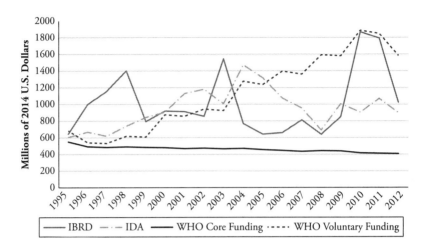

FIGURE 4.14 Comparison of annual disbursement from the IBRD, IDA, WHO core budgetary funds, and WHO extrabudgetary fund, 1995–2012. IHME, *Financing Global Health 2014: Shifts in Funding as the MDG Era Closes.*

2000s and 2010s, tracked the Bank's greater focus on the connection between health and poverty alleviation (the Bank's core mission). The global financial crisis that began in earnest in 2008 also played a role in the Bank's magnified commitments to health (and many other areas). As countries struggled to find commercial options to secure funds for capital-intensive projects, whether in health, infrastructure, or elsewhere, many turned to the World Bank. Given the softening of commitments to health and other social services in 2012 and 2013, it is likely that the upsurge in 2009, 2010, and 2011 resulted more from the financial crisis than the new 2007 World Bank Strategy. In that document, the Bank focused on health systems strengthening and health financing for its HNP portfolio, in an explicit effort to complement the funds lower- and middle-income countries receive from vertical funds, principally Gavi and the Global Fund.[67]

In the *1993 World Development Report: Investing in Health*, the World Bank made clear why it had amplified its health funding (and was planning on continuing to do so). Yet, it was far from the only public declaration of the Bank's engagement in health, before or after its publication, as the more recent 2007 strategy exemplifies. Throughout the 1980s and 1990s, the Bank published various policy and research pieces articulating the clear linkages between investing in health systems and fighting diseases as necessary components of fighting poverty.[68] It also joined efforts that were making the case for the linkages between development, poverty alleviation, and health, like WHO's 2000–2001 Commission on Macroeconomics and Health.[69]

With the advent and then growth over time of Gavi and the Global Fund, the Bank even more narrowly defined its work within health. In 2013 the World Bank's core budget (HNP) reflected these priorities, with a clear focus on health care systems (see fig. 4.15). The major priorities were health systems performance (50 percent), food security and nutrition (14 percent), injury (12 percent), child health (11 percent), and population and reproduction (6 percent).[70] In 2015, the Independent Evaluation Group (IEG) of the World Bank published the percentages of Bank loans by health-related MDG from FY2002 to 2014, and it largely tracks the snapshot data from 2013. Over those dozen years, 45 percent of the Bank's lending went to health systems, 19 percent to infectious diseases (including HIV/AIDS), 12 percent to child health, 9 percent to population and reproductive health, and 7 percent to nutrition.[71] The share of funding for disease-specific programs (the majority

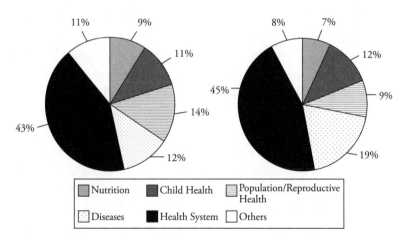

FIGURE 4.15 Composition of HNP commitments, FY90–FY01 (left); composition of HNP commitments, FY 02–FY14 (right). HNP thematic lending by theme and region raw data, available at "World Bank HNP Lending," http://datatopics.worldbank.org/hnp/worldbanklending.

of which focus on HIV/AIDS, malaria, and tuberculosis) fell from 19 percent of total HNP commitments from 2002 through 2007 to less than 2 percent in 2012, a level that did not change significantly in 2013.[72] As we argue in chapter 6, it is probably the growing financial heft of the Global Fund that precipitated this contraction in Bank commitments.

If we include World Bank trust funds in calculations of total World Bank funds, the picture changes dramatically, particularly in terms of annual funds committed and disbursed in global health (and also in climate change–related work). Trust funds are a financial arrangement set up with contributions from one or more donors and in some cases from the World Bank Group itself for a particular purpose. A trust fund can be country-specific, regional, or global in its geographic scope, and it can be freestanding or programmatic. We include a brief discussion of trust funds as their management has become an increasingly significant part of the Bank's work. It spends more than $200 million per annum to manage its more than one thousand trust funds of varying sizes and durations.[73] The World Bank itself has raised the question of what the proliferation of trust funds means in terms of aid harmonization (or lack thereof), country ownership, and also transaction costs.[74]

Trust funds are such a significant part of the Bank's business that they merit their own annual report from the Bank. As of June 2013, the World Bank Group held $28.9 billion across 1,030 trust-fund accounts.[75] The Bank charges administrative fees for trust funds to assist in covering costs such as administration, supervision, and oversight. Fees typically include an annual fixed fee, a start-up fee for new trust funds, and other fee arrangements that are ultimately negotiated and agreed upon with trust-fund donors.[76] A flat percentage fee for any personnel working on a trust fund is also being considered.[77] In 2012 and 2013, the Global Fund, the Climate Investment Fund, and the Global Environmental Facility were, by far, the largest trust-fund accounts held and managed by the Bank.[78] In contrast to HNP's focus on health systems, the trust-fund portfolio as relates to health is largely focused on disease-specific strategies including, and in addition to those mentioned earlier, the Global Partnership to Eradicate Poliomyelitis, Programs for Onchocerciasis Control, the Avian and Human Influenza Facility, and the Global Partnership for TB Control. Even the so-called

Health Results Innovation Trust Fund (HRITF) has a particular focus on reducing maternal mortality and reducing child mortality.[79] The Global Fund is the largest trust fund, accounting for 29 percent of 2012 contributions to Bank trust funds.[80] Adding in trust-fund monies, total Bank commitments to health increased from $3.1 billion in 2003 to $6.5 billion in 2013.[81] While growth has occurred in both types of funding, it is the trust-fund portfolio for health that has experienced the most dramatic growth from $1.3 billion in 2003 to $4.2 billion in 2013, in large measure due to the Bank's stewardship of the Global Fund's monies.[82] Given its role as the Global Fund's fiduciary and banker, the World Bank holds an ex officio seat on the Fund's Board.

From a principal-agent standpoint, we would expect principals to try to exert more control over the Bank's health work over time as its health lending and engagement increased and evolved, even with the challenge inherent in the Bank's vast portfolio of thematic areas, geographies, and lending groups, as well as its rather striated governance. Given those contextual and structural constraints, we would expect principals to then look elsewhere for greater oversight and even control into global health investments. Unlike WHO's experience, it is hard to see evidence of greater principal control in the patterns of IBRD and IDA funding—or in how the Bank then chose to allocate those funds. Excluding financial intermediary funds, like those the Bank holds for the Global Fund and others, $5 billion (or more than one-third of donor disbursements the Bank received in 2012) was earmarked by donors for specific uses, through trust funds and other mechanisms.[83] While not an insignificant percentage, it is a far lower percentage than WHO confronts annually. Not surprisingly then, donor control is more evident in the trust-fund portfolio. Arguably the origins of Gavi and the Global Fund lie in a persistent belief that WHO was unable to steward big global health programs any longer and that the Bank was either insufficiently focused or donors were insufficiently able to have transparency into the Bank's activities and influence.

The Global Fund to Fight AIDS, Tuberculosis and Malaria

A core difference between the "old" institutions, WHO and the World Bank, and the "new" ones, the Global Fund and Gavi, is that WHO and the World Bank provide technical assistance (and the Bank's significant levels of funding), while the Global Fund and Gavi provide funds and rely on others to provide technical assistance. Unlike WHO or the Bank, the Global Fund relies entirely on voluntary contributions. Even for its de facto permanent Board members like the United States, China, and the Gates Foundation (each of whom has held a formal Board seat at every Global Fund Board meeting since inception), there is no formalized expectation of funds. Similar to IDA, the Global Fund relies heavily on replenishment as its principal fund-raising mechanism, although it also solicits funds on an ongoing basis and receives funds from its (RED) partnership. While its governance differs significantly from that of the Bank's, at replenishment time it is still the donors alone who take center stage similar to IDA. Absent the addition of the Gates Foundation, the composition of the Fund's major donors closely resembles IDA's major donors.

In its first thirteen years, the Fund received $29.6 billion in financial contributions from donors, with $27.9 billion coming from donor countries, including both Board members and nonmembers, and from a small number of implementing countries largely through debt swap arrangements with donor governments.[84] These were not common arrangements. When swap agreements were struck, donor governments would forgive part of a loan repayment if developing countries would invest a commensurate amount in the Global Fund. Through the end of 2013, the Fund had received $75.8 million from five swap agreements across four implementing countries and two donors. For purposes of our analyses, we include those debt swap arrangements as donor contributions under the relevant donor. As was true for many public health concerns in the early twenty-first century, the only significant nonbilateral donor to the Fund was the Gates Foundation. The Gates Foundation donated more than $1.1 billion to the Fund in its first thirteen years, accounting for two-thirds of all nonbilateral funds the Global Fund received over that time period (fig. 14.16).[85]

Under principal-agent theory, we would expect the Secretariat to concentrate on securing pledges and contributions beyond the Board, to constrain the institutional power donors generally have derived from their financial support of international organizations through voluntary contributions. This likely would be particularly true in the Fund's

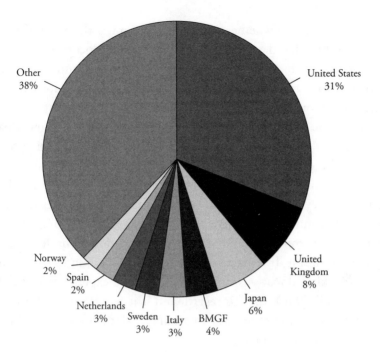

FIGURE 4.16 Top donors, Global Fund 2000–2013, total = \$29.6 billion. Global Fund, Total Pledges to Date, 2000–2013.

context given the its highly concentrated donor population. We would also expect the Secretariat to focus such efforts on the private sector and individuals given the early aspirations around each as potential significant sources of support.[86] We would then expect the Board to support such fund-raising diversification only if success would not pose a significant threat to its funding hegemony. In theory, the Global Fund would have more options given it is not constrained by the membership rules, assessment fees, and subscription expectations that arguably restrict both WHO and World Bank leadership in their fund-raising options. Although there is some evidence of the Global Fund Secretariat reaching out beyond the Board, it was clearly not a core area of focus in the Fund's first decade-plus of existence. The most significant non-bilateral and non–Gates Foundation funding source to the Fund over this period was (RED), originally Project (RED), which accounted for .75 percent of total Fund donations through 2013 (discussed later in this chapter). It is hard to know whether greater attention to fund-raising diversification would have changed the overwhelming bilateral donor presence—or whether a lack of attention was the result of a clear understanding that despite the Fund's framework document and early rhetoric trumpeting a more diverse funding base, it was unlikely to materialize. From 2000 to 2013, bilateral donors accounted for 94.3 percent of the monies the Global Fund raised.[87]

Unlike the World Bank's IBRD or Gavi, the Global Fund Board never seriously considered and certainly never approved raising funds through the capital markets.[88] In addition, the Board's inability for much of its first decade to determine protocols for accepting in-kind donations may also help explain why private support never materialized at substantial levels.[89] Even for WHO, which has long-standing protocols governing in-kind donations, such donations have never proven significant. It remains to be seen, given the Fund's newer policies on in-kind donations, whether the Fund's experience will differ from that of WHO's in this regard, and if it will be successful in the longer term in attracting and managing in-kind resources from its donors and for its grantees.

Yet, despite the absence of a diversified funding base, the Fund clearly succeeded in raising significant sums, as measured against any yardstick. An independent High-Level Panel, convened to examine allegations of fraud and misappropriation of Fund grant monies, referred to the Fund's first decade as "the halcyon days" when "donor governments competed with each other to demonstrate their compassion in the face of an accelerating emergency caused by HIV/AIDS, tuberculosis (TB), and malaria in the developing world."[90] The Global Fund did not ignore private sources of funding altogether. From its inception, the Fund embraced (RED), by far the most significant source of private-sector support for the Fund. Founded in 2006 under the rock star Bono's ONE Campaign, it raised more than $221 million through 2013 to support the Fund in its first decade, an amount that surpassed $350 million by the end of 2015.[91] Companies, including American Express, Gap, and Apple, sell (RED) products and then donate a portion of those proceeds to the Fund. For years (RED) donations were the only earmarked donations the Fund accepted. All (RED) monies support grants working to eliminate mother-to-child HIV/AIDS transmission in six designated African countries. The Fund generally has eschewed earmarked donations, but perhaps the uniqueness of (RED)'s private-sector position, and the hundreds of millions of dollars raised (accounting for .75 percent of total Fund donations through 2013), helped secure such a unique commitment from the Fund.

Particularly throughout the Fund's first decade, a variety of voices, largely from NGOs and advocates and strongly supported by Global Fund's watchdog Aidspan, routinely called for an "equitable contributions framework" whereby bilateral donors would contribute to the Fund a set percentage of their respective economies' size.[92] Other voices, including on the Board, argued instead for an annual contribution model (similar to WHO's), while the Secretariat, whenever engaged in the debate, proposed a spectrum of options without expressing an opinion.[93] Instead, the Fund adopted and retained replenishment as its primary funding mechanism. The Board convened three replenishment meetings in its first decade, with different degrees of success, particularly in terms of non-bilateral donor support. Yet, the close to $28 billion raised from initial pledges through the third replenishment likely goes a long way to explaining why, despite the advocacy for different fund-raising approaches and the unpredictability of replenishment meetings' results, the Board never moved from its voluntary contribution approach, never invested in developing an alternative or complementary mechanism to replenishment, and never formally tethered Board seats to minimum contribution levels.

Fund-raising never became a delegated power to the Secretariat, and it does not appear the Secretariat ever advocated that it become so.[94] This differs from WHO in which the Secretariat can—and does—solicit voluntary contributions and tries (and repeatedly fails) to secure higher regular budget fund rates. The continued lack of attention by the Global Fund Board to fund-raising is a classic example of agency slack. Fund-raising would seem to have created an opportunity for the Secretariat to advance its own agenda through establishing direct relationships with key donors, particularly through innovative fund-raising models. The fact that innovations were occurring elsewhere, most prominently at Gavi and UNITAID (the International Drug Purchasing Facility, largely financed by a levy, or tax, on airline tickets), both of which originated with government proposals and then developed their own distinct characters, could have been exploited as providing cover for such Secretariat actions.[95] On the other hand, what attention the Board did dedicate to fund-raising was done to ensure it remained firmly in control, through maintaining authority over the process and by continuing to provide the bulk of the Fund's monies. The United States accounted for close to 31 percent of total monies the Fund received in its first thirteen years, France close to 13 percent, the United Kingdom and Germany more than 7 percent, and Japan more than 6 percent. The top five donors to the Fund accounted for almost 65 percent of its fund-raising over the period.[96]

It is clear that from a funding perspective, the Global Fund is rather conventional. Its monies unmistakably and overwhelmingly come from traditional bilateral donors. This arguably was not inevitable as Gavi's experience demonstrates. Gavi was able to obtain a greater share of nonbilateral capital, although probing deeper arguably belies that observation given Gavi's financial reliance on the Gates Foundation. As another example, the International AIDS Vaccine Initiative (IAVI) receives approximately a quarter of its funding from a more diverse set of nonbilateral sources.[97]

The early expectations that the Global Fund would catalyze new sources of funding and spark innovative financing to a significant degree to support its own innovative model did not meaningfully materialize in its first decade. As Global Fund's Executive Director Dr. Mark Dybul points out, corporate social responsibility budgets in the private sector are limited and the private sector generally, in the Fund's experience, prefers to make in-kind donations of expertise from their core competencies, such as supply chain optimization or quality assurance, rather than cash contributions.[98] Given the volatility in the Gates Foundation's support for the Fund and the reticence of the private sector to provide cash contributions, one could argue that early hopes of a coalition of bilateral, private, and foundation funders were misplaced. Yet, the Fund continues to look beyond its traditional bilateral funding base for support, now in 2016, to high-net-worth individuals as well as to further support from (RED).[99] At the Fund's beginning, there were great expectations that a broader coalition of funders would lead to a more data-driven and accountable organization. As we discuss in chapter 5, the Fund has made a concerted effort over time to be more transparent and accountable to its Board as well as to the broader public, even without a multi-stakeholder funding base.

From a principal-agent perspective, it is not surprising that a broad coalition of funders did not emerge for the Fund, particularly given how significant the United States has been to the Global Fund. In most years, the United States accounts for one-third of the Fund's total donor base. Following every Global Fund Board meeting, the United States publishes its points of view on Board decisions and debates. Analyzing every such document through the first twenty-eight Board meetings yields few disagreements and arguably no significant disagreements between the decisions of the Global Fund Board and the organization's largest funder.[100] The United States also maintains a staff presence in Geneva with the sole purpose of liaising with the Global Fund. The greater density of interactions that likely result from such an arrangement may help explain the congruence between the Fund and the United States, or it may be explained by the fact that Americans have led the Fund longer than non-Americans have. Or the explanation may lie in the dependence of the Fund on US funds, a not implausible conclusion to draw, particularly from a principal-agent perspective.

Gavi, the Vaccine Alliance

Gavi and particularly the Global Fund benefitted from the robust ODA environment coincident with their first few years. Although Gavi raised significantly smaller amounts than the Fund, its experience of how it raised those funds contrasts sharply to the Fund's—even if the source of those funds does not dramatically differ. Unlike the Fund and World Bank/IDA, Gavi came relatively late to replenishment as a means to marshal donor funds. Prior to its first pledging conference in June 2011, all donor contributions to Gavi were made on an ad hoc basis, not as the result of a replenishment mechanism or part of levied membership dues or expected contributions. At that first pledging conference in London, donors committed $4.3 billion for Gavi for 2011 through 2015, significantly adding to the $3.4 billion already pledged.

Through December 2013, Gavi received $8.3 billion in direct donor contributions. Its most significant source of funds, by far, was the Gates Foundation, which contributed $2.1 billion. Most notable is that the Gates Foundation's contributions were effectively synonymous with nonbilateral support. Contributions from the Gates Foundation, both through direct unconditional funds and through matching funds, comprised 97 percent of nongovernmental and nonintergovernmental (e.g., the OPEC Fund and the European Union) support.[101] Yet the Gates Foundation's support, and by extension nonbilateral support, became less important on a percentage basis in Gavi's early second decade than had been true in its first ten years.

In Gavi's first decade, 2000–2010, 39 percent or $1.24 billion of Gavi's funding came from nonbilateral sources, with the Gates Foundation providing 97.7 percent of that nonbilateral support. The first few years of Gavi's second decade saw a decrease in the percentage importance of nonbilateral funding. Looking from 2000 to 2013, a slightly different picture emerges with nonbilateral support accounting for $2.15 billion of Gavi's total $8.32 billion of funding (see fig. 4.17), or just over 25 percent of Gavi's funds with the Gates Foundation remaining central to what nonbilateral support Gavi received. In total, over

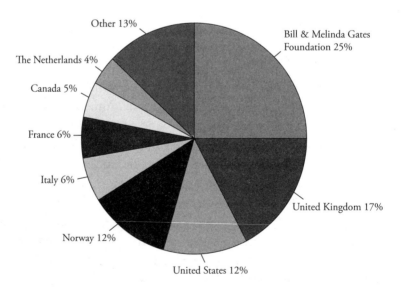

FIGURE 4.17 Gavi donors, 2000–2013, total = $29.6 billion. Included only donors at or above approximately 3%. Based on author's calculations using annual donor contributions to Gavi 2000–2013; Gavi, the Vaccine Alliance, accessed 31 March 2015, http://www.gavi.org/funding/donor-contributions-pledges/.

Gavi's first thirteen years, the Gates Foundation accounted for 96.8 percent of all nonbilateral support.[102] Clearly, in Gavi's case, nonbilateral and Gates Foundation were synonymous.

Additionally, one of Gavi's innovative mechanisms accounted for an additional 15 percent of the monies it raised in its first thirteen years. Gavi received $1.24 billion from the International Financing Facility for Immunization (IFFIm), which effectively securitizes long-term pledges from bilateral donors, converting the pledges into usable cash resources by selling bonds in the capital markets. Through the end of 2013, the United Kingdom, France, Sweden, Norway, the Netherlands, Spain, Italy, and South Africa had provided support to Gavi through IFFIm. Collectively they had pledged $6 billion over twenty years that had translated into $4.5 billion of bonds sold.[103] Only South Africa is an unusual suspect in that list (the others appearing on top donor lists elsewhere in this chapter). Perhaps the other countries were also induced to provide greater support to Gavi given the long-term bond option than they would have via shorter-term conventional cash commitments.

Over the same time horizon, Gavi raised $581.8 million through the Advance Market Commitment (AMC), a mechanism through which donors committed to purchase new pneumococcal vaccines at a price that covers development costs and provides some profit for the drugs' manufacturers with the provision that they be distributed only in low- and middle-income countries (to preserve the relatively higher prices in relatively higher-income countries).[104] The donor composition for the AMC (fig. 4.18) differs a bit from that of Gavi as a whole, including Italy, the Gates Foundation, Russia, Canada, Norway, and the United Kingdom, with Italy accounting for more than 40 percent of the total AMC-related funds through early 2015.

Still, for all of its mobilization of funds through innovative mechanisms and the strong, even foundational support of the Gates Foundation, Gavi too is largely dependent on bilateral donors and a conventional bilateral donor list. Moreover, Gavi is even more dependent on the Gates Foundation than the Global Fund is. Gavi and the Fund are hardly alone in continuing to rely on bilateral donors. Even the International AIDS Vaccine Initiative and related HIV/AIDS-vaccine initiatives are largely funded by governments, despite the strong business case for the private sector investing its work; 83 percent

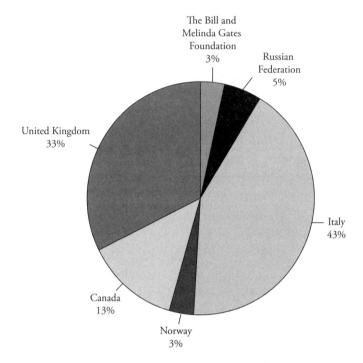

FIGURE 4.18 2010–2015 Donor composition of the advanced market commitment for Gavi. GAVI Alliance Secretariat, "Advance Market Commitment for Pneumococcal Vaccines" (annual reports, June 2009–March 2015).

of aggregate funding for a HIV/AIDS vaccine in 2011 came from the public sector, 13 percent from the philanthropic/foundations sector, and only 4 percent from the private sector.[105]

Of the four organizations we focus on, Gavi arguably has the most diverse funding base, if only assessed by percentage of funds originating outside of traditional bilateral donors. Yet, as mentioned earlier, most of Gavi's nonbilateral funds originate from the Gates Foundation. It also must be noted that Gavi is itself a significant funder of WHO as seen in the extrabudgetary fund analysis earlier in the chapter. According to Desmond McNeill and Kristin Sandberg, 25 percent of WHO's vaccine budget does indeed come from Gavi.[106] In other words, is it fair to think of WHO as a Gavi subcontractor? Likely so, and although lengthy ruminations on such questions do not belong in this chapter, we hope that other work will examine the convoluted relationships emerging between WHO and other actors in global health such as Gavi, the UN Development Programme (UNDP), and the UN High Commission for Refugees (UNHCR).

Gavi is often viewed as the multilateral most connected to the Gates Foundation and to Bill Gates personally. Out of all the organizations we discuss, the Gates Foundation is more important on a percentage basis over time and, in most individual years, to Gavi's coffers rather than to those of WHO or the Global Fund. Through 2013, the Gates Foundation provided more than $1.1 billion to the Global Fund, or 3.8 percent of the total contributions the Fund had received up to that point. In 2005, the Gates Foundation gave no money to the Global Fund. We are unable to discern the reasons for this—because neither the Gates Foundation nor Bill and Melinda Gates personally—commented at the time or have commented since on why funds were withheld from the Global Fund that year. One set of possible explanations relates to the Fund itself—a lack of confidence in its approach, its grant decisions, or its leadership. Another set of explanations relates to a greater focus by the Gates Foundation on Gavi and other global health investments that year. Regardless, the larger story remains the consistent support of the Fund and Gavi by the Gates Foundation and more traditional bilateral donors alike rather than one in which other, newer donors play—at least so far—meaningful roles in either.

If Gavi's and the Global Fund's stories evidence donor support and confidence (even if largely from conventional donors), WHO's narrative contrasts over the past few decades with continual donor skepticism. As judged by dollars (or euros) commanded, WHO is far from the most significant multilateral player in global health. Even the US Centers for Disease Control (which has a mandate inclusive of global health research and concerns albeit one also focused on domestic health), had in 2013 an annual budget of about $6 billion. That was three times that of WHO's ($3.98 billion over two years, 2013/14).[107] In addition, WHO donors' preferences for voluntary contributions not only constrain WHO's discretion to determine and respond to global health priorities it sets in a current budget cycle, it also constrains WHO's ability to plan for the future. With donors exerting strenuous control over now 80 percent of WHO's budget, perhaps the most apt question would be why WHO might invest time in strategy and planning based on its budget today, when ten donors can change more than 65 percent of its financing base tomorrow. There is no simple answer to this question. What is clear is that major funders exert significant influence over the health priorities, governance, and/or work of WHO, the Global Fund, and Gavi, albeit in different ways. The same may also be true at the Bank through trust funds, but if so, it is more difficult to prove based on information in the public domain.

The next chapter discusses the issue of information in the public domain. We move to examine what these organizations choose to publish, in what form and how frequently, and what such choices elucidate about the principal-agent dynamics within each.

5

Twenty-First-Century Governance

IF WE HAD WRITTEN this book twenty years ago, we likely would not have had even a paragraph dedicated to this chapter's focus. Historically, multilateral organizations have been viewed as accountable only to their member states and disproportionately accountable to the prevailing hegemons; organizational power followed political power. During the Cold War, the United States and the Soviet Union held that status, and in the 1980s and 1990s, during the twilight of the Cold War and dawn of the post–Cold War era, that position of preeminence belonged to the United States and, to a lesser extent, the so-called G7 countries, the seven biggest economies in the world. Indeed, the Global Fund first emerged as a codified proposal at the 2000 G7 Okinawa summit.

In the twenty-first century there is now an expectation that nonstate actors, whether from civil society or the private sector, will at least have direct visibility, even insight, into what happens in multilaterals' boardrooms, if not an actual seat at the table. These expectations are particularly robust in global health given the strong presence of nonstate actors providing money, technical assistance, and direct services. For example, the Gates Foundation is the second largest overall donor to WHO while Médecins sans Frontières or Doctors Without Borders (MSF), an international NGO, is the most notable and extensive provider of health care in emergency situations.

Even when nonstate actors are not enfranchised in decision-making, norms have evolved over the past decade and a half that knowledge about organizations' decisions and decision-making needs, at a minimum, to be accessible to those with relevant interests, such as international NGOs, as well as the broader public. Over the past couple of decades, a broadened view of accountability for multilateral organizations has emerged, moving accountability beyond donor governments and even beyond donor and recipient governments alike.[1] Different views exist about whom that accountability should be broadened to include and how such inclusion should be achieved. And, what a broadened definition of accountability means in practice varies. For example, it could mean access in real time to all meaningful information, or full access on a delayed schedule, or limited access with clarity around what is being provided to experts, the public at large, and what is not being provided. Or none of the above. Whatever one's position may be on questions of information access, affirmative answers around transparency increasingly are key to an organization's perceived legitimacy among civil society and the broader public alike.

Our four principal case studies have taken different approaches to whom they are formally accountable and who has access to information about their finances, decision-making, and ultimate policy and programmatic decisions. Margaret Chan has said boldly of WHO, it is "a servant of its member states" alone;[2] as of September 2015, WHO does not have a public information policy. The origins of both Gavi and the Global Fund reside in part in the broadening view of accountability—and its corollaries, membership and transparency. Both provide meaningfully more transparency than does WHO. Equally plausible is that both Gavi and the Global Fund's broader membership and commitment to a minimum level of transparency helped catalyze later choices on this issue by other international organizations, including the World Bank (even if not, as of yet, WHO).

The wider discussion about the legitimacy of multilateral institutions remains a contested one, with little agreement on what constitutes or conveys legitimacy and what the best mechanisms are for making sure that institutions remain legitimate even as norms and expectations evolve. We do not seek to answer those questions in a normative or even strategic sense for global health. Rather, we recognize what new norms have already emerged around participation and transparency, and we examine how each of our case study institutions has responded to these shifts.

This chapter builds on the work of the previous chapters by looking at how WHO, the World Bank, Gavi, and the Global Fund have dealt with: first, enfranchisement of nonstate actors, and second, transparency around financial flows, decisions, and decision-making. Ultimately, this chapter aims to answer a few key questions: How are nonstate actors included, both as formal observers and actors enfranchised in decision-making in the four institutions? What are the organizations' respective public information policies? What other steps have these institutions taken to provide the public with better visibility into their funding and decision-making? Again, we employ principal-agent theory to help explain why different organizations may have made different choices (as they did) in these different areas and what the implications of those different choices are.

WHO'S IN AND WHO'S OUT?: MEMBERSHIP AND MORE

Determining who belongs in, and out, is a classic way of controlling, or dispersing, power. All four of the organizations we study were constituted with very specific parameters around who would qualify for membership at their respective moments of creation and in the future. In the early twenty-first century, organizations with more diverse members tend to be viewed by the public more positively than those with more homogenous memberships, and yet, two of our four organizations have remained steadfastly member state driven.[3] This may partly be explained by a countervailing belief that great value still resides in forums in which only national governments can participate in debates and collectively make decisions.[4] In the view of some scholars and activists, organizations designed along that principle are more democratic in nature and therefore more legitimate. The reasoning goes that even in a world in which slightly less than half of the world's population lives in a democracy, democratic governments are more representative (and can be held more accountable) to their populations than philanthropic foundations, private companies, and civil society organizations, including NGOs, which are bound to their funders, their own Boards, or their own members.[5]

"Democratic deficit" is a term and framework generally applied to international organizations such as the World Bank or the UN system, including WHO, or regional organizations such as the European Union. It holds that organizations such as these are fundamentally less democratic than a national government. A democratic deficit, the theory holds, results from the lack of direct election by an international public for an international organization's leadership; member states (not their people) elect or select international organizations' executives, not those same member states' publics.[6] The inclusion of civil society, in particular, in international organizations could be viewed as shrinking the democratic deficit (by including more voices) or as widening it (civil society leadership, unlike leadership in a democracy, is not the product of open democratic elections). There are different ways then for membership—who's in and who's out—to answer questions of organizational legitimacy (table 5.1).

The "old" players

The World Health Organization

From its birth, WHO has comprised member states and member states alone. This is a position fiercely defended by recent WHO leadership, even as pressures for greater inclusion have intensified. Dr. Margaret Chan, WHO's Director-General (as of March 2016) has asserted repeatedly that the institution she leads is owned by member states, positioning the WHO Secretariat as the "servants" of those same member states, both in her speeches and in official WHO documents during her tenure.[7] Yet, Dr. Chan as well as previous WHO Director-Generals and the World Health Assembly itself have all recognized the important role nonstate actors play in global health. However, the World Health Assembly has repeatedly stopped short of granting them voting rights or finding other formal ways for them to influence and drive WHO's overall agenda—beyond, of course, the significant amounts of earmarked discretionary spending WHO accepts annually. Many of the largest voluntary contributors to WHO are not themselves member states as we highlighted in chapter 4.[8]

Formally, WHO has a process to determine and grant what it calls "official relations" status for NGOs that support WHO's "policies, strategies, and programmes."[9] To gain such official recognition from WHO, NGOs must be international and have the ability to speak authoritatively on behalf of their own staff and membership. These NGOs can apply once a year, with a committee of the Executive Board making decisions as to whether prospective NGOs meet WHO's criteria. The World Health Assembly delegated such decision-making authority to the Executive Board, and it retains discretion over the continuance or termination of official relations between WHO and NGOs.

As of January 2015, there were 202 NGOs in official relations with WHO.[10] The Gates Foundation, the largest nonmember state funder of WHO, is not included on the list, likely because it is a funding, not a programmatic, foundation. In contrast, Rotary International, another significant provider of voluntary contributions to WHO, is on the official NGO list. Those organizations that are included are granted access to nonconfidential materials (that presumably are also nonpublic) at the Director-General's discretion and participation at the World Health Assembly and other forums at the Assembly chairperson's discretion.[11]

There are other mechanisms through which nonstate actors can and do engage with WHO, such as through partnership arrangements. The most prominent of these are those that WHO hosts and to which it provides administrative, legal, fiduciary, and other resources. Notable examples of such partnerships include Roll Back Malaria (RBM), which until recently was hosted by UNITAID, the health commodity purchasing fund largely financed through airline ticket levies, and WHO.[12] However, these have distinct governance structures with their own Boards, and therefore are not central to understanding how WHO engages with nonstate actors. While WHO will participate on other Boards with nonstate actors (through RBM or Gavi, for example), it continues to eschew similar arrangements for governing itself.

Additionally, WHO has a formal policy governing any interactions with private-sector companies, a group it refers to as commercial enterprises. Unlike with NGOs, there is no official list of such interactions but rather guidelines on acceptable interactions—including addressing specific health issues, exchanging information, shared research and development efforts as well as cash and in-kind support from such enterprises to WHO—provided no actual nor perceived conflicts of interest exist between a company's core business and WHO's constitution and work. Specifically, WHO prohibits accepting cash donations from any private-sector company with business directly related to WHO's work (because of the possibility of a conflict of interest) or which is incompatible with its overall aims (e.g., the tobacco and arms industries). Specific guidelines also exist for areas of special vulnerability to conflicts of interest, for example around clinical trials. For all donations, WHO publicly discloses all cash and in-kind donations from the private sector and does not accept anonymous donations.[13] While WHO makes public that it, as of 2015, actively engaged with hundreds of academic institutions and two dozen philanthropic foundations, it does not disclose the specific entities it has engaged with nor what forms its engagement has taken.[14] There is not the same formality—or disclosure—around those groups as around commercial entities or NGOs.

The last time WHO updated the parameters surrounding its official relations with commercial enterprises was in 2000 at the 107th Executive Board meeting. The last time it did the same regarding NGOs was in 1987 at the 40th World Health Assembly.[15] There have been efforts, ultimately unsuccessful, to update both of these policies in the intervening years. Particularly in the past few years, the WHO Secretariat, the World Health Assembly, and the Executive Board have all taken up the question of WHO engagement with nonstate actors. Historically, nonstate actors were organized by type, as seen in the varying approaches mentioned earlier. Recent proposals have instead offered a typology for nonstate actors organized along type of interaction—financial, consultative, nonstate actors in WHO governance, and WHO in nonstate actor governance (e.g., Gavi)—rather than the identity of the actor.[16]

At the 68th World Health Assembly in May 2015, members voted to postpone finalizing a new policy for WHO's official engagement with NGOs, foundations, private-sector entities, and other nonstate actors.[17] Various reports from the meeting pointed to a continued lack of consensus around whether to treat all nonstate actors unitarily or to have different guidelines for WHO's engagement with NGOs versus private foundations versus private-sector companies. Additional rumored disagreement surrounded whether to accept financial contributions from all of those various groups and, if doing so, when caution or conflict of interest policies would be needed before entering into specific financial arrangements (e.g., with the food and beverage industries).[18]

Not surprisingly, opinions on such proposed policies were not confined to WHO member states; NGOs and others also offered pointed thoughts on everything from whether WHO was positioning relationships with nonstate actors for maximum public health benefit to whether conflicts of interest were adequately addressed.[19] The frustration in the long delays to updating WHO's governing and operational approach likely has contributed to WHO's decreasing resource pool as competition has emerged from better-funded bilateral programs, philanthropic foundations, and the new multilaterals of Gavi and the Global Fund (which include nonstate actors on their Boards). These are not merely rhetorical or philosophical inquiries. If WHO had been forced to listen to MSF's persistent and urgent calls to mount a strong response to Ebola in early 2014, would WHO have acted more strongly, much sooner, and with more conviction? Earlier action could have saved thousands of lives and untold millions, if not billions, of dollars.[20] An expert panel convened by WHO to evaluate its Ebola response called out WHO's "poor partnerships" with nonstate actors as contributing to the slow and inadequate response to the outbreak.[21] It urged WHO to ensure that whatever new policy it adopted defining potential relationships during an outbreak between it and others, nothing should interfere with the vital work nonstate actors undertake during an emergency, including private sector–driven research.[22]

WHO's continued state-centric approach juxtaposes strongly to Gavi and the Global Fund, which include NGOs engaged in program delivery and advocacy as well as technical partners like WHO in the boardroom (the Global Fund and Gavi) and with an actual Board seat (Gavi). For WHO to play the global coordinating role that it has historically viewed as uniquely its own in global health, and for the agency to be able to assert authority, possess legitimacy, and be effective as such a coordinator, it must significantly rethink how to engage nonstate actors in meaningful ways. Looking at the vital work of nonstate actors in combating HIV/AIDS and in beating back the 2014/15 Ebola outbreak, this is truer now than ever before. At a theoretical level, the continued hold that states exert as principals over WHO makes sense from a principal-agent perspective—why dilute control by bringing in more principals (or empowering your agent)? However, an addendum needs to be added to that question: member states are being forced to do so. Given the competition for resources and credibility in the global health arena, member states need to find ways to maintain the unique identity of WHO as a convener of member states while complementing that with meaningful roles for entities that deliver on parts of WHO's mandate (like MSF or pharmaceutical companies) and help fund its work (like the Gates Foundation).

The World Bank

No international organization in health has come under as much scrutiny and censure by NGOs and civil society than the World Bank. The only possible contender for equal criticism since World War II would be its sister international financial institution, the International Monetary Fund (IMF), which sits across the street from the Bank in Washington, DC.[23] In 2014/15, WHO arguably wrested this unenviable crown from the Bank and IMF given the widespread condemnation of its failures to respond quickly and effectively to the Ebola crisis. In the face of these external pressures, the Bank and WHO have taken drastically different approaches to including nonstate actors while equally remaining member state–based organizations. In contrast to WHO, the World Bank has no formal list of NGOs or private-sector companies with which it has an official relationship. This absence should not be taken as a lack of engagement. In fact, it is arguably the extent of such engagement that would make any definitive list impossible to keep accurate. The Bank estimates it engages with thousands of NGOs or civil society organizations (CSOs), the Bank's preferred nomenclature, every year, at the international, regional, country, and local levels while calling out, in various publications, a number of organizations by name with which it has ongoing work, including joint operational programmatic work.[24]

The Bank has two main vehicles for engaging nonstate actors, through discrete projects and through its Civil Society Policy Forum, with a myriad of additional efforts focused on specific issue areas (e.g., in 2011/12, there were four civil society consultations across the health, nutrition, and population portfolio), areas related to Bank management (e.g., on the Bank's access to information policy), and research studies (e.g., on climate change).[25] Additionally, the Bank in recent years has invited CSOs to be formally engaged in certain funding decisions, albeit of relatively small dollar amounts.

In 1970, the year the Bank made its first family-planning loan to Jamaica (and its first health-related loan), 20 percent of Bank projects had NGO involvement.[26] Today, the Bank uses CSOs as a broad term to mean traditional NGOs, faith-based organizations, philanthropic foundations, and any entity that is not part of a national government or private-sector company. From 1970 on, NGO involvement across the Bank portfolio climbed steadily, reaching 50 percent of newly funded World Bank Group projects by 1994 and subsequently staying above that threshold.[27] Yet by the early twenty-first century, the World Bank itself recognized that such percentages obscured whether NGOs played a meaningful role in shaping, implementing, or providing on-the-ground oversight for World Bank–funded projects. The Bank also acknowledged it had not invested in building internal staff and competencies to enable it to meaningfully engage NGOs.[28] Currently, the World Bank tracks the specific ways in which CSOs engage in Bank-financed projects to assess whether such engagement is substantial. From 2010 through 2012, CSOs participated in 82 percent of newly financed Bank projects.[29] We know this level of detail because every three years since 2002, the Bank has published a review of its engagement with civil society, including NGOs, labor unions, and philanthropic foundations, among others. Building and tracking such relationships is clearly part of the work of the now 120 Bank staff in more than one hundred country offices formally tasked with engaging local CSOs and the local offices of international CSOs.[30] We make no claim that such increased Bank focus has translated into meaningful engagement by CSOs. Rather, the Bank's investment globally contrasts to that of WHO's. Indeed, it is not clear from any official WHO documentation if WHO has even a de facto or implicit similar approach through its regional or country offices regarding fostering CSO/NGO relationships and involvement in its work. Certainly WHO has no such explicit approach and publishes no analogous triennial document.[31]

Another difference from WHO is the Civil Society Forum the Bank convenes in advance of its Annual Spring Meetings every year. WHO has no such analogue alongside its World Health Assembly meetings. The Bank has taken a "demand-driven" approach to the Forum, with CSOs generally determining the areas of focus and the Bank staff then joining. In 2014, more than six hundred CSOs participated.[32] While the Civil Society Forum and percentage of projects with NGO engagement may attract the most attention, it is the inclusion of CSOs in the funding decisions of the Bank's Global Partnership for Social Accountability (GPSA) that is most notable. The Bank set up the Global Partnership in 2012 to fund CSOs working to improve public services—including health—and to support and promote good governance practices. For the Global Partnership, the Bank constructed a multi-stakeholder Board inclusive of donor governments, recipient governments, and CSO representatives. While the total dollar amount is tiny relative to the Bank's overall portfolio—$15 million supporting twenty-three grants in seventeen countries, as of September 2015—it is clearly significant that the Bank has enfranchised CSOs in making decisions about how to invest Bank resources.[33]

In contrast to the careful tabulation of World Bank projects that involve CSOs and the number of CSOs that attend the Bank's now-annual Civil Society Forum, the Bank does not disclose aggregate participation levels by the private sector. This may be the inevitable result of how embedded multiple private-sector actors of various sizes and scope are across Bank projects. In other words, the Bank itself may not know. This is not surprising for several reasons. The Bank has a long-stated explicit focus on cultivating private-sector development and a thriving business environment, including in the health space.[34] It also recognizes (and repeatedly notes in various reports and analyses) that in many developing countries significant percentages, even the majority of key social services, including health care, are financed and even delivered through the private sector.[35] If the Bank wants to help nurture better health-care delivery and deliver better health outcomes, in many countries it must engage with the private sector. This recognition does not discount the criticism of the Bank that it has a philosophical bias (and even a blind spot) toward the private sector.[36]

If we reflect on the intense criticism of the World Bank by CSOs in the past several decades and the passionate protests seen outside Bank Annual Spring Meetings in certain years, it makes sense the Bank would find ways to bring more CSOs into its processes rather than persist in an antagonistic dynamic. The Civil Society Forum, the Bank staff around the world who are responsible for engaging with CSOs on the ground, the ongoing consultations, and the Global Partnership are examples of how the Bank has worked to involve CSOs in a way that is—hopefully—meaningful to its work and feels like a worthwhile effort for CSOs, even if at times such engagement also entails compromises for such CSOs. From the Bank's perspective (presumably), an additional benefit in the last few years is a decline in protests outside of its Annual Spring Meetings, possibly because those who were protesting are now "inside," possibly because Dr. Jim Kim, the current president of the Bank, started his career with an NGO, or possibly because CSO collective attention has moved on to other concerns. Regardless, CSOs are far more visible and are involved in far more parts of the Bank than is true at WHO. Yet, the member-state principles retain ultimate decision-making authority at the Bank, from big questions of resource allocation to determining Bank leadership. The World Bank has gone much farther than WHO, but still resides closer to it on the continuum of nonstate actor inclusion than to Gavi or the Global Fund.

The "new" players

As discussed extensively in chapter 3, both Gavi and the Global Fund, in contrast to WHO and the World Bank, have formally included nonstate actors on their Boards since inception. For each, nonstate actors incorporate NGOs/CSOs as well as the private sector, with Gavi granting Board seats specifically to pharmaceutical companies as well as to independent research institutions, which do not necessarily have a presence on the Global Fund Board. To complement the work in the previous chapters, we examine here the additional ways Gavi and the Global Fund look to engage a broader constituency of nonstate actors beyond the Boardroom.

Gavi

Turning first to the question of civil society participation, Gavi's CSO Board member provides leadership for the Gavi CSO Constituency, supported by a nineteen-person steering committee representing, as of September 2015, more than 250 CSOs.[37] In certain Gavi countries, CSOs deliver up to 60 percent of vaccines, making engaging with these organizations core to its business model.[38] Indeed, in some countries, Gavi directly funds CSOs to provide vaccine delivery support services.[39]

In others, CSOs are part of the delivery platform that Gavi funds, working alongside governments. In 2015, CSOs were part of grant recipients in twenty-two countries, a diverse group from India to South Sudan.[40]

To support its CSO partners on the ground, Gavi invested $28 million between 2007 and 2012 to strengthen CSOs' ability to engage in implementing Gavi grants. Additionally, CSOs in ten Gavi-eligible countries received support to facilitate their involvement in national health-sector planning and priority setting.[41] Gavi subsequently decided to subsume this funding stream into its Health Systems Funding Platform. This decision was an effort to harmonize funding streams, not to defund CSOs involved with delivering on Gavi's mission to close the vaccine gap.[42] One example Gavi cites to explain why it directs support to CSOs is the role these organizations play in vaccine delivery in Afghanistan and other fragile states.[43] Another is the crucial role CSOs play in many countries' health systems planning work, and Gavi has provided targeted funding to support such CSO engagement.[44]

In this arena, as in those discussed in previous chapters, the Gates Foundation looms large at Gavi. Bill and Melinda Gates provided the initial impetus and tranche of funding for Gavi, and the Gates Foundation holds a permanent seat on the Gavi Board. Additionally, the Gates Foundation has used its support to encourage other philanthropic and private companies to provide financial support to Gavi, albeit with limited success as we note in chapter 4. While more partners for Gavi's work are meaningful in terms of providing more diverse support, their collective pledges rarely reach even a small percentage of Gates's financial support in a given year.[45]

Yet, Gavi's relationship with the private sector stands as unique among WHO and the Global Fund, and is more intensive than anything we have observed or could find related to health at the World Bank.[46] Gavi, from the beginning, has included private-sector representatives from the vaccine industry. Strict conflict of interest policies are intended to prevent those same Board members from distorting debates around which vaccines to focus on or how hard to push industry for price concessions based on precommitted higher vaccine-purchase volumes. At times, the existence of such policies has not provided Gavi sufficient protection from criticism of the inevitable appearance of conflicts of interest, whether they materialize or not. For example, in 2011, when Crucell, a vaccine company, was tapped to take one of the two Board seats reserved for pharmaceutical companies, significant criticism was levied at Gavi. In 2010, previous to its appointment, nearly 60 percent of Crucell's revenue came from Gavi for sales of its pentavalent vaccine. In an interview with the *Financial Times*, a MSF representative said, "We think some conflicts are too big to manage. If you look at the agenda of the board meetings at Gavi, almost all issues impact Crucell's bottom line." The *Financial Times* article goes on to point out that most of Gavi's then Board members had potential conflicts, either as countries receiving funds, donating funds, or organizations such as WHO and UNICEF that similarly receive Gavi funds for technical assistance or to procure vaccines. In this instance, as in others when scrutinized, Gavi defended its conflict of interest policy and adherence to it.[47] Still, even Gavi recognized in its 2010 evaluation report that while it had made progress in affordability for some vaccines, it had not yet in others (though it did not link this to its relationship and work with the pharmaceutical industry). Pentavalent was one area in which Gavi acknowledged it had not yet made that particular vaccine, along with others, more affordable.[48] Shortly before Crucell joined the Board, pharmaceutical companies, including Crucell, began publishing for the first time what Gavi paid (and bought) from UNICEF for their vaccines. From 2014 to 2015, the weighted average price for pentavalent vaccines dropped 36 percent.[49] This resulted in part from Gavi incentivizing increased production and key suppliers significantly dropping their prices. Perhaps Crucell being in the room made a difference. Or perhaps not. Clearly Gavi believes working with industry translates into more sustainable gains, even if the timeline is longer than civil society (or Gavi itself) may expect or hope.

Yet for all the furor in 2011 around Crucell's Board appointment and at other junctures for similar concerns around Gavi's perceived inherent conflict of interest in its work with pharmaceutical companies, much of the criticism levied at Gavi is based in critiques that it is distorting health-sector priorities through the sheer volume of vaccine-related aid.[50] The concern, once again, is that highly targeted, vertical aid of any variety, vaccine-related or disease-related, leads to fragmented health services less able to meet a population's basic needs. Gavi's approach has been criticized for contributing little to strengthening countries' health systems.[51] One paper evaluating Gavi's earlier health systems strengthening decisions called them "the Gates approach," not in a complimentary way.[52] Gavi has responded to these and similar critiques over the years by introducing and then amplifying its formal funding commitments to health systems strengthening. From 2007 (the first year Gavi disbursed funds specifically targeting health systems) to 2015, Gavi invested more than $856 million in Gavi countries' health systems programs or approximately 10 percent of total Gavi funds disbursed over the same period.[53] The comparable percentage of total Global Fund disbursements directed to "other" areas besides HIV/AIDS, TB, TB/HIV joint work, and malaria (the Fund does not break out health systems in its data), through 2015 was less than 2 percent.[54] We will engage more with the horizontal versus vertical debate in chapter 7, but here we wanted to highlight that Gavi receives at least as much scrutiny, and likely more, for its disease-specific approach than its private-sector inclusion, even as it has broadened its relationship with the private sector and broadened its areas of investment.

In early 2015, Gavi launched a partnership with the International Federation of Pharmaceutical Wholesalers to strengthen the vaccine supply chain through supply-chain management-focused training programs across Gavi-supported countries. Additionally, Gavi works with private companies on logistics training programs and with medical supply companies on syringe development and injection safety campaigns.[55] The announcement of many of these partnerships shortly before the replenishment meeting in Berlin in late January 2015 likely was not coincidental. What some critics see as a conflict of interest, Gavi clearly views as a source of strength. Private-sector cash donations, in-kind support, and formalized partnerships across the private sector and with CSOs are all welcomed. From a principal-agent perspective, such a strategy makes sense for the agent to increase its autonomy and discretion. The more cooks in the kitchen, the easier it is for an organization's Secretariat (versus its principals through the Board) to set priorities and drive the agenda. Although, if one believes that greater inclusion of stakeholders equals greater organizational legitimacy, then it is good for both Gavi's principals as well as for the Secretariat.

The Global Fund

The Global Fund has more Board seats reserved specifically for CSOs than Gavi does (three versus one) but fewer seats reserved for private companies (one versus two). The different approaches each takes to engaging with nonstate actors stretch far beyond the boardroom. Until Merck was elected to take the private-sector Board seat starting in 2013, no health commodity company, pharmaceutical or otherwise, had ever held the Board seat at the Global Fund.[56] In terms of private-sector health commodity engagement, for most of its existence the Global Fund took a different approach than that of Gavi's. Repeatedly, over its first decade, the Global Fund Board voted against accepting any in-kind health commodities donations from the private sector and from meaningfully engaging with health commodity companies. Even when the Global Fund Secretariat mounted arguments that in-kind donations would increase the Global Fund's ability to support its grantees and that it itself would not need to manage any such donations, and the United States and others suggested that the Fund accept such donations at least in emergency situations, the Board voted not to support such policy changes. Similarly, in the Global Fund's first decade, its Board repeatedly decided against extensively using its potential purchasing power to drive down the per unit costs of treatment or prevention interventions, again out of concern that such market-shaping agreements would move too far away from country-ownership and possibly drive out generic competitors.[57] The Global Fund remained concerned about any possible conflicts of interest and wanted to avoid even the appearance of the Fund compromising its guiding principles of being a financing entity and country-driven by accepting in-kind donations of medicines or bed nets, for example, or working too closely with health commodity companies.[58] Additionally, much of the fund-raising attention in the Fund's first decade focused on a hoped-for, yet never materialized, high level of financial support for the Fund from the private sector. Chapter 4 discussed the Global Fund's disconnect between financial aspiration and reality. One analysis traced the Fund's unwillingness to accept in-kind contributions from private companies as likely hindering its ability to attract financial support from those same companies.[59]

Over time, the Secretariat came to define the private sector more as an in-country partner, publishing reports on private-sector representation in country-coordinating mechanisms (CCMs) or private-sector cofi-nancing pledges made to CCMs as part of their grant applications.[60] Eventually, the Global Fund Board itself moved its aspirations away from the private sector as a source of significant financial support. Perhaps this is seen most clearly, albeit implicitly, in the independent High Level Panel convened by the Board in 2011. In 2010, the Fund's inspector general identified fraud in multiple grants in Mali and Mauritania, and suspected fraud in additional countries.[61] Even though a subsequent full inquiry discovered relatively low levels of fraud in re-lation to the Fund's total grant portfolio, the Global Fund's Board launched the High Level Panel, charging it with conducting a serious inquiry into the Fund's business model and operations. Its final report contains neither discussion on nor recommendations for strengthening the relationship between the Global Fund Secretariat, or CCMs, and the private sector, not as related to cash fund-raising, in-kind support, or any other dimension.[62]

The Global Fund's approach to the private sector changed signifi-cantly in 2013. Previously, the Global Fund largely eschewed its pur-chasing power, not working with CCMs and Principal Recipients to pool together grant funds designated for purchasing mosquito nets, di-agnostic tools, or medicines. In 2013, the Fund committed to using its new pooled procurement mechanism to buy ninety million bed nets; this saved the Fund and its grantees an estimated $140 million over two years.[63] The Board's decision for the Global Fund to engage in such bulk-volume purchasing for lower unit prices more closely resembles Gavi's historic business model than the Fund's. Indeed, the Fund has made clear that the bed-net purchases are only the first phase of its new approach. Yet, unlike Gavi, participating in the Global Fund's pooled procurement program is voluntary for CCMs and Principal Recipients.[64]

While the Global Fund did not meaningfully engage health com-modities companies on its Board or in its business model until its second decade, from inception it has been highly focused on civil soci-ety engagement. From the Fund's beginning, the Northern and Southern NGO representatives each had a Board seat. The Affected Communities' representative also had a presence from the Fund's be-ginning in the Boardroom, first as an observer and then with full voting rights starting in 2004. Examining the few Board reports in which comments are identified by Board members, it is clear, at least in those meetings, that the Affected Communities' member (representing people affected by HIV/AIDS, TB, and/or malaria) was an active participant in Board discussions.[65]

Beyond the boardroom, the Global Fund's founders intended its Partnership Forum to play a meaningful role in informing the Fund's strategic direction. As conceived, the Forum was intended to provide an opportunity for all Fund stakeholders, and particularly civil society, to discuss the Fund's governance and operations and then offer direct feedback to the Fund's Board and management. Through 2014, the Global Fund had convened four Partnership Forums. Although between three hundred and five hundred participants attended various forums and hundreds more joined the Fund's e-forums, there is no evidence from the Board record that the voices the Partnership Forums included influenced Board decisions, beyond those related to the Partnership Forum itself.[66] Similarly, there is little evidence that the nonstate Board members, private-sector and NGO members alike, have swayed meaningful debates, even if at times they have participated vigorously. There is evidence, as we saw in chapter 3, that suggests that the views of government representatives, particularly those from its largest donor, the United States, continued to heavily influence key Global Fund decisions.[67]

The Gavi Secretariat (the agent) has asserted itself through the cacophony of different constituencies on the Board and more broadly in the Gavi ecosystem. The opposite seems to have occurred in the first decade of the Global Fund. The Global Fund's Secretariat perspectives are rarely evident in key debates behind closed doors or in the public domain; the in-kind donation debates mentioned earlier at the Fund Board are the exception. It is impossible to have a real sense of what the Fund Secretariat's positions were regarding the Fund's enfranchisement of nonstate actors, including civil society. That is surprising. We would expect an agent to look to build relationships with arguably more friendly principals as well as with friendly constituents beyond the boardroom, to counterbalance strong principals. Considering the marked influence of the United States in the Global Fund Board's decision-making, as seen in the paucity of examples of the Board ever voting against the US positions cited in chapter 3, we would expect the

TABLE 5.1 Membership: Who's In and Who's Out

	Board Inclusion	Nonstate Actor Inclusion: Financial Engagement	Nonstate Actor Inclusion: NGO/CSO Engagement	Nonstate Actor Inclusion: Other Means
World Health Organization	Member states only.	Nonstate actors do not have voting rights or other formal ways of influencing the WHO's overall agenda, except for the financial contributions they can make through earmarked extrabudgetary contributions as well as non-earmarked extrabudgetary contributions (though in practice the latter are an insignificant portion of nonstate contributions to WHO).	WHO can grant "official relations" status for NGOs that support WHO's "policies, strategies and programmes" through approval by the Executive Board. Official relations status grants NGOs privileges including approval to attend meetings of the Executive Board and World Health Assembly, the right to make a statement at these meetings, and access to nonconfidential documents.	1) WHO can engage in partnership agreements such as Roll Back Malaria (RBM), to which it provides administrative, legal, fiduciary, and other resources. 2) WHO has formal guidelines on acceptable interactions with private-sector companies, known as "commercial enterprises" 3) WHO also "engages" with academic institutions and philanthropic foundations, but there are no formal guidelines regulating this.

| World Bank | Member states only. | The World Bank has recently invited civil society organizations (how it refers to NGOs) to be formally engaged in certain funding decisions (though of relatively small dollar amounts). Civil society organizations increasingly participate in Bank-financed programmatic delivery. Over the period 2010–2012, civil society organizations participated in 82% of newly financed Bank projects. The World Bank also engages the private sector through the International Finance Corporation, which finances investment in developing countries and provides advisory services to their businesses and governments, and as partners in delivering programs financed by the IBRD and IDA. | The World Bank has no formal list of NGOs with which it has a relationship, unlike WHO. From 1970 onward, NGO involvement across the Bank portfolio increased steadily, reaching 50% of newly funded World Bank Group projects by 1994. | 1) The World Bank primarily engages with nonstate actors through two vehicles: projects on the ground in countries where IBRD and IDA provide financing and its Civil Society Policy Forum.
2) The design of the World Bank's strategic priorities, laid out in its Country Assistance Strategies (CASs) for low-income countries or Country Partnership Strategies (CPSs) for middle-income countries, reflects the input of a variety of stakeholders, including civil society organizations and the private sector.
3) The World Bank has additional efforts focused on specific issues areas that engage nonstate actors (e.g., research studies, civil society consultations, etc.). |

(Continued)

TABLE 5.1 Continued

	Board Inclusion	Nonstate Actor Inclusion: Financial Engagement	Nonstate Actor Inclusion: NGO/CSO Engagement	Nonstate Actor Inclusion: Other Means
The Global Fund to Fight AIDS, Tuberculosis and Malaria	The Global Fund has formally included nonstate actors on its Board since inception: three seats for civil society organizations (a Northern NGO, a Southern NGO and one for organizations that represent people living with HIV/ AIDS, TB or malaria); one seat for a private company; and, one seat for a private foundation (held since inception by the Gates Foundation).	In its first decade, the Global Fund Board repeatedly voted against accepting any in-kind health commodities donations from the private sector. However its approach changed in 2013, when it committed to engaging the private sector through bulk volume purchasing (à la Gavi). Private and NGO partners have contributed over US$1.69 billion to the Global Fund, including substantial commitments from the Bill & Melinda Gates Foundation and US$300 million raised through (RED).	The Global Fund has engaged CSOs heavily since its inception. One example of this is the Partnership Forum, a venue through which civil society stakeholders have the opportunity to discuss the Fund's governance and operations and then offer direct feedback to the Fund's Board and management. Private sector and nongovernment partners are also involved in Country Coordinating Mechanisms (CCMs) in many countries. In fact, having processes for electing a nongovernment CCM member is one of the six Eligibility Requirements that CCMs must comply with in order to be eligible for funding.	1) In addition to the participation of CSOs at the country level through CCMs, private-sector companies also serve as Principal Recipients or subrecipients of grants at the ground level, thus allowing them to implement interventions. 2) As a funding entity, the Global Fund does not have presence in country, and so CSO partners also work to support the Fund's awareness and advocacy efforts on the ground.

Gavi, The Vaccine Alliance	Gavi has formally included nonstate actors on its Board since inception: one seat for a civil society organization and two seats for private companies, which can include representatives from the vaccine industry as well as research and technical health institutes. The Board also consists of nine independent or "unaffiliated" individuals who are not directly involved in Gavi's work. UNICEF, WHO, the World Bank, and the Bill & Melinda Gates Foundation hold permanent seats.	With a $750 million contribution, the Gates Foundation provided the initial impetus and funding for Gavi, and has a greater influence over it than WHO does. Today, foundations, corporations and organizations contribute 22% of Gavi's funding, and the private sector contributes 1%. These contributions can be made in four ways: direct funding (including multi-year grant agreements and pledges), the Gavi Matching Fund, the International Finance Facility for Immunisation (IFFIm) and through long-term pledges to the Advance Market Commitment (AMC).	Gavi supports CSOs by encouraging their engagement in national health policy processes in Gavi-eligible countries and through direct funding via the Health Systems Funding Platform (HSFP). CSOs also receive direct funding to provide vaccine delivery support services and provide up to 60% of immunization services in some countries.	1) Gavi's CSO Board provides leadership for the Gavi CSO constituency. 2) Gavi has a uniquely strong relationship with the private sector, from which it receives cash donations and in-kind support.

Secretariat to redouble such efforts. Similarly, the presence of strong developing countries on the Board, notably China, might add further impetus to such efforts by the Secretariat. Yet, the ongoing preeminence of the Board in setting and driving the agenda is less surprising when considering how significantly the Fund relied on the United States as its primary financial supporter, and on China and other developing country Board members to be part of the work on the ground that the Fund financed.

We are able to probe into the questions tackled in this book because of the information that each institution shares. Similarly, we are hindered, as are other academics, journalists, and a curious public, by the information these institutions choose to keep internally, or to not keep at all. It is to questions of transparency that we now turn.

QUIS CUSTODIET IPSOS CUSTODES? WHO WILL WATCH THE WATCHMEN?: TRANSPARENCY

Sometimes this quotation is translated as "who will guard the guardians?"[68] Although an early satirist coined the quote, it is often used to question how those with power—political, financial, moral—can be adequately held accountable for how they use that power. It is an apt epigram to begin this section given our case-study institutions' command power flowing from political, financial, and moral sources. It recognizes that "watching" encourages playing by the rules, whatever those rules may be. In other words, the theory holds, people (and institutions) under scrutiny are more likely to uphold their duties than those left unexamined. The public, including our students, tend to have high expectations about transparency and low expectations of their own ability to influence any major institution, whether an international organization or international NGO. Their interest tends to focus on what organizations disclose, what they do not disclose, and what explains the difference. Certainly in the twenty-first century, publics across the world expect to be part of the collective watchmen, holding those with power accountable for their use of that power.[69]

Transparency is often discussed in terms of offering protection against corruption rather than increasing participation and legitimacy. Some have gone so far as to frame transparency as what institutions must do to manage the politics of the mistrust and cynicism that the public has for any concentration of corporate or political power, particularly when at great remove from an electorate (as all four of our institutions are as none of their Boards or management rose to their positions through broadly democratic elections).[70] Yet, this is not all that is expected of transparency today. Without shared internal transparency (equal access to equal information) between agents and principals, agents will always possess an asymmetrical informational advantage given they are closer to the organizations' work. Without shared internal transparency among principals, all principals cannot equally participate. An absence of external transparency, clearly defined by institutions themselves, to CSOs, for example, constrains those same organizations from meaningfully participating in the various civil society/NGO arrangements that international organizations have created to help deliver against their missions and objectives.

Recognizing that transparency facilitates both participation and accountability does not provide an immediate answer to any of the "who" or "to whom" questions. Who should be allowed, even expected, to participate in the governance of multilateral organizations? That question was addressed in the first part of this chapter. Now we turn to such broad questions as the following: How should organizations like the World Bank or WHO, which are composed solely of member states, think about transparency in terms of accountability beyond their member states to the broader public? Would accountability to select CSOs be sufficient (as deemed by the organizations or an independent watchdog)? And who would formulate such a list? The organizations themselves? An independent entity of experts? Who would constitute such an independent entity, define what constituted an expert, and determine who could be considered truly independent? What are legitimate justifications for keeping certain information, whether intellectual property or decision-making criteria, private (and who determines what constitutes legitimate reasons in those cases)? We hope this brief cascade of derivative questions helps illuminate why—even in an age of online databases, instantaneous communications, and increasing expectations of transparency by the media and the public—institutions answer these questions differently and the different answers themselves continue to evolve. We are taking a snapshot in time (summer 2015) and the history before it to elucidate the ways WHO, the World Bank, Gavi, and the Global Fund have tackled at least some of the questions.

Today, broadly speaking, there are two categories of transparency. Internal transparency aims to close the asymmetry gap between principal and agent, whether at the instigation of the principal, the agent, or both. Such internal transparency is also an expected (though not always realized) benefit of organizational membership. External transparency aims to close the asymmetry gap between institutions and the public, including organizations and companies who work with but are not part of the institutions themselves. In theory, external transparency enables the public to understand the motivations of the institution alongside its actions, building a set of shared norms and expectations over time. Particularly today, transparency and the act of being transparent are fundamental to credibility, the lifeblood of an organization. As Robert Keohane and Joseph Nye summarized, "Credibility is a crucial resource, and asymmetrical credibility is a key source of power."[71] Pursuing that logic, institutions that are more credible with the public will have more power to act on their mandates over time (and likely more resources from those publics' treasuries to fund their work). In this view, principals and agents alike have a shared interest in finding a set of transparency policies and practices that are acceptable both to the public and themselves.

We are going to examine each institution for how transparent they are to their principals and how transparent they are to the public. In chapter 6, when we turn to organizational reforms, we will look at what, if any, the effects of such transparency have been on engagement beyond the organizations' member states and nonstate actors. While the World Bank and its "sister" institution, the International Monetary Fund (IMF), have come under significant scrutiny and criticism by civil society for their "democratic deficits" and their overall lending approaches and methodologies, engaging in those debates lies outside the scope of this book, except insofar as relates to the Bank's health work.[72] Whether more transparency facilitates greater understanding and public engagement is important, in part because more data and information alone do not necessarily advance those objectives. Indeed, a deluge of data can have the opposite effect. As Joseph Nye has pointed out, "A plenitude of information leads to a poverty of attention."[73]

Joseph Nye's quote may sound anathema to those who think more information is always better and who prize transparency as an unalloyed good and goal. Yet, there are equally compelling, if not stronger, arguments that full and immediate transparency is not always in the best interest of protecting public health. During public health crises when an organization is trying to determine what is happening, it might be best for such a determination to be made first, and then subsequently shared with clear, action-oriented public health directives rather than sharing real-time incomplete information untethered to specific recommendations, a volatile combination that may lead to panic. The reality or even specter of greater transparency can have a chilling effect on the candor and quality of public health debates. During politically fraught negotiations around health issues, transparency may lead those at the table to be less likely to find workable compromises when their constituencies may view any compromise as a weakness.[74] There are also legitimate concerns of compromised security, privacy, and intellectual property, all particularly important when thinking about an individual's right to privacy regarding one's own health information and how that information might be used and to what end.[75] For our purposes, we examine each institution along two dimensions related to public access to knowledge: transparency into where their monies are going, and transparency into how key decisions are made and by whom (table 5.2). We do not look here at transparency into how the organizations themselves receive funding because we documented in chapter 4 that each organization is transparent about its donors.

The World Health Organization

As of September 2015, WHO is the only entity we examine that does not have a transparency, public information, or open-information policy. It does have an open access policy, but at the moment that applies only to WHO-authored or coauthored articles and papers. As WHO says itself of that policy, "it does not apply [even] to ... conference proceedings."[76] The absence of any umbrella-access policy means that there is no shared understanding between WHO and the public as to what the public has the right to know about WHO's decision-making, programs, and operations. But that does not mean WHO is monolithically opaque. For example, resolutions and supporting documents submitted to the World Health Assembly as well as to WHO's Executive Board are available online. Significantly, many are available in all six UN languages (Arabic, English, French, Mandarin, Russian, Spanish). In contrast, neither the Global Fund nor Gavi provide materials online in all six UN languages, and the World Bank's provision of materials in the UN languages varies by topic (as of 23 October 2015). Therefore, member states, civil society, and the public—at least those who read one of the six UN languages—have the ability to access information on the major decisions of the World Health Assembly and Executive Board. The Executive Board meetings' proceedings are now made available in real time through WHO's website in all six UN languages.[77] Yet, the Executive Board and World Health Assembly are not the only decision-making authorities within WHO. So too is the Director-General a significant decision maker.

WHO's Director-General has exclusive control over whether to declare an outbreak a Public Health Emergency of International Concern (PHEIC). When considering whether to declare a PHEIC, she must convene a committee of public health experts to help inform her decision.[78] The most recent full PHEIC declaration concerned the Ebola outbreak in Guinea, Liberia, and Sierra Leone in August 2014; WHO declared a more limited PHEIC in February 2016 concerning the possible (and by April 2016 the confirmed) link between Zika and microcephaly, as well as other neurological disorders.[79] While membership of the Emergency Committee is in the public domain, as relates to the Ebola decision, there is no public record of what documents and evidence the committee consulted or what options it considered and discounted before recommending to Director-General Chan that she declare a PHEIC. All that was disclosed to the public was the committee's unanimous recommendation and her ultimate PHEIC declaration.[80] This is a classic example of transparency about a decision but a complete lack of transparency into decision-making: WHO's posture around the PHEIC process, and Ebola specifically, has not changed, even in the months following Dr. Chan's declaration in November 2014 that WHO would share information about WHO's Ebola response in a "transparent and accountable manner."[81]

It is not that WHO does not have an interest in transparency. In April 2015, for example, WHO called for more transparency into medical research, specifically that all medical trials be registered, rather than the current practice in which pharmaceutical companies, government researchers, and others report only successful medical trials.[82] What is notable is that this occurred less than a year after the Ebola PHEIC declaration (though more than a year after the first calls for it to do so). WHO is now asking for more transparency from government and privately funded research entities relating to their core business model than it itself has been willing to provide.[83]

In terms of funding flows, WHO makes publicly available its forward-looking programmatic budgets as well as its retrospective audited financial statements. However, these two resources together provide less useful information than the more specific and granular information the Global Fund and Gavi provide around their respective grant portfolios and investments. We are hardly the first to notice that the information WHO discloses around where it spends its money does not provide meaningful insight into how that money is spent or necessarily to what end. The UK Multilateral Aid Review 2013 update noted that one of WHO's three core weaknesses was that it had "no clear and transparent system to allocate aid."[84] The earlier 2011 UK Multilateral Aid Review similarly observed that WHO was weak on disclosures.[85] Roughly 75 percent of WHO funds are spent by regional offices, which have varying levels of transparency, adding to the difficulty in tracking funds by the interested public as well as WHO member states, including donors.[86]

As of 28 December 2015, WHO is the only one of our four focal institutions that does not report to the International Aid Transparency Initiative (IATI). The IATI's stated mission is to close the information gap between donors and recipients, and between donors and citizens, in their own countries and around the world. Bilateral and multilateral donors that report to the IATI do so in a standardized format to make simpler comparisons across donors, by year, and other variables.[87] Similarly, WHO does not participate in the Aid Transparency Index, an initiative of Publish What You Fund: The Global Campaign for Aid Transparency, while the other three do. While WHO is not a financing entity as the World Bank, Gavi, and the Global Fund are, UNICEF is similarly not predominantly a financing entity, and it submits data to the IATI and is part of the Aid Transparency Index.[88]

WHO is also unique compared to our other focal institutions in its lack of a programmatic or projects database to provide visibility into various projects' funding flows over time or the results that WHO garnered, or didn't, for its investments. Funding flows, at least, can be aggregated together from individual WHO biennial budgets; there is no analogous raw data on programmatic performance, as judged by WHO itself or through independent evaluations.[89] As we discuss later in this chapter, the World Bank, the Global Fund, and Gavi each have online portals to enable anyone with curiosity and sufficient Internet access to track investments by country and thematic health area, as well as to varying levels, in order to monitor the results and assessments of the institutions' investments. In contrast, WHO has only individual web pages dedicated to topical areas of its work, for example addressing violence and injury prevention. Still, the information shared on each webpage varies widely in scope, detail, and timeliness, and generally does not contain the results of WHO's work in a given area. This may be inevitable given WHO's focus on determining and tracking health challenges across the globe, setting standards around how best to address such challenges, and providing technical assistance to countries that need help in meeting those standards. Given that no two national and subnational contexts are identical, the health challenges and their recommended responses all vary around the world. Recognition of this dynamic makes the evident idiosyncrasies in WHO's reporting across health areas less surprising. Nevertheless, the absence of performance ratings and assessments of WHO programs, by WHO or independent evaluators, on the WHO website is out of alignment with current expectations of transparency and with the choices other multilateral organizations increasingly are making.

Returning to the specific example of WHO's work on violence and injury prevention, and looking at traffic injuries in particular, we find a substantial number of publications relating to WHO's work in this area, including fact sheets, media briefs, the most recent global status report on road safety from 2013, epidemiological data on traffic injuries by WHO regions that track such data, and even the staff list of the WHO department. Yet, while WHO provides country profiles as relates to traffic injuries, WHO does not provide any transparency into how it—or anyone else—views its convening, norm setting, health tracking, or technical assistance work as relates to traffic injuries or how much it has invested in the area.[90]

While WHO provides a consolidated data repository through its Global Health Observatory (GHO) portal of various health indicators by country, it offers no consistent view or performance indicators of its own work on the same health topics or in the 178 countries or areas that report data to WHO. Nor, again, does it provide a sense of how much it is investing along the dimensions of health topic or country.[91] In 2010 and 2011, the WHO Secretariat considered whether to begin posting reports on progress against country-level indicators specifically relating to the health workforce, including reports from nonstate actors, moving away from an exclusive reliance on member state reporting. Reports from nonstate actors would have shed additional light on the activities of both member states and WHO, at least as relates to health workforce programs, as well as other multilateral and bilateral actors. However, in 2012 the Secretariat decided against such disclosure and against the broader transparency that had been under consideration.[92] In addition to the opacity around the PHEIC process, the continued lack of transparency into how WHO tracks its own progress (versus that of its member states), and the challenge of comparisons across programmatic areas or funding streams over time helps explain why transparency remains such an area of particular focus for those calling for WHO reform.[93]

The World Bank

Concerns over the lack of transparency by the Bank have been voiced for relatively longer than the other three institutions, in significant part due to its close but strained relationship to its largest shareholder and donor, the United States. Starting in the 1970s, the US Congress began to engage more with the Bank, pressing for more information about its activities and expressing opposition to loans the Bank made to particular countries, such as Vietnam and India.[94] Civil society and NGO criticism historically focused on the lack of visibility into what and who influenced Bank decisions, as well as the specifics of those decisions, relating both to loans and to any contracting relationships within loan arrangements. Particularly in the 1990s, mutually aware of these criticisms, the Bank's principals and interested external parties alike hoped greater transparency would collapse the information gap between those "inside" and "outside" the Bank.[95] In addition, the Bank in more recent years has attracted scrutiny for its own transparency policies and practices due to the Bank's focus on good governance and transparency by borrower governments and companies.[96]

By 2015, the background of these debates had changed dramatically, not because of shifting norms as much as significant rearrangements in Bank policy. In 2010, the Bank introduced a formal access to information policy, outlining what information it would make publicly available, what information the public had a right to ask for, and what information the Bank would withhold. The policy's default on transparency is that information will be disclosed unless it is on the policy's (not short) exceptions list. It went into effect in 2011.[97] In 2012, the World Bank launched Open Contracting to facilitate more competitive bidding for contracts, and it increasingly has made available data on Bank-financed contracts, including data subsets organized by issue area, such as road costs across Bank contracts.[98] The Bank does not publish what influences its decisions to reward contracts to one entity over another, again an example of decision transparency but not decision-making transparency. From the Bank's perspective, doing so might compromise the Bank's subsequent ability to negotiate in that issue area or with the previously losing contractor. Given the lack of transparency into Bank decision-making around these policies, it is not clear what rationale was used in any given decision.

Additionally, the Bank publishes extensively on the results of its programmatic investments, as assessed by the programs themselves, certain internal assessments, and through the Bank's Independent Evaluation Group (IEG). The Bank's projects database includes information on more than ten thousand individual projects the Bank has supported since 1947, as well as various publications on countries receiving Bank funds, areas of focus by the Bank, and reports on the Bank's own operations.[99] For the Bank's Health, Nutrition, and Population (HNP) portfolio, raw data on grants, particularly relevant financial information, is also available from 1970, the year the Bank began its health portfolio.[100] Additionally, the Bank provides a database of all approved current HNP projects, both those ongoing and those pending. Along with financial information, each project's page includes any reported results against the project's baseline and performance targets and its implementation ratings, as judged by the Bank. As one example, as of December 2015, the page dedicated to the Additional Financing for the Health System Improvement Project in Uzbekistan contains status reports and results from as recently as the previous June and July. Certain indicators show significant improvement from baseline, such as health personnel receiving additional training, while other indicators show no progress, such as hospital management staff receiving additional training. The Bank rated the overall implementation progress in July 2015 as "moderately unsatisfactory."[101]

It is evident from what the Bank has recently shared that it is not selectively providing access to favorable project evaluations or favorable reports on the Bank more broadly. As one example, the IEG found that between 1997 and 2008, $18 billion of the Bank's loans rarely led to highly satisfactory program outcomes with moderately satisfactory or better outcomes in only two-thirds of all projects.[102] As another, an internal 2009 review of the Bank's health strategy reported satisfactory outcomes in only 52 percent of its projects.[103] In fact, in 2014, the UK House of Commons International Development Committee said, "We welcome [the] Bank's commitment to improve but are concerned that significant expansion of the Bank's work in health is commencing without evidence that the major failings detailed in a number of internal and external reports have been addressed."[104] Such an opinion would have been impossible to voice before the Bank's significant programmatic-related disclosures. The Bank's policies since 2011 facilitate understanding of what decisions were made but not why they were made, or who participated in making them. Similarly, while the Bank is committed to greater transparency, it does not bind its contractors to the same level of disclosure. Third parties have the right to prevent the release of any information they provide to the Bank, even if it relates to the success or failure of a given program.

Despite the Bank's move toward more openness in what it funds, the Bank's Board of Directors and Executive Directors have continued to preserve their own confidentiality. The Bank does not publish meeting agendas, resolutions, or the record of their meetings, as the Global Fund does. In policy and practice, the Bank shares nothing it considers internal communications; not surprisingly, this posture continues to attract scrutiny and criticism from the media and activists alike.[105] It also does not publish the fees it charges to each trust fund for its management, even though trust funds are an increasing part of the Bank's funds and business. Even so, the Bank is far more open than WHO is and has been recognized as such.[106] Unlike WHO, parts of the Bank report to both the International Aid Transparency Initiative and the Aid Transparency Index. In 2014, the latter rated the World Bank's IDA "very good" on transparency and open data; the IBRD did not report to the Transparency Initiative.[107] Transparency International, the global transparency watchdog, said of the World Bank, it is "a bank others look up to" in terms of transparency.[108]

Gavi

Since the financial crisis of 2008/9, significant attention has been paid to the role of trust in the financial system and how transparency can validate or invalidate that trust. Perhaps that zeitgeist has contributed to the increased scrutiny the World Bank has received and its credible steps toward greater transparency, as well as to the attention to fraud in Global Fund grants in 2010/11, as we discuss in chapter 6. Questions broadly related to the democratic deficit have also propelled studies of trust between various publics, in donor and recipient countries, and international organizations.[109] In 2014, such a study focused on Gavi was published, but nowhere in it was transparency mentioned.[110]

Gavi introduced its first transparency policy in 2009, updating it in 2013. Gavi's policy actually couples transparency and accountability, making clear that its commitment to transparency around cash and vaccine support (financial transparency) is important both for its relationships with recipient countries as well as its stewardship for broader aid accountability and harmonization (accountability).[111] Gavi makes available, by country, estimates of Gavi's grant approvals as well as its commensurate financial and in-kind commitments and disbursements. It also provides relevant mortality and vaccine coverage statistics by country (when available), as well as all Gavi publications organized by country.[112] Gavi's approach is a good example of avoiding the plenitude Joseph Nye warned about. It does not inundate the public with information yet still provides useful transparency around decisions and financial flows by country and type of work it supports within each country.

That does not mean that Gavi does not provide extensive information. It does. Gavi provides raw financial and in-kind commitment and disbursement data by type of support (e.g., measles or pentavalent vaccine programs), by year, and by country.[113] While it historically did not publish grant-specific or country-specific programmatic information, it began to publish such information alongside its full country evaluations project that it launched in 2013, in partnership with the IHME and others. The first wave is focused on Bangladesh, Mozambique, Uganda, and Zambia. Gavi has also committed to publishing results across its programs and grants, including as relates to CSO partners. The first such reports are expected following the end of the 2011–15 cycle.[114] While these may be less intensive than the full country evaluations, they will certainly offer relatively greater visibility into the Gavi portfolio. In the interim, approved grant applications proposals available by country indicate what Gavi expects from each of the CSOs (and other partners) it provides vaccine-related or health system–related funding to around the world.[115] It is important to acknowledge that while publishing such grant-focused performance results as expected in 2016 or subsequently may be new to Gavi, it has always published various evaluations, for example on its initial health systems strengthening funding or its support to CSOs.[116] Looking at Gavi's policies and practices around disclosure, in 2014 the Aid Transparency Index ranked Gavi fourth overall, awarding it the same "very good," its highest ranking, that it provided the World Bank's IDA.[117]

In terms of accessibility of information, Gavi (unlike WHO and the World Bank) provides broad information access to its policies, financials, and specific country pages only in English and French (as of 28 December 2015). It provides application guidelines, depending on the type of vaccine support, in English, French, Spanish, and Russian. However, Gavi works to increase internal transparency among principals and between principals and the Gavi Secretariat, across languages. A key way Gavi does this is through facilitating and financing additional opportunities for recipient country governments on Gavi's Board to meet with one another and Gavi staff.[118] This is not the same as public transparency. Still, additional efforts toward shrinking internal asymmetries of information among principals, and between principals and their agent, is crucial to ensuring more stakeholders beyond donor states can meaningfully engage in Gavi governance.

In contrast to the World Bank, Gavi publicly provides the materials the Board considers, at least in its formal meetings, as well as the minutes from its committee meetings. While not the same as providing real-time online access such as WHO's Executive Board, it is a significant level of openness, particularly given that the level of shared documentation from Gavi goes farther than WHO's practices.[119] The Aid Transparency Index scored Gavi at 100 percent for its public sharing of financial information and organizational level data. It scores less well on the sharing of performance indicators, a shared, albeit varied, challenge across all of our case studies.[120] Gavi tracks its aggregate performance across vaccine coverage of new and underused vaccines, DPT3 coverage, equity in vaccine coverage within countries, change in price of vaccinating one child for its key vaccines, and resource mobilization for its work. It publishes updates to these indicators periodically. At the start of 2016, its most recent update was from April 2015.[121] It is not clear, at least from looking at what Gavi publishes, how much of a country's vaccine coverage rate could be attributed, in whole or part, to Gavi's funding. An inability for any interested person to consistently link Gavi funding to specific outcomes by country likely explains the relatively lower ratings Gavi receives for transparency around performance data.

Gavi seems to have recognized that the significant investment donors made in creating an institution focused on closing the vaccine gap indicated a high degree of trust that such a new, focused entity could deliver on that mission. Indeed, the study mentioned earlier on Gavi and trust focused on the role that a lack of trust in the late 1990s among vaccine-interested donors played in Gavi's inception. It also highlighted the role that the resulting trust in Gavi by donors played in securing Gavi's mandate and funds, particularly in its early years. Perhaps Gavi's efforts to shrink information asymmetries between its principals and agent, among principals, and between it and the public were all driven by recognition that trust is an asset to be preserved and one vital to its survival.

The Global Fund
The Global Fund's origins are inseparable from a narrative of trust lost among donors in existing structures to respond to HIV/AIDS and the

subsequent granting of trust by donors and civil society for an innovative and well-financed response to HIV/AIDS, as well as to tuberculosis and malaria.[122] From the Fund's beginning, it has published on its website all approved proposals, signed grant agreements, and grant-performance reports. The grant-performance reports are self-reported by grantees in line with the grant agreements' articulated key performance metrics, programmatically and financially. The Fund does not publish reports from Local Fund Agents (LFAs), often accounting firms; in 2015, PricewaterhouseCoopers, one of the world's largest accounting firms, served as the LFA in 85 of 144 countries with active Fund grants.[123] As the Global Fund does not have staff in-country, LFAs function, and have long been billed as, their "eyes and ears on the ground."[124] Local Fund Agents assess proposed Principal Recipients for new grants and for renewed funding, as well as work to verify grantee's self-reported progress reports for data quality and results. They are advisory to the Fund and do not have any decision-making or fiduciary responsibility, possibly explaining why the Fund does not publish their advice and recommendations. However, LFA reports are often referenced in the Fund's inspector general reports and elsewhere, meaning at least selectively that LFAs' work is visible to the public.[125]

Similar to Gavi, the Global Fund publishes all financial information not only by grant but also by country, disease area (though it does not break out health systems support), and year of funding, providing significant transparency into what it disburses to its grantees.[126] The Global Fund also publishes those proposals that were not successful in receiving grant funding, including the specific rationale for why the TRP recommended against providing Global Fund support. No other organization we study publishes so extensively on unsuccessful funding or programmatic applications.

Within global health institutions, only the Gates Foundation has a similar policy, albeit one narrowly focused on research. In 2014, the Gates Foundation announced it would begin publishing the results of research it funded in whole or part, even that which proved unsuccessful.[127] *Nature* called this move the "world's strongest policy on open access research."[128] While Gates's policy does not yet encompass unsuccessful grant applications, it is a move toward transparency from the largest nonbilateral and nonmultilateral funder of global health, and one of the major stakeholders and principals of both Gavi and the Global Fund.

Unique among our case studies, the Global Fund also makes publicly available all reports from its inspector general. The Board established the inspector general's office in 2005 and approved the policy of timely public disclosure of its findings and reports in 2007.[129] Putting this policy into practice is what led to the crisis of confidence around the Fund in 2011 as donors and the media reacted to an inspector general's report of identified and suspected fraud. The Global Fund's defenders were quick to point out that the Fund's unusual level of transparency enabled such public scrutiny of its practices and that low levels of fraud and misuse of funds were common—and arguably unavoidable—across multilateral institution working around the world.[130] Global Fund supporters also feared the Fund would pull back from its commitment to transparency and stop disclosures from the Inspector General's office or the boardroom. This did not happen.

The Global Fund, like Gavi, makes publicly available all nonexecutive session documentation considered by the Board and the minutes of Board and Board Committee meetings. It has done so since inception. This means that we know more about what WHO says (or does not say) in the Global Fund Board meetings than in WHO's own meetings on potential infectious disease emergencies.[131] Similar to Gavi, the Global Fund now provides support to its implementing country Board members to facilitate their ability to meet outside of Board meetings and to be able to afford to come to Board meetings, whether in Geneva or elsewhere. However, the support provided to the implementing country Board members by the Fund, both financial and otherwise, historically has been far less than what Gavi provided, making shrinking the informational asymmetry among principals at the Fund relatively more difficult. Gavi has long paid for developing-country Board members and alternates to attend the Board meetings as well as for their advisers to come to Geneva a month before meetings for briefings to help prepare their Board members in advance of Board meetings.[132] It was not until 2009 that the Global Fund Board approved financial support to facilitate implementing countries' participation at Board meetings and between Board meetings; the policy went into effect in 2010.[133] Implementing countries were not unaware that the absence of such support had historically impaired their ability to engage meaningfully with the Fund or at level equal to that of donor

TABLE 5.2 Transparency: Policies and Practices

	Financial Information	Governance Information	Contract/Grant Information	Language Availability	Transparency Policies
World Health Organization	WHO makes publicly available its forward-looking programmatic budgets as well as its retrospective audited financial statements, though largely at an aggregate level. For example, this includes budget projections broken down by categories of prioritized investments or by level of organization (country offices, headquarters, and regional offices).	Resolutions and supporting documents submitted to the World Health Assembly as well as to WHO's Executive Board are available online. Documents or evidence consulted in committees convened by the Director-General regarding the declaration of a Public Health Emergency of International Concern (PHEIC) are not publicly available.	No programmatic or projects database is available to provide visibility to funding flows and assessment of individual program efforts over time.	All official WHO documents are available in all six UN languages: Arabic, English, French, Mandarin, Russian, and Spanish. However, this is not true for program-specific technical reports and clinical guidelines which are often available only in English, or in English and French.	WHO is the only one of our four focal institutions that does not have a transparency nor open information policy as of September 2015. It is also the only one of these four that does not report to the International Aid Transparency Initiative (IATI) and does not participate in the Aid Transparency Index. However, transparency measures do exist in the form of livestreaming of Executive Board meetings, as one example.

(*Continued*)

TABLE 5.2 Continued

	Financial Information	Governance Information	Contract/Grant Information	Language Availability	Transparency Policies
World Bank	The World Bank's projects database includes information on projects the Bank has supported since 1947, including financial information. The Bank continually adds new historical data to the project database. For the Bank's HNP portfolio, raw data on grants, particularly relevant financial information, is also available.	Meeting agendas, resolutions, or minutes from meetings of the Secretariat, the Board of Directors, and the Executive Directors are not publicly available. The Bank shares nothing publicly that it considers "internal communications."	The World Bank launched Open Contracting in 2012 to facilitate more competitive bidding for World Bank contracts. Of the average 20–30,000 contracts that result yearly for World Bank–financed projects, about 7,000 are reviewed by World Bank staff and information about the winning contracts is made publicly available after contract signature. The World Bank's Contract Awards Database is updated weekly.	Varies by topic. All materials are available in English. Certain materials, depending on project or meeting location, are also available in Albanian, Arabic, Bulgarian, Cambodian, French, Hindi, Indonesian, Japanese, Macedonian, Mandarin, Mongolian, Polish, Portuguese, Romanian, Russian, Spanish, Thai, Turkish, Ukrainian, and Vietnamese.	The Bank introduced a formal access to information policy in 2010, which outlined what information the Bank would make publicly available. It does not publish decision-making criteria for contractor selection. The Bank was named "a bank others look up to" in terms of transparency by Transparency International in 2012.

| The Global Fund to Fight AIDS, Tuberculosis and Malaria | The Global Fund publishes all financial information by grant, country, disease area, and year of funding. | All nonexecutive session documentation considered by the Board and minutes of Board Committee meetings are made publicly available. | Since its beginning, the Global Fund has published all approved proposals, signed grant agreements, and grant performance reports on its website. The Global Fund regularly updates its "Funding Decisions" webpage, though noting that the information may be incomplete if there is a time lag between the approval of a grant and the signing of that grant. As of February 8, 2016, the grant information for the newest grant, approved on January 17, 2016, was available. Notably, the Global Fund also publishes unsuccessful proposals and the rationale behind the Board's ultimate funding decisions. | All Board documents, grant portfolio information, funding, and performance-level data are published only in English. Certain materials are also available in French, Russian, and Spanish. | The Global Fund's Board established the Inspector General's office in 2005 and approved the policy of timely public disclosure of its findings and reports in 2007. Overall, we know more about what the Global Fund decides and how it has made its decisions over time than the other three focal institutions. |

(Continued)

TABLE 5.2 Continued

	Financial Information	Governance Information	Contract/Grant Information	Language Availability	Transparency Policies
Gavi, The Vaccine Alliance	Gavi makes available all grant approvals, as well as commensurate financial and in-kind commitments and disbursements information, organized by country, year, and type of support.	All materials considered by Gavi's Board (at least in its formal meetings), as well as the minutes from its Committee meetings, are made publicly available.	Gavi publishes grant-specific and country-specific programmatic information alongside its Full Country Evaluations project. This project, running from 2013 to 2016, engages local research institutions in Bangladesh, Mozambique, Uganda and Zambia, in partnership with IHME and PATH to collect real-time data on country immunization programs. Findings are to be made available on the Gavi website throughout this period.	All materials are available in English and French.	Gavi introduced its first transparency policy in 2009, updating it in 2013.

countries.[134] It is important to note that neither WHO nor the World Bank provides any financial support to facilitate their developing-country Board members' participation at or between Board meetings.

Another complicating factor in the Global Fund's Board dynamic is the substantial involvement of the United States with the organization, including having two designated personnel at the US consulate in Geneva dedicated to maintaining the US relationship with the Global Fund. That level of engagement is far beyond any other donor or Board member with the Fund and likely enables the United States to possess an informational advantage among its fellow principals. Additionally, as of early 2016, the Global Fund publishes all Board documents only in English making meaningful engagement by non-English speakers with Board decisions and decision-making challenging. Certain Global Fund information is available in French, Spanish, and Russian. However, similar to a lack of accessibility beyond English into Board proceedings, grant portfolio information, funding, and performance-level data are also available only in English. These are not the reasons, however, that the Aid Transparency Index awards the Global Fund a "good" rating, one level down from what Gavi and the World Bank IDA received. Rather, a lack of subnational data and technical reasons drove its relatively lower rating. Overall, at least in English, we know more about what the Global Fund decides and how it has made its decisions over time, than Gavi, the World Bank, or WHO.

CONCLUSION

When organizations expand their stakeholder engagement and enhance their transparency, they are attempting to increase their own legitimacy and to build trust among donors and the public. This is not only a normative concern but also one tied to political and public authority as well as to funding. In data on developing-country perceptions on development partners, the Global Fund, Gavi, and the World Bank rate the highest across the development aid landscape, on usefulness of advice, agenda-setting influence, and helpfulness.[135] The Global Fund rates highest on frequency of communication, Gavi on usefulness of advice (the Global Fund ranks third here), and the World Bank first on agenda-setting influence; WHO does not rate in the top ten in any of those areas.[136] Perhaps this is a reflection on the greater funds that the Global Fund, Gavi, and the World Bank invest in countries in global health, or perhaps on the diversity of stakeholders that formally influence the policies and practices of all but WHO, and the confidence that developing countries can gain through more shared information from all but WHO.

What is clear, particularly in the aftermath of Ebola, is that the "older" institutions in global health—WHO and the World Bank—must increase both stakeholder engagement and transparency to regain their legitimacy and public trust; this is particularly true of WHO. We discuss their efforts to remain relevant in chapter 6.

6

Disruption and Reform

IN THIS CHAPTER WE draw together lessons from the previous chapters on the governance of global health. First, we discuss what possible consequences may emerge—or may already have emerged—from the arrival of the Global Fund, Gavi, and other more focused, vertical funds. Second, we assess whether these "new" models have lived up to the expectations of their founders, both as relates to their own achievements as well as to their ability to more readily reform than "older," more traditional state-based international organizations. Finally, we examine the impact of the "new" models on WHO and the World Bank and their efforts to reform in order to remain purposeful and relevant. Comparing the reform trajectories of the four institutions provides insight into whom each is accountable to and what, if any, are the consequences of failure.

THE "NEW" MODELS: POSSIBLE CONSEQUENCES
FOR MULTILATERALISM

In this book we have argued that cooperation in global health in the late twentieth and early twenty-first centuries has been realized in part through new vertical initiatives, and through increased multi-bi funding. Coming to the fore is an approach to cooperation, which is:

- Disease or issue-specific
- Governed by a small group of stakeholders
- Funded in a discretionary way (as opposed to long-term commitments).

We draw on Sridhar and Woods's work that highlights three important risks emerging from these three changes.[1] A first important concern is *normative*. The convergence of new disease or issue-specific initiatives like the Global Fund and Gavi creates enormous momentum behind treatments (or preventions) of specific diseases. But not all diseases, or causes of premature mortality, are included. Some international partnerships and campaigns are more successful than others—and what defines success is not often universally agreed upon. Critics allege that global health pursued through coalitions of the willing (either in vertical initiatives or in discretionary special funds in international organizations) imposes the priorities of powerful donor states and philanthropic organizations on less developed countries, whose populations have little recourse to demand accountability or to influence such organizations' priorities today or in the future. Put simply, the democratic deficit of global health governance could be viewed as increasing through the confluence of vertical initiatives and increased voluntary contributions to WHO and the World Bank.

A second possible consequence concerns *efficiency*.[2] The risk is that the new health funding may be creating mechanisms that encourage donors to favor short-term priorities, even important ones, over longer-term public health goals. The theoretical advantage of traditional multilateral organizations is that their greater representation and relative autonomy permit them to bring a clarity and discipline to difficult choices: the rationale for creating WHO was to ensure that nations would "compromise their short-term differences in order to attain the long-run advantages of regularized collaboration on health matters."[3] Multilateral forums such as UNAIDS have also been important in the area of HIV/AIDS treatment to bring evidence-based policies to the fore, rather than short-term politically popular policies in any one country or with any one constituency. An example of the advantage historically offered by traditional multilateral forums is the WHO Framework

Convention on Tobacco Control, which strengthens the hand of Health Ministries to fend off the agendas of those in their government who would prioritize commercial tobacco interests over public health concerns.[4]

A third consequence of these shifts in global health governance is that they possibly erode important public capacities in global health: in terms of knowledge and information derived from global monitoring today, and in possibly underinvesting in areas of expertise that may be needed in the future because they are not currently fashionable.[5] The erosion of capacity is particularly evident in outbreak prevention and response. When donors use discretionary funding to effectively conduct bilateral (or multi-bi) activities under a multilateral aegis, they implicitly benefit from the core multilateral funding and commensurate work of previous decades. They benefit from a wider, previously built technical expertise in agencies such as the World Bank or WHO.

Global monitoring may be a casualty of the new health funding if it diminishes the capacity of multilaterals effectively to monitor and disseminate information. Here, the relative autonomy or independence of global agencies is important.[6] As we discussed in chapter 3, one reason that states form international agencies is so they can pool or analyze information. Subsequently, this internationally gathered and analyzed information enables (at least in theory) more effective multilateral action. In health we sometimes see this sharing of information, for example around outbreaks and disease incidence, and collaboration in analysis of such data by qualified epidemiologists. The benefits of sharing and pooling information and expertise accrue to all countries including to governments which have built their own extensive public health expertise and information sources, such as the United States' Centers for Disease Control.

The impartiality of the international agency pooling information is vital for monitoring. Countries need to trust an international agency in order to give it information and to respect the integrity of the information it, in turn, provides its members and the broader public. The most recent International Health Regulations (IHR), enacted in 2007, are instructive here. The IHR require countries to report certain disease outbreaks and public health events to WHO. WHO member states adopted the IHR by consensus, reflecting a desire to balance their sovereignty with a shared commitment to prevent the international spread of disease. Building on WHO's competence in global disease surveillance, alert, and response, the IHR define the rights and obligations of countries to report public health events and establish a number of procedures that WHO must follow in its work to protect global public health security. The IHR also require countries to strengthen their existing capacities for public health surveillance and response to be able to meet their end of the bargain. In the IHR context, again, WHO draws on its technical expertise to work closely with countries and partners to provide technical guidance and support to mobilize the resources needed to implement the new rules in an effective and timely manner. Notably, the regulations do not include enforcement mechanisms for states that fail to comply. They rely instead on the potential consequences for countries of noncompliance—for example, a possible devastating epidemic—to provide a sufficient incentive. The Guinean government's delay in reporting suspected Ebola cases revealed the challenges in this approach.[7]

The importance of international collaboration on disease control was also highlighted in 2007 when Indonesia's health minister Siti Fadillah Supari drew attention to the fact that developing countries were supplying H5N1 virus samples to WHO Collaborating Centres for analysis and preparation for vaccine production, but that the resulting vaccines produced by commercial pharmaceutical companies in the developed world were unlikely to be available to developing countries such as Indonesia. Supari called this system "unfair."[8] Her point was that actions taken by developing countries for the public good were being exploited by pharmaceutical companies (outside Indonesia) for subsequent profit. Yet, if developing countries or any country were to withhold flu or any other virus samples from WHO Collaborating Centres, a threat would be posed to global health security as well as to the ongoing risk assessment for influenza, including as relates to already affected developing countries.

For these reasons—and recognizing the real tensions that Supari's critique exposed—the design of international institutions for collecting and sharing information and knowledge is vital to protecting public health today and in the future. Likewise, the expertise of international organizations and their capacities to compile, analyze, and monitor information are central. All of these could have been corroded by the shifts in global health governance over the past fifteen years.

On the more positive side, the new health funding has focused attention on how and where international organizations, such as the World Bank and WHO, might do better while also maintaining pressure on the Global Fund and Gavi to live up to their founders' expectations, including their nimbleness to reform when necessary. The tough competition for available resources and attention is forcing these institutions to reflect on how to reform in order to remain more appealing to the wider set of principals: governments, the Gates Foundation, the private sector (including pharmaceutical companies), NGOs, and even the public.

GAVI AND THE GLOBAL FUND: ACHIEVEMENTS, LIMITATIONS, AND REFORM

We consistently refer to the Global Fund and Gavi throughout as "new" institutions, because of their age relative to WHO and the World Bank. However, each has lived now, as of early 2016, for more than a dozen years. Yet the label of "new" still resonates because a core impetus of the creation of the Global Fund and Gavi was, in the words of Gavi CEO Seth Berkley, "to challenge conventional wisdom around AIDS and vaccines in particular as well as to change the conventional way of doing business in global health."[9] Indeed, supporters of the Global Fund and Gavi alike point to this broader disruption as being part of their core missions. Part of the disruption was expected to be in the monies galvanized toward their missions, and part in how they conducted business. Arguably nothing captured this latter motivation more succinctly than the Fund's inaugural Executive Director Richard Feachem's oft-repeated mantra: "Raise it, Spend it, Prove it" and his oft-added addendum, "for those who need it most."[10] And while these organizations emerged from a desire to reform specific areas of global health as well as the global health ecosystem, each has also confronted moments of significant reform in their relatively short lives. We examine, briefly, the records and reforms of each and then, in the conclusion, query whether Gavi and the Global Fund are currently structured to meet a post-MDG world and whether more reforms are, or should be, on the horizon.

Gavi, the Vaccine Alliance

While Gavi's founders hoped it would positively disrupt and reshape the vaccine paradigm—and the broader aid landscape—it has experienced substantially less internal disruption and reform than the Fund (as will be subsequently discussed).[11] This is not to say Gavi did not carry a heavy mantle of expectations. It did. The aspirations for Gavi centered on the meaningful inclusion of the private sector at all levels of its work, the reshaping of the vaccine market from a high-price, low-volume dynamic to a high-volume, low-price dynamic, and the raising of substantial funds to help incentivize and capitalize on that shift.[12] Together, these new approaches, alongside an upsurge of resources, were intended to help narrow the vaccine gap between children who lived in wealthier countries and children who lived in low- and middle-income countries. Unlike the Global Fund, at inception Gavi did not include performance-based funding or an independent review of grant applications. In its early years, Gavi was found to be "hesitant" in requiring recipient countries to consistently measure and track grant performance.[13] In the past few years, likely in response at least in part to such critiques, Gavi has both adopted performance-based funding and introduced guidelines around performance tracking.[14] As more data on each becomes available, it will provide rich material for scholars to compare Gavi's decisions pre and post those changes, as well as Gavi's experiences relative to those of the Global Fund.

While the Global Fund has only recently adopted a more open and collaborative approach to pharmaceutical companies and health commodities companies more broadly, such collaboration and partnership have been core to Gavi from inception. A few factors influenced this approach, seen as radical at the end of the twentieth century when the private sector was largely viewed more as an antagonist than a partner. Likely the most important factor explaining this dynamic was the recent history of the Children's Vaccine Initiative (CVI). Launched in 1990, the CVI brought together WHO (lead agency), UNDP, UNICEF, the World Bank, and the Rockefeller Foundation to accelerate vaccine development and increase the effectiveness and efficiency of WHO and UNICEF's vaccine delivery efforts. There was significant hope that this multiagency effort with a strong private foundation partner would catalyze vaccine innovation from development to delivery and increase vaccine coverage around the world.[15] Ten years later, however, vaccine rates had not significantly changed and some had even declined; as one example, DPT3 (the three-dose combined diphtheria, pertussis, tetanus) vaccine coverage rates dropped slightly from 1990 to 2000.[16] Additionally, the pharmaceutical industry agreed to partner with CVI, to deliver a temperature-stable polio vaccine. Frustration mounted when the CVI later rescinded its engagement and did not use the solutions it had originally requested.[17] It was not unreasonable that Gavi's founders hoped it could improve on CVI's experience.

A second factor precipitating Gavi's embrace of the private sector was the Gates Foundation's (and Bill Gates's) commitment to new vaccine research and development. The Foundation recognized that working with the branded and generic pharmaceutical companies, rather than being at loggerheads with them, would likely yield results more quickly.[18] As seen in chapters 3 and 5, it is certainly true that private pharmaceutical companies have long been engaged in Gavi's governance as well as its strategic planning. Given that, Gavi's success as judged against meaningful inclusion of the private sector is clear.

In terms of its market-shaping work, Gavi's success in this area has accelerated over time as it has continued to attract more resources to increase its negotiating leverage for preexisting vaccines—individual vaccines and in bundles—as well as to incentivize the development of new vaccines. As one example, the total cost to immunize a child, inclusive of vaccine purchase price and delivery, with the pentavalent (Hib, pertussis, tetanus, hepatitis B, diphtheria), pneumococcal, and rotavirus vaccines dropped from $35 in 2010 to $22 in 2013.[19] Pneumococcal vaccine third-dose coverage increased to 28 percent in 2014, significantly below the 40 percent target for 2015 but well above the 1 percent levels in 2010. The UN Interagency Working Group on Child Mortality (UN-IGME) estimates that across Gavi-supported countries, child mortality fell from 77 deaths per 1,000 live births in 2010 to 69 deaths per 1,000 live births in 2013, with vaccines, including the pentavalent, pneumococcal, and rotavirus ones, cited as playing an important role in that more than 10 percent drop in child mortality in less than five years.[20] While Gavi is generally recognized as being a driving force behind rising vaccine rates around the world, including the impact recognized by the UN-IGME, it is not clear what portion of that success Gavi specifically could claim, and for what specific reasons (in addition to or across its infusion of funds into vaccine purchases and distribution). In late 2015, Dagfinn Høybråten, Chair of the Gavi Board, attributed Gavi's success to its work with the public and private sector, including in its governance.[21]

In chapter 4, we saw that Gavi's goals of attracting a diverse funding base met with greater success than did the Global Fund's. It can claim a greater proportion of funds from nonstate actors, albeit the majority of such funds originates from the Gates Foundation as a single donor, with additional meaningful support from nontraditional donor governments through its International Financing Facility for Immunization (IFFIm) bond program. There is no PEPFAR analog in vaccines and immunizations, so it is also easier to claim, though difficult to prove, that Gavi deserves credit for the upsurge of resources dedicated to vaccines. In 2014, Gavi disbursed $1.1 billion to procure new and underused vaccines.[22] In 2000, UNICEF's entire budget was $1.1 billion, and it spent less than $150 million on purchasing vaccines and immunization equipment.[23] Clearly, Gavi played a significant role in the swell of vaccine-targeted funding in the twenty-first century's first fifteen years.

One significant difference between Gavi and the Global Fund is that Gavi began not as one entity, but as two. In Gavi's first incarnation, the Gavi Alliance oversaw vaccine policy development and implementation, with a Secretariat based in Geneva and housed at the UNICEF office, with staff seconded by UNICEF.[24] Its Board resembled Gavi's Board today, including permanent members UNICEF, WHO, the World Bank, and the Gates Foundation, plus rotating seats among an equal number of donor and developing country governments, industrialized and developing country vaccine companies, along with representatives from civil society and from a technical or research institution. Generally, this was the entity referred to as Gavi. However, the Gavi Alliance initially had no legal status and was frequently referred to as a "coordinating" mechanism or "informal" institution. The World Bank referred to it as "an informal alliance of partners with a shared mission."[25]

The Vaccine Fund was constituted as a purely financial entity to raise and steward funds in support of the work of the Gavi Alliance in Gavi-eligible countries. Its Board was initially comprised of global luminaries and experts in economics and finance, with the former South African president Nelson Mandela serving as Chair with Board members such as the former US Treasury Secretary Larry Summers and the Nobel Prize–winning economist Amartya Sen.[26] The initial executive leadership of each also differed significantly. Tore Godal, the first head of the Gavi Alliance, came from WHO, while Jacques-François Martin, the inaugural head of the Vaccine Fund, came from a pharmaceutical background.

When the Boards of the Gavi Alliance and the Vaccine Fund decided to merge in 2007, they mutually agreed to reconstitute into a Swiss foundation, in the model of the Global Fund, under the banner of the Gavi Alliance, with the Vaccine Fund remaining to focus solely on raising funds within the United States to support Gavi's work.[27] The administrative functions that UNICEF had performed were moved to an independent Gavi Secretariat.[28] The reasons cited publicly for the merger aligned closely to those discussed more privately: greater efficiency in fund-raising and operations, more coherent brand awareness, and strengthening of the partnership between the public and private constituents engaged in Gavi's work, including among the financial and pharmaceutical sectors as well as developing and donor countries.[29] It was viewed as a relatively easy decision, from a Board and staff perspective.[30] Julian Lob-Levyt, then Gavi Alliance's Executive Director, framed the merger at the end of 2007 as a "decision that draws on our ability to grow through change."[31] One example of this was the expansion of the presence of independent Board members. It is challenging to envision a similar statement emerging from the Director-General of WHO or the president of the World Bank, or their institutions making similar decisions. Indeed, it is possible that one of the reasons the Global Fund and Gavi have both remained relevant and significant players in global health is that their core principals have continued to shape their priorities and their structures, rewarding them with funding and mandate—and legitimacy—in return. In the creation of these "newer" institutions, the United States, the Gates Foundation, and others wanted alternatives to WHO and the World Bank. In the continued evolution of the Global Fund and Gavi, it is clear they still do.

The Global Fund

In addition to making a significant impact on the number of people infected and vulnerable to HIV/AIDS, TB, and malaria, the Global Fund's founders harbored many other hopes for its ultimate performance. These included catalyzing more funding from more diverse sources for its three constituent diseases; making funding decisions in an identifiable evidenced-based way (known as performance-based funding or PBF); and giving developing countries "ownership" of the Fund through providing a vote and voice on the Fund Board equal to that of donors and, of equal importance, "ownership" of the grant process from conception to implementation (reflected in the use of the term "implementing" country instead of "recipient" country by the Global Fund).[32]

According to multiple independent studies ranging from the Institute of Medicine's audits of PEPFAR to the World Bank Independent Evaluation Group's examinations of the Global Fund to scholarly work focused on a subset of Global Fund grants, the Global Fund monies have made a significant impact in the fight against the Fund's three diseases.[33] It is fair to say that there is no real dispute of the Global Fund's impact claims from either the few scholars that have examined groups of Fund-financed grants or from the more numerous partners of the Global Fund that have done the same. If we then accept the Global Fund's assertions that in addition to statistics cited at the beginning of the book, there are one-third fewer deaths from HIV/AIDS, TB, and malaria in the countries where the Global Fund has financed grants than would have been true absent the Fund's financing, then the central questions shift. We turn, once again, to whether the Fund raised as much money as possible to have as much possible impact and whether that money was allocated to its best use, as determined by previous performance by implementers and engagement by the countries and constituents most affected.

The Fund's creation helped focus funding for HIV/AIDS, TB, and malaria, but whether those resources still would have flowed to those diseases or broader health concerns remains an open question, particularly given the advent of the United States' PEPFAR program in 2003 and the surge of interest in HIV/AIDS by the Gates Foundation. As discussed in chapter 4, almost one-third of the Fund's funding in a given year comes from the United States; the proportion from 2000 to 2013 is similar (just under 31 percent). The Gates Foundation accounts for two-thirds of nonstate funding the Global Fund received from 2000 to 2013;[34] the Gates Foundation first meaningfully gave to AIDS research in 1999 and to HIV/AIDS treatment programs in 2000. It is hard to determine whether the Fund precipitated larger donations from the United States and the Gates Foundation or was an almost accidental beneficiary of the decisions of each to move more aggressively into HIV/AIDS. Government donations comprise more than 94 percent of the monies the Global Fund received in its first thirteen years and, adding in the Gates Foundation's contributions, account for more than 98 percent of the total. While securing close to $30 billion in cash contributions is extraordinary for any institution, certainly a relatively new one, the Global Fund did not meaningfully diversify its funding base more than its predecessors did, particularly given the Gates Foundation's current importance to WHO's budget. That observation does not detract from the millions raised through (RED), but rather highlights once again that while the Fund may have raised more money than would have been directed to its diseases in its absence, its funding base more closely resembles a traditional institution.

The Global Fund did not invent performance-based funding, but it was the first significant international institution to make a constitutional commitment to it.[35] Performance-based funding is when institutions make future funding decisions based in part or entirely on the applicant's previous performance. During its first decade, the Fund issued calls for proposals from applicant country-coordinating mechanisms (CCMs) through what was known as a "Rounds-based" approach, occurring approximately once a year. The independent Technical Review Panel (TRP) would then review applications on technical merit and make funding recommendations to the Board, which the Board would then accept, amend, or reject. As mentioned briefly in chapter 3, the TRP is composed of experts across the diseases, across interventions, and across geographies, and while it answers to the Board, it appoints its own members and so can fairly be considered relatively free of political influence, at least from the Board.

From what data exists from the Fund's first decade (when it made funding decisions in a Rounds-based funding approach), the Board made nonpolitical decisions for initial funding, as seen in the perfect approval rate of its TRP's funding recommendations.[36] It is harder to know if decisions to continue funding particular CCMs were made in a similar depoliticized and even performance-based mind-set. There are examples of the Board pushing back on suggestions to discontinue funding of grants in the first decade, often citing reasons of force majeure for poor grant performance, such as a resurgence of violence.[37] Insufficient data exists in the public domain to evaluate whether grant performance prevailed as the sole, main, or only one criterion of many when the Board made decisions to continue funding grants. In other words, whether the Fund lived up to its performance-based funding ethos in its first decade remains uncertain; the picture on initial funding is much clearer. At the end of 2013, the Fund introduced a New Funding Model, which we describe in detail later in this chapter. While it remains too soon to determine with confidence whether performance is the dominant factor in recent Fund financing decision-making, performance-based funding remains a focus, at least in theory, for the Fund and its Board.

A big question also surrounds whether the Fund's methodology of tracking performance was sufficient to inform funding decisions. A persistent criticism of the Fund throughout its first decade, including in the independent Five-Year Evaluation it commissioned[38] and in AusAid's March 2012 assessment,[39] as only two examples, was that it relied more on process measurements (e.g., frequency of on-time Principal Recipient reporting) and inputs or outputs (e.g., number of bed nets procured or distributed) rather than outcomes or impact (e.g., number of malaria cases averted or related number of additional school days attended).[40] The Fund, as mentioned previously, has now shifted in how it defines and tracks performance, including using lives saved through the interventions it funds as an important metric. Yet, whether these new approaches are already impacting funding decisions or will lead to better funding decisions remain open questions. As more data emerges about the Board's decisions related to initial and ongoing funding under the New Funding Model, a clearer picture of the Fund's commitment (or lack thereof) to performance-based funding will emerge.

Perhaps the heaviest expectation at the Fund's inception was that it would be a different type of international organization from the World Bank or even UNAIDS. The equal balance between donors and implementers on the Fund's Board was intended to give equal voice and influence to implementers, a first for formalized international cooperation, and in line with donor rhetoric on country ownership. If meaningful enfranchisement of the vaccine industry and related constituents in its governance was most important to Gavi, this would have been an animating force for the Fund. Equal votes, however, did not mean equal influence or participation for implementers and donors.

Country ownership was built into the Fund through the creation of a Secretariat rooted firmly in Geneva without a country presence, which also lessened concerns about the Fund engaging in supply-driven technical assistance. Previous research from one of us (Clinton), "The Global Fund: An Experiment in Global Governance" (2014) reveals that the Secretariat's absence in-country and in the provision of technical assistance created space for donors to fill the roles that Secretariats in other organizations traditionally do. Still, donor engagement through technical assistance, actively encouraged by the Secretariat, was only one channel of influence for donors. Conceivably a stronger channel was their presence on grant-country coordinating mechanisms (CCMs), which were created to write Global Fund grants and then oversee their implementation. Close investigation reveals a heavy donor presence on CCMs. As of 2012, more than 60 percent of active CCMs included at least one Global Fund donor.[41] The United States had a presence on more than 50 percent of active CCMs. Arguably, donors circumvented the Secretariat, and even the Board, over funding rounds, across diseases and around the world.

When the Global Fund initiated its reform program in late 2011/early 2012, questions persisted as to whether the Fund would survive the crisis of confidence that precipitated the reforms. Yet, it was not core questions of financing, performance-based funding, or developing country enfranchisement that precipitated the crisis of confidence or identity. Rather, the spotlight was on fraud and whether those concerns might be indicative of larger challenges at the Fund. Allegations of corruption, cronyism, and inefficiency were reminiscent of many past critiques, well founded or not, of WHO and UNAIDS, the Global Fund's direct predecessors.[42] Many of those same critiques were used as justifications, albeit quietly, for the Fund's creation, making their resurfacing around the Fund particularly troubling.

Although European bilateral donors and the European Commission were among the Fund's largest financial contributors in its first decade, they were also among its greatest skeptics early on. Similarly, they were among the Fund's harshest critics when significant questions about the misuse of funds identified by the Fund's own Inspector General were disclosed to its Board and other major stakeholders in late 2010 and broke publicly across the world in late January 2011.[43] The events precipitated the Board calling for an independent review. The *Economist's* headline a few weeks later summed up questions being asked in newspapers, in blogs, and on news channels from London to Windhoek, from Dublin to Delhi: "Can the Global Fund to Fight Aids, Tuberculosis and Malaria Restore its Reputation as the Best and Cleanest in the Aid Business?"[44]

Lost in the media frenzy was that the findings of fraud were known only because of the Fund's commitment to transparency as mentioned earlier (see chap. 5). In contrast, in most other multilateral and bilateral organizations, fraud often goes unnoticed or unreported. Traditional supporters pointed out the Fund was being punished for its transparency, and that the fraud itself, while troubling, occurred in a relatively small number of Fund grants. Despite these arguments, the damage was done.[45]

The Fund responded to the crisis by releasing "Results with Integrity: The Global Fund's Response to Fraud" in April 2011 (see fig. 6.1), which included details of the identified fraud. The report also disclosed the actions the Fund had already taken in response, from seeking restitution to supporting criminal prosecution efforts in certain countries, including against organizations and individuals who had served as Principal Recipients or on CCMs.[46] By the end of 2011, all donors who had frozen donations to the Fund following the fraud disclosures had reinstituted their pledges, at least in part. Throughout this time, the United States, the Fund's largest donor, repeatedly and forcefully supported the Fund.[47]

By mid-2012, Gabriel Jaramillo, the Fund's new General Manager, had deployed, for the first time, a majority of Secretariat resources—

COUNTRY	FRAUD (US$)	UNSUPPORTED (US$)	INELIGIBLE (US$)	UNACCOUNTED INCOME/DRUGS	OTHER (US$)	TOTAL (US$)
CAMBODIA	–	222,706	–	1,362,466	–	1,585,172
CAMEROON	33,455	2,199,530	3,370,322	–	–	5,603,307
CONGO (DEMOCRATIC REPUBLIC)	–	1,110,107	933,586	–	–	2,043,693
DJIBOUTI	145,893	4,262,288	857,827	–	–	5,266,008
HAITI	–	519,326	1,253,869	704,730	–	2,477,925
MALI	4,074,444	1,034,935	–	–	122,106	5,231,485
MAURITANIA	6,755,000	–	–	–	–	6,755,000
PHILIPPINES	–	–	2,021,280	–	–	2,021,280
RWANDA	–	–	–	–	–	–
TANZANIA	–	–	–	819,000	–	819,000
UGANDA	–	–	–	–	1,600,000	1,600,000
ZAMBIA	13,000	5,808,446	4,998,389	–	–	10,819,835
TOTAL (US$)	11,021,792	15,157,338	13,435,273	2,886,196	1,722,106	44,222,705

FIGURE 6.1 Identified fraud in Global Fund grants, as of April 2011. Global Fund, "Results with Integrity: The Global Fund's Response to Fraud," 2011, 5.

people and money—to supporting "impeccable grant management," with a high percentage oriented toward high-impact interventions in "high-impact" countries. Each grant across the entire portfolio received for the first time a dedicated point person at the Secretariat. Within three months of Jaramillo's arrival, 75 percent of the Secretariat staff was focused on grant management; previously, it had never exceeded 50 percent.[48] This shift brought the Fund closer to the 70–80 percent ranges common at other multilateral financing institutions.[49]

Still, for some early supporters of the Fund these changes were the death knell to the hoped-for newness of the Fund and broader systematic disruption its innovations would spearhead. Indeed, the Global Fund's Board's decision to appoint Jaramillo, a former finance executive who had served on the independent High-Level Panel, drew dramatic reactions across the public health landscape, with some heralding the arrival of a banker as "good for the Global Fund" and others warning that his appointment revealed a "crisis" in global health, signaling complacency from donors to the threat of AIDS and a focus on efficiency over impact.[50] In his first interview as General Manager, Jaramillo told the *Wall Street Journal* rather dispassionately: "There is nothing broken [at the Fund] that can't be fixed, but there's a lot of fixing to do."[51]

The changes at the Global Fund over the past few years have been either substantial or minor, depending on your perspective. In our view, the changes, while significant, have been understandable evolutions of the Fund's long commitment to country-ownership, metrics-driven funding decisions and to remaining a financial, grant-making entity, not a programmatic one. Recent key changes at the Fund include the reorientation of Fund staff toward grant management and empowering the Executive Director to negotiate agreements with potential partners (not grantees) to advance the Fund's work. Additionally, the Fund put in place more stringent requirements for CCMs, Principal Recipients, and, for the first time subrecipients (effectively the subcontractors that PRs rely on to deliver the grant's work). It also largely standardized evaluation approaches and reporting across grants,[52] something that would have been inconceivable in the Fund's early years given a belief that country-ownership was incompatible with any standardization. Yet, such standardizations could be viewed as increasing country-ownership. For example, by defining the remit of CCMs more precisely, it may well limit, or at least constrain, the ways in which donors can engage on the ground through CCMs and through technical assistance.

Perhaps most significant is that the New Funding Model provides for a continuous dialogue with a CCM, rather than the episodic one that occurred during a grant application and negotiation during the Fund's first decade. Notably, now the Fund, not applicants, takes the first step in projecting the total resources available to an applicant over a standardized three-year horizon. The previous two-phase funding model was supposed to be a linchpin for performance-based funding, but there is little evidence if that occurred in practice. What is clear is that during the Rounds-based funding approach, the TRP did not consider past grant performance in making funding recommendations to the Board with each new round. Currently, under the New Funding Model, the TRP takes into account grantees' past performance on delivering Global Fund grants in assessing an applicant's technical robustness and feasibility. Based on its assessments, the TRP then makes funding recommendations, the classic definition of performance-based funding (provided the recommendations are ultimately accepted). The Secretariat is also significantly more engaged in the grant process than was true historically. The TRP makes its recommendations to the Secretariat, which then negotiates grant agreements, pending Board approval. The Board then approves or declines grant agreements.

Nonetheless, for all those changes, the fundamentals remain the same, at least when we look at the Fund's principals. The individuals sitting on the Board have changed over time, but the constituencies remain the same and many of the Board members remain constant, such as the United States, the Gates Foundation, and China. The only replenishment the Fund has convened (as of early 2016) since the reforms were first introduced in late 2013, yielded a similar group of major supporters as had been seen in previous replenishments.[53] The High-Level Panel convened after the findings of fraud and ensuing furor noted that various implementing country health and finance ministers saw the Fund as no different from other international institutions.[54] It is likely that the reforms introduced did not change the dynamic of a strong donor presence. Donors remain on many CCMs and continue to provide direct technical assistance to grantees. In addition, the main donors to WHO and other multilaterals largely continue to be the main donors to the Fund's coffers. The Global Fund's experience bears out some of the concerns catalogued earlier in this chapter: it likely enabled strong principals to retain even greater control than would have been possible in a traditional multilateral. Over time, the strong principals likely evolved an asymmetrical informational advantage over the Secretariat, through their roles on CCMs as well as through their other global health programs in implementing countries; the latter would be as true for the Gates Foundation as any bilateral donor. Arguably, this broad-based perspective across implementing countries also increased strong principals' informational advantage over their fellow developing-country Board members as well. The governance of the Fund made reforming the Secretariat more straightforward than with the "older" institutions given the influence that strong principals (United States, Gates Foundation, and others) could exert across the organization at all levels.

THE REFORM AND RELEVANCE OF WHO

One of the side effects of the move of resources and political will toward public-private partnerships—and their clear claims of "credit"—has been for the "old" agencies to reflect on how they can remain relevant and adapt to the changing political environment. However, it is not an easy task for these institutions to change the way they do business. We now reflect on some of the key challenges for WHO and ways in which the agency and its principals (member states) are attempting to address them.[55]

Include nonstate actors in a meaningful way

As a UN agency, WHO is composed solely of member states, which govern through the World Health Assembly and its Executive Board. This governing structure affords WHO legitimacy and influence, standing alone among large global-health focused international organizations as the voice of the community of nations in global health. Yet, as discussed in chapter 5, this state-centric focus often sidelines valuable stakeholders—public, private, and philanthropic.

Because nonstate actors have not been given a voice in WHO, they have redirected their energies elsewhere. This process has been gradually "hollowing out" WHO, as resources and influence move to partnerships such as the Global Fund and Gavi where they have more input. Nonstate actors play no formal role in WHO governing structures (see chap. 5). The Assembly and Board do not fully recognize stakeholders beyond states. This contrasts with UNAIDS, which for twenty years has included civil society on its governing board, although with non-voting status. More recent partnerships, like the Global Fund and Gavi, seat civil society, businesses, and private foundations as voting Board members. Nonstate actors have gained prominence in these new models. In December 2015, the Gavi Board reconstituted its Executive Committee to include a civil society organization for the first time, along with donor countries, developing countries, the Gates Foundation, independent Board members, and two from UNICEF, WHO, or the World Bank.[56]

Currently, at WHO, there is no single platform for dialogue among international organizations, states, partnerships, foundations, businesses, and civil society. Recognizing this, the Director-General proposed in 2011 a World Health Forum: multi-stakeholder meetings under WHO auspices to increase effectiveness, coherence, and accountability, and reporting to formal governing structures.[57] Member states, however, rejected the Forum, while some civil society groups feared it would advance corporate interests over their own. These fears were largely based on the documented efforts by the tobacco industry to influence WHO policy and recommendations.[58] In response, the Director-General more recently proposed stakeholder forums targeted to key policies, including separate consultations with different constituencies, and web-based and in-person meetings.[59] Little progress so far, at least as of the end of 2015, on this front means that it is unclear whether real change will materialize.

To be effective, these forums must visibly influence WHO's agenda, priorities, and governing structures. For example, Larry Gostin has proposed that the agency create a meaningful platform for developing an innovative "Framework for Global Health," adopted by the Board and Assembly, monitored by civil society, and with genuine accountability mechanisms.[60] A group of scholars and diplomats has proposed a Committee C of the World Health Assembly made up of major stakeholders, such as international organizations, foundations, multinational health initiatives, and civil society.[61] The objectives are to increase transparency, coordination, and engagement across stakeholders with WHO. The two extant World Health Assembly committees are composed solely of states, and their business is concerned mostly with governance and financing of the agency. Yet, the Assembly's mandate extends beyond WHO in any one incarnation, granting WHO authority to "direct and coordinate" global health activities, while also collaborating with specialized agencies, governments, professional groups, and other actors (WHO Constitution, art. 2). The constitution grants the Assembly power to establish additional committees and to invite nonvoting representatives (art. 18). A Committee C would debate health initiatives, give stakeholders a venue to present their activities and plans, and discuss harmonization of activities. This proposal has not moved forward and currently appears unlikely to gain traction.

In addition, as touched on in chapter 5, WHO makes it very difficult for NGOs to gain "official relations" status, which is a prerequisite for nonvoting participation in WHO meetings. NGOs with this status may attend Executive Board and Assembly sessions and make prepared (but not extemporaneous) statements. With limited exceptions, to enter into official relations, an NGO (1) must be international, representing "a substantial proportion of the persons globally organized" in the field; (2) must have a constitution, governing body, and administrative structure, with a voting membership; and (3) must have major activities relevant to WHO's "health-for-all" strategy. Even then, most

NGOs must have two years of informal relations with WHO prior to applying for admission into official relations.[62] This burdensome process often excludes NGOs that are domestic, poorly funded, small, or have a specific mission—even if they are influential and even if they work alongside WHO in-country, including on WHO programs as well as through Gavi or Global Fund grants. Given how onerous the application process is, it is not surprising then that most NGOs currently in official relations are donor country-based.[63]

The Executive Board and Assembly could lower the bar to NGO participation while still ensuring the NGOs that are granted official relations status are meaningfully engaged in work alongside WHO or in service to the shared mission of health for all.[64] They could offer financial support to developing country NGOs to facilitate participation; this could be similar to the financial support that the Global Fund and Gavi provide to developing country delegations to ensure they can substantially participate in their respective Board meetings by facilitating intraboard meeting conversations (similar to what donors traditionally have done).[65] They could also expand opportunities for civil society input, such as by allowing extemporaneous statements, facilitating NGO side sessions at the Assembly annual meeting, and conducting open hearings on priorities and programs. In 2004, the Assembly postponed for "further study" a proposal to simplify the process for nonstate participation.[66] The proposal is still pending (as of early 2016) with little prospect of success. It is worth noting that the absence of NGO voices has led to poorer decision-making. While we mentioned this example earlier, we believe it bears repeating: If WHO had given greater heed to MSF's consistent and unequivocal calls for a strong response to Ebola, the outbreak might have been stopped before it spun out of control.[67] Failing to provide an effective participatory forum for those working on the ground impoverishes global dialogue and risks decisions being made on the basis of an incomplete picture—or not at all.

The main resistance to including nonstate actors can be traced to concerns over conflict of interest, as perceptions of probity underpin the confidence and legitimacy others bestow on the agency. We agree that WHO must be careful to make sure that cooperating entities, from any sector, are genuinely devoted to advancing public health, without pecuniary or other competing interests or with such interests clearly disclosed and ring-fenced.[68] Although true for all groups, it is especially pertinent when engaging the private sector, such as the food, alcoholic beverage, pharmaceutical, and biotechnology industries (WHO already has strict rules to exclude tobacco companies or those funded by them). This is in part because WHO has a duty to set and oversee health and safety standards for businesses. Several types of conflict of interest are possible. First, for example, it would be inappropriate for the alcoholic beverage or marketing industries to fund the development of alcohol-related guidelines. Second, voluntary contributors to WHO generally finance areas of their own interest, and companies, NGOs or individuals may profit or increase their visibility by influencing WHO decision-making or policy positions, if only by what they are providing funds for and then what is left unfunded. Third, private-sector companies and NGOs alike that provide donations to WHO may at some point look to provide services to it, whether commercial or sub-contracting in nature; arguably the latter is already happening with WHO and certain NGO partners. The Executive Board could overcome these challenges by designing a clear, transparent process for managing potential conflicts, including through stringent disclosure, monitoring, and enforcement.

Private foundations also exercise considerable influence shaping institutions' agenda. Wealthy philanthropists such as Bill Gates and Michael Bloomberg donate vast resources to global health, and it is both through their donations as well as the attention they command that they have demonstrated an ability to shape the world health agenda, elevating causes as diverse as vaccines (Gates) and traffic-related injuries (Bloomberg). Indeed, Gavi's creation followed an initial $750 million grant from Gates. Given the paucity of resources to vaccines when Gates made its foundational grant to Gavi, and the resources that Gavi commands today, it is clear that the Gates Foundation monies were transformative. Given this influence, questions of intent relating to private foundations arise.[69] For example, the Gates Foundation and other undisclosed sources helped fund the WHO blueprint for reform, raising the question of whether there is sufficient separation between the interests of WHO and wealthy donors, even if broad agreement exist around donor-financed objectives, like WHO reform.[70] This only further supports the contention that future WHO conflicts of interest policies and practices must be both robust and inclusive of potential private sector, NGO, private foundation, and other partners for the institution.

Improve transparency, performance, and accountability

As an intergovernmental agency, WHO must be open to scrutiny, with its evidence and reasons for policies as well as its dealings with outside parties plainly disclosed. Once again, we are not the first to point this out.[71] Disclosure is a necessary but insufficient condition of sound governance, as WHO must also competently manage potential conflicts of interest, both financial and nonpecuniary. Most importantly, good governance requires tangible results with clear targets and plans for their achievement. The Director-General's proposal for a "results-chain"— standard indicators to measure outputs and impact—is an important step. WHO's proposed 2016–17 budget included numerical indicators for each program area and deliverables at country, regional, and headquarter levels.[72]

In the aftermath of the Influenza A (H1N1) pandemic in 2009, an independent IHR review committee suggested two years later that WHO establish a $100 million reserve fund for public health emergencies, as well as an emergency workforce that could be deployed quickly in case of an epidemic.[73] Neither was implemented. Commissioning reports is only the first step to accountability, and an insufficient one if it does not lead to meaningful reform. WHO must also follow through on recommendations and adjust in response to past failings. Had WHO followed the recommendations of the H1N1 Review Committee, the response to the Ebola epidemic would likely have been quicker, less costly, and more effective—and most importantly, more lives would have been saved. Following the January 2015 Executive Board resolution, WHO now seems committed to implementing versions of both of these recommendations. We know we are not the only ones who will be watching closely what happens on this front in 2016 and beyond.

Stakeholders demand clarity on how their resources will achieve improved health outcomes. Yet, an independent evaluation graded WHO as "weak" on key parameters, such as cost-consciousness, financial management, public disclosure, and achievement of development objectives.[74] The 2011 reform agenda promised to establish independent evaluations of WHO's work.[75] This would then be in line with the independent evaluations the Global Fund has periodically both commissioned and participated in, as well as the increasing openness of Gavi and even the World Bank, at least around the grants and loans each finances.

Any WHO reform agenda also must stress human capital, which is at the heart of WHO's strength and credibility. WHO, like most UN agencies, has struggled in its ability to recruit top talent given its bureaucratic and long hiring process, to monitor the performance of staff through a robust annual appraisal process, and to fire staff that are underperforming. This is true at all levels of WHO, from global to regional and country offices, from the Director-General to entry-level positions.[76] The World Health Assembly and Executive Board must also address this core challenge to ensure that WHO Secretariat can deliver on its responsibilities.

Exercise closer oversight of regions

WHO's decentralized, regional structure poses a significant challenge to demonstrate results and deliver on priorities. This is not a new challenge for WHO. As described in chapter 3, the six WHO regional offices are uniquely independent within the UN system, with full power over regional personnel, including appointment of country representatives. Regional committees meet annually to formulate policies, review budgets, and review activities. The Health Assembly and Executive Board formally approve decisions, but in practice they do not provide tight policy and budgetary control.

WHO headquarters is currently discussing how it can exercise more oversight and control over regional personnel and decision-making.[77] The agency could start by fully disclosing the funds held within each regional office and how regions invest those funds to meet health objectives, with monitoring and benchmarks of success also shared. Even if decentralized decision-making remains the norm, WHO could apply the same yardstick across regions to assess efficiency and effectiveness. In addition, the performance of regional and country representatives, who are often political appointees with little knowledge of public

health, too often results in the prioritization of local economic and political interests over public health needs as well as general incompe-
tence. In January 2015, the WHO Secretariat articulated a series of new
measures that aim to tackle these two problems. A central one requires
that WHO representatives be public health experts who must pass examinations and undergo training in outbreak recognition and management, the provisions of the IHR, and a number of other key WHO
priorities.[78]

Employ adequate and predictable financing of core functions

By its own admission, WHO is "over-extended and overcommitted,"
with insufficient resources to meet expanding needs, and resources not
fully within its control.[79] The annual disbursements of the Global Fund
(>$3 billion in 2014), US government funding for global health (>$10
billion in 2014), and the Gates Foundation's total grant support (almost
$4 billion in 2014) at least equal if not overshadow the $4.17 billion
biennial budget that the Director-General proposed for 2016/17.[80]
Despite a quadrupling of global health funding for the decade ending
in 2010, and a doubling of WHO's budget, the agency finds itself in
fiscal crisis, a state indicative of a larger crisis of donor and partner
confidence.

   The agency, relying on projected contributions, ran a budget deficit
of at least $300 million in 2010/11. To close the deficit, members set
WHO's 2012/13 budget at $3.96 billion—nearly $1 billion less than the
Director-General sought, with three hundred headquarters staff members (>10 percent of personnel) losing their jobs. A combination of
unfunded mandates from its members, growing health challenges, a
long-term rise in the value of the Swiss Franc (while WHO assessments
are generally in dollars), and poor fiscal controls all contributed to the
current predicament. Budget cuts—and the lack of donor trust those
cuts reflected—severely undermined WHO's ability to respond to the
Ebola epidemic. For example, the team that manages emergency response was "whittled to the bone"—reduced from ninety-four staff to
just thirty-four.[81]

   The agency's dire financial position is not due solely to insufficient
funds, but also its lack of flexibility in investing resources. In chapter 4

we note that while thirty-five years ago half of WHO's budget was from discretionary sources—voluntary funds—by 2014 it had grown to nearly 80 percent.[82] Having voluntary funding represent such a disproportionate amount of the agency's total budget is untenable for any organization. Voluntary contributions have inevitably transformed WHO into a donor-driven organization, with donors, not the World Health Assembly or Secretariat, setting much of its agenda.

WHO's reform plan proposes broadening the funding base by attracting donations from foundations, emerging economies, and the private sector. Although worthwhile, these stakeholders are unlikely to behave differently than traditional donors and will prefer to control their funds through earmarks. To be fair, why should new donors to WHO expect a different "deal" from the agency than what preexisting donors have received? Reliance on philanthropic and corporate funding, moreover, opens the agency further to the charge that it is not fully independent. Finally, the Global Fund's experience indicates that hoping for and even investing in recruiting broad private sector and philanthropic support does not necessarily yield a broader base of financial support.

To increase WHO's control over its budget and better align financing with World Health Assembly–determined organizational priorities, the 2013 World Health Assembly gave itself the power to approve the budget in its entirety, rather than only that portion funded by assessed contributions. A financing dialogue, concluded in 2014, aimed to increase predictability and alignment of WHO's financing with the organization's program of work. It, along with more realistic budgeting, was designed to reduce the impact of drastic fluctuations in voluntary allocations, while trying to curtail the ability of individual donors to sway WHO's agenda through earmarked contributions. The dialogue's final report offered a series of recommendations, including introducing a coordinated resource mobilization approach across WHO and incorporating prospective donors and scientists in future financing dialogue meetings. WHO has not yet implemented most of these recommendations and shows little sign, at least as of early 2016, of doing so.[83]

Ideally, member states would give untied voluntary contributions above their assessed dues and provide longer-term commitments to invest in WHO's long-term health; others too could provide such funding. WHO could also consider charging an administrative fee for voluntary contributions to supplement its core budget. Although over-heads are a familiar model in academia and for NGOs, WHO would have to guard against the risk that charges might drive donors toward other agencies, particularly as it would be clear that they would be used to support, even subsidize, WHO's core work. In return for this flexi-bility and predictability, the agency could scale back on activities agreed by the Executive Board to its core functions and in areas where it possessed both a unique comparative advantage and sufficient donor funding dedicated to those areas – and stop work in those areas that did not meet such standards.

WHO's unique feature as a legal authority

WHO possesses a unique feature among all institutions active in global health. Its constitution grants the agency extraordinary rule-making powers to create both soft and hard law.[84] No other institution in global health has ever been granted similar authority: WHO was formed as a normative institution, charged with directing and coordinating global health activities, including through binding rules. Norm development can set the global health agenda, guide priorities, harmonize activities, and influence the behavior of key state and nonstate actors. The justifi-cation for WHO's norm-creation role is not simply that it is embedded in its constitution but that there is also a belief that shaping norms will support positive change far better than scientific and technical support could alone.

If WHO is to reassert its constitutional authority as a normative in-stitution, then what principles should it adopt? What is the most effec-tive combination of hard and soft norms? And how can it facilitate implementation of, and compliance with, health norms? WHO's his-tory and constitutional design point to human rights—and the right to health—as a primary source for norm development. What is strik-ing about the postwar consensus is that the United Nations envisaged health and human rights as intertwined social movements, with the UN Charter, the Universal Declaration of Human Rights, and the WHO Constitution as the defining instruments. The first two sentences of the Constitution's preamble define health expansively and proclaim "the highest attainable standard of health" as a fundamental human right.

The agency was intended to be the vanguard of the right to health and at times, such as at the Alma-Ata Conference in 1978 and through the resulting declaration, positioned itself as such.[85]

Yet despite notable achievements, WHO has been reticent to venture into norm-development, and it rarely invokes the right to health. It certainly has not been a leader in the health and human rights movement, leaving that space to civil society and the UN Special Rapporteur on the right to health. The Assembly in sixty-five years has not passed a single resolution on the right to health. Exemplifying states' reluctance, the United States in 2008 strenuously objected to an innocuous WHO/OHCHR (Office of the High Commissioner for Human Rights) fact sheet on the right to health, emphasizing "the seriousness of our concerns" and reiterating "our request that it be rescinded."[86]

WHO has rarely exercised its law-making powers, negotiating only two major treaties—the IHR and the Framework Convention on Tobacco Control. This represents a missed opportunity, as law can be a powerful public health tool.[87] Just as the Framework Convention and IHR were justified by the fact that tobacco and health security as relates to infectious diseases transcend borders, so too do a range of major health challenges, including alcohol overconsumption and antimicrobial resistance, both areas that WHO has called greater attention to in recent years.

Soft norms complement international law—a fact that WHO increasingly realizes with codes of practice, action plans, and global strategies.[88] Indeed, states are more likely to buy into expansive standards if they are not legally bound, providing WHO with an opportunity to issue bolder guidance on highly consequential issues, such as health systems, access to essential medicines, and socioeconomic determinants of health. The agency could go beyond declarations, reports, and commissions by negotiating normative standards for adoption by state and nonstate actors, for example to ameliorate the risk of even greater drug resistance than what the world currently confronts. Soft instruments, moreover, can become the building blocks for subsequent treaties, with greater enforcement and ultimately, accountability.

Legal agreements could have made for a stronger and more efficient response to Ebola. An agreement on the equitable sharing of experimental drugs and other therapies could guide fairer distribution, an issue of

significant concern during the Ebola outbreak as experimental therapies were only made available to citizens of richer countries. (WHO
does have one such agreement, the Pandemic Influenza Preparedness
Framework, but it applies only narrowly to the flu.[89]) A biomedical research and development agreement could accelerate the development
of safe and effective treatments and vaccines, particularly for neglected
diseases like Ebola.

If norms are to have "bite," they must include effective mechanisms
for accountability. Although WHO's comparative advantage is not in
policing, and we would never recommend that it develop such capa-
bilities, the agency is well constituted for convening, monitoring, and
reporting. The convening process itself could lay the groundwork for
gaining stakeholder "buy-in." Once a normative instrument is adopted, ongoing monitoring could provide a "feedback loop," with actors
reporting on progress. Weak health systems in certain developing
countries remain a key challenge, requiring innovative financing and
technical assistance such that countries can meet the needs of their
people and provide requisite reporting back to WHO.

Traditionally, international instruments have been directed primarily at states, leaving out multiple stakeholders. Extending normative
influence to businesses, foundations, the media, and civil society could
help ensure compliance. Advocates could exert political influence and
rally public opinion. For example, NGOs with relevant expertise could
issue "shadow reports," holding stakeholders to account for failing to
live up to their promises, and WHO could create private-sector "Codes
of Conduct" for NGOs and private companies alike. Given the pressures outlined in the earlier part of this book, WHO must recognize
the important role nonstate actors play in global health today and
reform to stay relevant in the current and future health landscape.

THE REFORM AND RELEVANCE OF THE WORLD BANK

We now look at some of the key challenges for the World Bank and
ways in which the agency and its principals (member states) are attempting to address them.[90] Given that the Bank's mandate is far
broader than just health, we identify reforms both within the health
sector and for the institution as a whole.

The largest challenge facing the Bank is a structural one: IBRD financing has collapsed as fee-paying clients, the emerging economies, no longer rely on the Bank for support but instead turn to alternative sources of finance.[91] Put simply, the World Bank is running out of countries to lend to.[92] Its major borrowers, such as India, China, Brazil, and South Africa, often prefer to access resources through global capital markets, foreign direct investment or regional banks. Indeed, middle-income countries generally now have several possible income streams and depend less on the funds of the Bank. As the International Development Association (IDA) finance thus grows in relative importance, not only to support low-income borrower countries but for the Bank in itself, the entire mechanism of the Bank comes into question. A side effect of the increasing importance of IDA versus IBRD is the greater visibility and emphasis on social-sector lending, including for health, within the Bank. Such loans are largely financed through IDA, which operates through a replenishment model where donors make pledges for a fixed amount of time. As the data in our book shows, IDA's budget has been contracting and is likely to further contract as overseas development aid budgets flatline and regress and regional banks look to grow in prominence as a source of financing for middle income and lower income countries alike.

Shorten approval process for loans

Not unaware of these challenges, the leadership of the Bank has made several attempts to keep the institution relevant to a broad group of countries. The first is to address one of the key factors driving borrowers away—the lengthy process for approval of loans. As a result of the heavy scrutiny by NGOs of the Bank's lending operations (e.g., protests against the Narmada dam), the Bank since the 1990s has increased the conditions put on countries before they can receive loans.[93] Borrower countries must ensure in their loan applications that a range of issues are taken into consideration such as potential environmental damage, the resettlement and compensation of indigenous people as well as the establishment of safeguards to protect against corruption. If countries have access to other funds, the past ten years have shown that they predominantly prefer private markets. Competition has also been heightened with the creation of the China-led Asian Infrastructure Investment Bank set to start lending to developing countries in 2016 without the same stringent conditions often required by the World Bank. These trends are unsettling for the World Bank, which is essentially a bank whose future funding comes in part from the current interest payments on IBRD loans to middle-income countries. If there are a decreasing number of IBRD loans taken, the World Bank must look for alternative funding sources (e.g., increased donor contributions) or it will have to downsize. Some say that the Bank is sliding into irrelevance and without reform, its time is coming to an end.[94] Others such as the former Bank president Bob Zoellick and the former president of the Center for Global Development Nancy Birdsall argue that a refocused Bank is needed, driving forward the beyond-aid development agenda and investment in global public goods, such as managing the health and environmental risks of climate change.[95]

One World Bank staff member recounted the difficulties with how the Bank "thinks." In his words, "The Bank likes to think big, because otherwise it is not worth the time of staff if they're not going to move lots of money."[96] In addition, as the Bank runs out of borrowers, he noted that the Bank is forced actively to "sell" projects to governments. And, in fact, the workload on staff has been steadily increasing over the past half century. More than thirty years ago, in 1981, a Bank staffer remarked:

> Every few years there is a new factor that we must take into account, but we are not given more time or staff to accommodate it. This makes me think that the Bank's senior management is responding to outside pressures by delegating the hard choices to us. I don't have any clear understanding of whether we are supposed to pay lip service to, say, the environment or the role of women in development, or to take them seriously. Even worse, I don't know to what extent the Bank wants me to take any one of these things seriously when they conflict with one another. I can make up my own mind on this, but am I supposed to?[97]

More recently, reflecting on the Bangladesh Integrated Nutrition Project, the former head of nutrition at the Bank noted:

I think, firstly, that it's clear from the ICR, the Implementation and Completion Report of BINP, discussions within the Bank that there's no doubt that with hindsight we all agree that moving forward with NNP too quickly was a mistake. The Bank has said so publicly, has written it down. There is no doubt about that. That there were very strong political reasons for doing that [moving ahead quickly] is also a reality, and I think understanding some of that, and acknowledging some of that, and how do we as technical people respond to those kinds of realities I think is something we all need to deal with.[98]

If a project takes too long or costs too much, it is often seen as a failure on the part of the staff. Spending too long on local complexities is at times considered as creating unnecessary work and hampering the real work of the loan point-person. However, whether local "complexities" are adequately consulted, included, and accounted for has enormous bearing on whether the funded program can be successful in meeting its health (or other) targets.

The Matrix Programme Cycle for a Health, Nutrition, and Population Sector Programme, as one example, is estimated to last ten months from project conception to approval although in reality it can take two to three years, and on average takes 25.2 months.[99] The first step is a Project Concept Note, which takes about a month to complete. The second step is the Preparation Mission, which lasts roughly a month. During this process, a mission led by the World Bank works with authorities in the borrower government and relevant local organizations for the preparation of the tentative project. Once the mission has returned, the aide-mémoire is circulated. It contains the main issues discussed and agreements reached during the mission between the borrower country and the World Bank mission. It outlines the next mission (pre-appraisal) and the next steps.[100] Approximately three months later, after a number of reports have been completed (e.g., Strategic Investment Plan, Environmental Assessment, Social Assessment, Land Assessment), the Pre-Appraisal Mission is sent to the borrower country. This mission usually lasts twelve to fourteen days and involves several meetings with the relevant ministries in the government. After its preappraisal aide-mémoire has been completed, a Quality Enhancement Review (QER) is conducted. Working together,

Bank personnel from the region (e.g., South Asia), the sector (e.g., HNP), and the Quality Assurance Group (QAG) undertake the QER to provide technical assistance to staff and managers working on a project. The time between the Pre-Appraisal Mission and the Project Appraisal is usually two to three months, including the QER. Once the Project Appraisal occurs, a revised Project Implementation Plan is sent for review to the borrower country. Another month is spent negotiating the terms of the loan and project before approval.

Two issues jump out from the schedule that a prospective borrower confronts. First, Bank loans take a long time, which leaves borrower countries unable to start important or time-sensitive projects, not to mention that by the time the first funds arrive, the project as conceived may not be a priority. Second, the timetable presented reflects the enormous amount of work given to Bank staff. Designing a project is a long and arduous process, and staff simply do not have time to put together a whole new project. A credible "shortcut" is to draw on Bank blueprints and project documents that can be exported to every country. Ngaire Woods notes:

> Junior officials are regularly sent to far-away places to analyze rather alien and difficult solutions. As mentioned above, a clear blueprint of models and policies provide the Fund and Bank staff with a well-structured starting point from which to define the problem, map out the stakes, prescribe the solution, evaluate the chances of success, and assess the implications of their prescription. Obviously, the simpler and clearer the model the more usefully it fulfills these functions. . . . The template is necessary because it guides staff working in countries all over the world, permitting them to act with the full backing of their institution and to put agreements in place with a minimum of time and resources.[101]

In a way, staff are forced to use a blueprint even if they acknowledge that the blueprint is flawed.[102] The challenge, if such templates are adopted, is to ensure that the local complexities—at times criticized as elongating World Bank loan time—are still given specific consideration. We hope that clarity around what is standardized and what must be customized can lead to loan agreements being struck more quickly, and also ultimately to more efficient and effective outcomes for borrower countries and their constituencies.

Improve transparency over financing, operations, and governance

A second way in which the Bank has attempted to remain relevant is to become even more transparent in its financing and operations (see chapter 5 for additional detail). As noted, the Bank has done relatively less well in increasing transparency in key governance decisions. To briefly recap, the World Bank consists of a president, an Executive Board (that votes on and elects the president), a Board of Governors, and vice-presidential units. The World Bank president is an American traditionally selected by the United States, although non-OECD countries have more recently challenged this informal citizenship norm. Conventionally, the American head of the World Bank "balanced" the European head of the IMF (currently a position held by Christine Lagarde, former French Finance minister). The World Bank presidential election process also has been criticized for not being transparent or following a set of clear selection guidelines.[103] The president serves an initial five-year term, which may be renewed by the Executive Board for five years or less, with no limit to the number of terms. He is chairman of the Bank's Board of Executive Directors and ex officio president of the Bank group: the IBRD, IDA, IFC, MIGA, and the International Centre for Settlement of Investment Disputes (ICSID).

The Executive Board, the "political heart" of the Bank, governs the World Bank and all member states are represented on it.[104] It consists of twenty-four elected and appointed Executive Directors who serve full-time in Washington and make decisions on the day-to-day operations. The representation on the Executive Board is not equal. Only large donor countries such as the United States, Japan, Germany, France, the United Kingdom, China, Russia, and Saudi Arabia have their own Executive Directors. The other sixteen seats are elected for two-year terms by groups of countries (constituencies) represented by just one position. This has been a large source of contention since power is shared unequally. For example, twenty-two African countries are represented by one Executive Director.

TABLE 6.1 International bank for reconstruction and development
(IBRD) voting power (percentage)

U.S.	15.99
Japan	7.41
Germany	4.34
Russia	2.8
China	4.78
All other countries	64.68

Source: World Bank, "International Bank for Reconstruction and Development
Subscriptions and Voting Power of Member Countries," accessed 13 January 2016,
http://siteresources.worldbank.org/BODINT/Resources/278027-1215524804501/
IBRDCountryVotingTable.pdf.

Although the Executive Board is supposed to work through consensus and discussion, voting power plays a significant role. With this background, it is important to note that not all countries have the same number of votes (see table 6.1). Each country has a weighted number of votes depending on its quota and commensurate capital contributions to the Bank. Quotas are established through a cumulative assessment of national income, foreign reserves, international trade, and political calculations. Reviews of these quotas are made every five years and are supposed to serve as a technical assessment. However, quota allocations and subsequent voting power are deeply political.

For example, as discussed in previous chapters, the United States is the only member to have individual veto power over major decisions. This is because an 85 percent majority is needed for such decisions. As the United States' share has dropped, it has always negotiated an increase in the majority needed so that it retains its veto power. Informally it has been noted that the United States is the most vocal member of the Board as well: "Representing the largest, most influential member, the US representatives speak on virtually every issue coming before the Board."[105]

Become more of a knowledge bank

The third major effort to keep the Bank relevant has been to reposition and rebrand itself as a knowledge bank whose greatest value resides in its knowledge and policy prescriptions rather than finance itself. Bank presidents have continued to oscillate between a strong technical core in Washington and empowered regional and country offices with decentralized solutions. In 1997, the Bank split into major geographical and network vice-presidential units, all based in Washington. Regional vice-presidencies include Africa, East Asia and the Pacific, Europe and Central Asia, Latin America, Middle East and North Africa, and South Asia. In addition, there were a number of network vice-presidencies such as Human Development, Financial Sector, Private Sector Development, and Infrastructure. Each network had many subthematic areas, or sectors, each in charge of its own recruitment and hiring. As a result of the new management structure, sector staff were also located in regional vice-presidencies and in the Bank's country offices around the world. A sector person in a country office would report to a sector manager (in Washington typically) and then to a sector director based in the respective regional unit in Washington.

In 2005, Jean-Louis Sarbib, the former senior vice-president for Human Development at the Bank stated: "Our presence everywhere in the world allows us to draw lessons and to share these lessons, from one place to the next... [we] help design evidence-based policies."[106] President Jim Kim has also stated his intention to make the World Bank more of a knowledge bank. Under his tenure, Kim has moved the Bank away from a structure centered on country units moving to one focused on fourteen Global Practices—knowledge-based sectors such as agriculture, health and education—so that "vast amounts of knowledge in our ranks can be spread and be used in any country that asks for our help in finding a solution to a development problem"[107] For example, recently the Bank expanded its service delivery activities, including expanding its work with borrower countries to achieve universal health coverage.[108]

A principal concern articulated by scholars has been whether the Bank has the authority and credibility to take on this role. Do developing countries trust the Bank's technical expertise and recommendations?[109] Within health, its legacy is controversial with academics and NGOs critical of its role in perpetuating inequality over time, such as through its former support of structural adjustment programs (part of the Bank's previous loan conditionality) and user fees for social

services, including in health care.[110] As has been recognized over decades of development work, for ideas to work in practice requires local
trust and ownership of both the problem and the solution.[111] This all
indicates a preference for decentralization and stronger country engagement, for example by moving staff out of Washington to country
offices. Such a shift might result in better tailored local solutions rather
than blueprints solely emanating from experts sharing knowledge—
even gleaned from country missions—at headquarters.

World Bank's unique advantage as an economic institution

What ultimately makes the Bank unique in global health? What distin-
guishes it from our other three case study institutions? At face value the
answer is quite simple: it is a bank that countries can rely on for financing
their health sector, both as it is today and as they envision it for tomorrow. The Bank has two official functions as a development bank: project lending and policy lending. Project lending is when the Bank disburses funds for a project with specific objectives and with the
government typically executing the mutually agreed-upon plan. Loans
are disbursed over a fixed period according to intermediate targets determined over specified project phases. Policy lending refers to lending
for budgetary support of governments' policy reform programs.
Borrower governments have varying levels of input in the design of
project and policy lending. The Bank's budgetary support can be significant. For example, India is the World Bank's largest borrower and the
recipient of the largest sum of interest-free credits from the IDA.
Between 1945 and 2015, the Bank committed $102.1 billion, of which
India received $73 billion and has repaid $37 billion already.[112] In 2013/14,
the Bank provided $5.2 billion including IBRD ($2 billion) and IDA
($3.1 billion) financing. In general, health and social service projects re-
ceive about 4 percent of Bank financing in India.

To identify the Bank's comparative advantage in the health sector it
is worth briefly reflecting on global health financing flows more
broadly. We have argued through the course of this book that most of
the interest, and financing, in global health has been driven by disease-
specific concerns and commodity-based solutions. Tied to the rise of
partnerships is the question of *why* most health aid flows to vertical

programs through these types of partnerships. We put forth several plausible explanations based on the literature and our own analyses. First, the recent shift to vertical health funding might be attributable to the values and business-like strategies of major philanthropic donors. These private donors, the Gates Foundation being the largest but far from the only, strive for timely and quantitative results, and often revise their grants based on performance indicators. For these donors, vertical funding mechanisms are often viewed as ideal to achieve their goals and to leverage concurrent investments from the public and private sector. Increasingly, bilateral donors are introducing significant (and some may claim onerous) reporting requirements on grant recipients, developing countries and NGOs alike. For some bilateral mechanisms, such as PEPFAR, a largely vertical program, such reporting has always been part of their business models.

In contrast, the difficulty in accurately monitoring and evaluating the impact of horizontal interventions (e.g., primary health care) results in little incentive for donors to fund broader health systems. The relative success, particularly in more recent years, in measuring the impact of Global Fund and Gavi grants further exacerbates this challenge, although the challenges in systems monitoring are very real. For example, the global health community does not have accurate nondisease-specific mortality estimates, which creates a lack of data to quantitatively assess the success or failure of horizontal funding approaches. Specifically, information is unavailable about the mortality rate due directly or indirectly to a lack of access to health systems. Previous efforts to generate agreed-upon systems-level metrics have not proven successful.[113] This insufficiency of current metrics to determine results of, and improvements to, horizontal health funding leads to considerable uncertainty among researchers and donors in deciding how best to invest monies. With the current global health system driven by data collection of disease-specific causes of death, investing in broader health systems is seen by certain donors as a bottomless pit, where there is no universally accepted proxy for the impact of health systems investment on mortality. However, when incentives (e.g., through data-driven feedback or widespread public advocacy) are aligned toward funding health systems, "vertical" donors have demonstrated a willingness to incorporate horizontal funding programs into their initiatives. The irony is that despite the proliferation of funds and the exponential increase in monies available since 2000 for global health, developing country governments still struggle to find external support for core health work.[114]

The above discussion on the drivers of vertical financing flows points to the important role the Bank can play in working with governments on the long-term financing necessary to build robust healthcare systems and to help finance recurrent expenditures such as health-worker training and salaries. The Bank is well-placed given its long-standing relationship with ministries of finance and its commitment to working with countries to find solutions to health-sector challenges in an ostensibly "demand-led" way. Thus to gain this kind of "horizontal" support that partnerships and bilateral donors are reluctant to fund, low-income countries still rely on the Bank for IDA grants—and this may create a space for the Bank to deliver real value to developing countries and prove its worth to donors. The Bank, under the leadership of President Jim Kim and Dr. Tim Evans in the Health, Nutrition and Population Global Practice, has taken up universal health coverage as a key issue, advocating that countries around the world move toward this goal,[115] while additionally working to strengthen health systems in specific contexts, for example in Guinea, Liberia, and Sierra Leone, the three countries hardest hit by Ebola.

The Bank has strict rules in regard to which projects and policies it can respectively support and prescribe. In both project and policy lending, the Bank's Articles of Agreement states explicitly that the Bank shall not be involved politically with member states and be motivated only by technical, economic considerations:

> The Bank and its officers shall not interfere in the political affairs of any member; nor shall they be influenced in their decisions by the political character of the member or members concerned. Only economic considerations shall be relevant to their decisions, and these considerations shall be weighed impartially in order to achieve the purposes stated in Article I.[116]

The former World Bank president Alden "Tom" Clausen established his position on poverty immediately stating in 1982, "The World Bank will remain a bank. It is not a Robin Hood...nor the United Way of the Development Community...it's a hard-headed, unsentimental institution that takes a very pragmatic and non-political view of what it is trying to do."[117] This approach arguably has resulted in reluctance to take on human rights, such as the right to health, or to ascribe any value to good health beyond economic gains.[118] Because IDA funds are given at donors' discretion, such an approach historically may have been the Bank's only option. It is hard to imagine, for example, the Reagan or Thatcher governments not retaliating through funding freezes had the Bank shown an interest in funding significant health-care risk insurance programs across the world.

Given the World Bank is indeed a bank, it is not surprising then that cost-effectiveness is the dominant and overriding concern for setting priorities for lending and approving loans or grants. In making the case for the Bank to start funding nutrition projects, the Bank health staff created a metrics of nutrition, reflecting the relationships between nutritional gains, labor, discount rates, and productivity. This approach remains the one that the Bank uses today. It can be viewed as an econometrics of suffering, in which mathematical analysis of production relationships is used to determine the magnitude of nutritional deprivation, providing justification for the spending required to alleviate it.[119]

This logic is troubling for many civil society members and academics alike as it appears to trivialize pain and suffering and treat health as if it is purely a commodity.[120] For example, Philip Musgrove, a former World Bank economist, said in an interview, "What's unusual about health is just that it's a peculiar asset, because you can't sell it, you can't give it away, you can't get many spare parts for it, and while your body is in the hospital, you can't go get a loaner body the way you can when your car is in the shop. The biology never goes away, but the economics has to be there."[121] Given that many who work in global health would say that health is exceptional and that the right to health should underpin any approach,[122] clear tension exists with the Bank's complete economic logic. For example, we would argue—as would many—that a human rights approach supports allocating resources to strengthen health systems and universal health coverage, both areas of current Bank investment.[123]

As is true in much of life and analyses, we have to know the past to understand the present. Despite its significant and influential role, there is little scholarly work on the Bank's history in global health, the impact it has had in this arena and on how its processes have supported or constrained those impacts. As we pass the fortieth anniversary of the Bank's first loan to health for the Onchocerciasis (River Blindness) Control Programme, now is a propitious time to examine three broad questions of relevance not only to international institutions but also to global public health policy. First, what has the Bank contributed over the past forty years to global health in terms of finance, ideas, and networks, and how effective have these contributions been? Second, how has the Bank's increasing involvement in health as an international financial institution transformed how we think about health (particularly given Gavi and the Global Fund are financing entities)? Finally, what have been the positive (e.g., quantifiable, measurable, relevance to ministries of finance) and negative (e.g., neglect of social justice, equity, and local concerns) aspects of this involvement? These are beyond the scope of this book, and we plan to investigate these issues together over the coming years.[124]

CONCLUSION

It is clear that both WHO and the World Bank must evolve if they are to maintain their global health leadership positions, in the view of donor and developing countries, as well as civil society and the public at large. It is also clear that the Global Fund and Gavi must continue to manifest their commitments to transparency and multisectoral engagement to maintain their relevance, and to hopefully motivate reform particularly by WHO in these areas. Even with such reforms as discussed and good stewardship by the individual institutions, what remains an open question is whether we will see broader progress in improving health beyond specific disease campaigns. Even in the aftermath of Ebola, amid the ongoing crisis of Zika, and with mounting evidence of the short- and long-term benefits of investing in health systems and health insurance, it does not appear as if ODA (Official Development Assistance) for health or developing countries' own domestic budgets are shifting to meaningfully incorporate such broader efforts. In other words, we have yet to see whether the post-2015 era with its emphasis on sustainable development will live up to its billing by yielding coalitions backed by meaningful financing committed to long-term broader-based health investments. We offer thoughts about what that might look like, for our focal institutions and beyond, in chapter 7.

7

Final Reflections

WHETHER CONFRONTING AND CONTAINING an Ebola outbreak originating in Guinea or a Zika outbreak originating in Brazil, whether deploying vaccines to rural India or getting insecticide-treated bed nets to Malawi, we hope our book has made a convincing case that governance matters. International institutions, bolstered by resources and norms, play a crucial role in organizing and structuring governments', and increasingly other actors' interests and actions. To really understand institutions means delving into how they are governed, how they make decisions, and how they are financed. We have taken a closer look at the four most important global health institutions, as determined by resources commanded, to provide a better picture of how the "system" works in global health, why it functions the way it does, and, hopefully, to illuminate how it could work better.

Stepping back, our book tackled several objectives: in chapter 3, we examined how the World Health Organization (WHO), the World Bank, the Global Fund, and Gavi are governed and how their different governance structures could influence their roles in the global health system. In chapter 4, we outlined how each is financed and how that might influence their agenda and priorities. In chapter 5, we compared the inclusiveness and transparency of our case study organizations. Finally, in chapter 6 we offered some thoughts on what reforms are needed to ensure these structures can tackle the major health challenges of the twenty-first century and are able to do so in part because of their perceived legitimacy from their members, partners, and the broader public around the world.

We highlight three key conclusions from our analysis. First, the past few decades have seen the consolidation of influence across three of our case-study institutions into a few principals' hands, namely the United States, the United Kingdom, and the Gates Foundation. This is clearly evident in the creation of Gavi and in the disproportionate role each plays from a financing perspective in Gavi, the Global Fund, and WHO, as well as global health broadly. Chris Murray has pointed out that these three donors accounted for more than 60 percent of the increase in resources flowing to global health from 2000 to 2014.[1] From a governance perspective, Gavi and the Global Fund have smaller groups of principals than do WHO and the World Bank. Yet, the growing importance of a small group of funders to WHO and the persistence of a small group of funders to the World Bank's IDA raise the specter that those institutions are, in reality, also beholden to—or at least accountable to—a small number of principals.

Additionally, the Gates Foundation has changed the nature of who is a principal, given it is a philanthropic entity, not a government and so shifts, at least in theory, the goalposts around the democratic deficit that international organizations inevitably contain. The significant role the Gates Foundation plays in global health makes it imperative that other major global health actors engage with it. It continually puts pressure on performance and results, and when unhappy, pushes for quick reform in whatever ways that it can (and for the specific reforms it believes should take shape). This is particularly true for the Global Fund, Gavi, and, to a limited extent, WHO. It is also crucial that those three institutions as well as the World Bank continue to engage with the nongovernmental organizations (NGOs) that the world increasingly relies on to provide health care, recognizing that the most significant NGO partners may vary from each and across geographies.

Second, the Global Fund and Gavi were established to meet specific and results-based missions, and were structured to make them more appealing to principals; as we discussed in chapter 3, their governance increases the likelihood that donor preferences would prevail, both in individual debates and structurally within the organizations themselves.

We believe that this type of governance would be hard-pressed to address nondisease-specific objectives such as noncommunicable diseases (NCDs), universal health coverage (UHC), and even global health security issues such as pandemic preparedness or health systems strengthening and resilience more broadly (all of which are interrelated). One common thread across nondisease-specific objectives is that all require even broader coalitions than those initially mustered around combating infectious diseases in both the Global Fund and Gavi, although both have incorporated more partners over time. Looking at pandemic preparedness, while medical and public health resources are obviously required, so too are logistics, supply chain management, financial, trade, communications, and even military expertise, particularly if we look at the lessons of what finally worked—a multisectoral partnership inclusive of all of the above—to contain the Ebola outbreak of 2014/15.

Third, the World Bank and WHO must reform to stay relevant, and reform must be driven by their principals in conjunction with their organizational management—in ways in which principals trust the respective agency and are willing to delegate. As we lay out in chapter 5, major issues that need to be addressed relate to membership and voting rights as well as transparency, all of which tie into both monitoring and accountability. The 2017 election of a new WHO Director-General creates opportunities for key member states to select a strong, outspoken, and reform-minded leader for the organization who can work with them to ensure suitable and substantial changes are undertaken.

"NEW" CHALLENGES IN GLOBAL HEALTH

While the primary aim of our book is to illuminate what motivates the behaviors of the institutions we focus on, we also hope to inform more recent debates in global health. To that end, we now briefly look at a few key challenges confronting global health in the next decade, doing so specifically in terms of institutional response and governance.

Noncommunicable diseases

As the 2010 Global Burden of Disease study confirmed, NCDs—primarily cardiovascular disease, cancer, chronic respiratory disease, and diabetes—are now the major cause of death and disability across the world.[2] This was not true even twenty-five years ago. In 1990, 47 percent of disability-adjusted life years (or years lost to early death, disability, or ill-health) worldwide were from communicable, maternal, neonatal, and nutritional deficits, 43 percent from NCDs, and 10 percent from injuries. By 2012, this had shifted to 34 percent, 55 percent, and 11 percent, respectively.[3] More than 80 percent of NCD-related deaths occur in low- and middle-income countries, with lower socioeconomic groups the worst affected in terms of morbidity, mortality, and loss of economic opportunity.[4] These figures do not account for the health and economic burdens of the wide range and prevalence of mental illnesses.

The shifts in governance and financing described in this book have clear implications for the NCD agenda.[5] First, NCDs are currently not a major funding priority for donors. According to the Institute for Health Metrics and Evaluation (IHME), only $185 million of the $28.2 billion spent globally on development assistance for health in 2010 was dedicated to NCDs.[6] Another way to look at this is on a comparative basis. That year, donors spent $300 for each year lost to disability from HIV/AIDS, $200 for malaria, and $100 for TB, but less than $1 for NCDs. Specifically analyzing WHO's expenditures shows a significant misalignment with the burden of disease, both globally and at the regional level.[7] Of WHO's regular budget in 2008/9, 25 percent of funds were allocated to infectious diseases, 8 percent for noncommunicable diseases, and roughly 4.7 percent for injuries. Additionally, close to 18 percent of the 2008/9 regular budget was allocated to WHO leadership and support functions, and 12 percent to health systems strengthening, with the remaining 30 percent plus funds targeting other health priorities.[8] Over that same period, donors allocated their extrabudgetary funding to WHO primarily to infectious diseases at 60 percent, while only 3.9 percent was used for NCDs and 3.4 percent for injuries. From 2004 to 2008, nearly half of the funding for NCDs derived from a single source: the Bloomberg Family Foundation.[9] If the Bloomberg Family Foundation were to make NCDs a priority in the same way that the Gates Foundation made closing the vaccine gap a priority, it would be interesting to observe what institutional shape, if any, such a commitment assumed and what exactly in return the Bloomberg Family Foundation expected for such investments and leadership.

Second, the drivers of many NCDs are intricately connected with government policies beyond the health sector, as well as in private-sector practices.[10] While this is also true in infectious diseases, such as HIV/AIDS, it is particularly true across heart disease and many cancers, the most significant NCDs in terms of health burden (although it is critical to recognize that a suspected, and in some cases known, risk factor for many cancers and other NCDs in the developing world are previous infectious disease incidences). Some countries have already begun to recognize the vital role government policy plays in constraining NCD risk and have introduced multisectoral participation on health issues through interministerial working groups focused on global health and the reduction of health inequities. This is similar to the many already existing broad-based public-private partnerships focused on HIV/AIDS prevention and treatment in different countries around the world. Australia, Canada, India, Norway, Sweden, Switzerland, Thailand, Uganda, the United Kingdom, and the United States are a few examples of where this type of work has occurred.[11] One lesson from these national (and subnational) government examples is the importance of incentives to encourage nonhealth sectors to participate, both from within the government as well as from the private sector. It is also important the health sector engage in relevant debates elsewhere. However, WHO and other global health institutions generally lack the resources and mechanisms to meaningfully participate in policy debates that involve trade, agriculture, security, education, and climate change, all of which have a direct impact on health. Currently, WHO relies mainly on its bully pulpit, which it has used to varying degrees of success depending on WHO leadership and the broader public health issue being addressed.[12] For NCDs in particular, the global response requires more than new funding or financing mechanisms; it requires new global norms and regulations around the key vectors of the epidemics and linkages to communicable disease efforts, particularly for individuals over their lifetimes. This points to the importance of WHO's continued involvement, the only global health body with the power to create international law, as well as that of the World Bank's, given its role in providing financing for countries to make long-term investments, its ability to be a direct broker with ministries of finance, and its track record as a key producer of knowledge that governments use to pass specific pieces of legislation—all useful when thinking about how to mitigate NCD risk factors across the world.[13]

Third, new institutions such as the Global Fund and Gavi herald a major shift in global cooperation, one in which voting rights and board membership are granted to the private sector and philanthropic organizations, and where legitimacy is claimed through improving specific measurable health outcomes. Given the aggressive tactics the tobacco industry has used to oppose regulation addressing a key NCD risk factor (tobacco use in any form), it will be difficult to have certain members of the private sector at the table while addressing key risk factors for continued rising NCD rates around the world (tobacco use, alcohol overconsumption, poor diet, lack of physical activity).[14] Indeed, during the negotiations around the Framework Convention for Tobacco Control, the WHO then-Director-General Dr. Gro Harlem Brundtland explicitly and consistently barred the tobacco industry from participating. Yet, it is much easier to imagine possible collaborative outcomes that could be win-wins for public health and the food-and-beverage industry around the world, given as a world we need more healthy food options at affordable prices (rather than tobacco for which there is no safe level of use). The WHO could lead work inclusive of industry to combat obesity, improve nutrition, and end chronic vitamin and mineral deficiencies, including anemia, while making clear that WHO, and WHO alone, sets standards and guidelines.

Finally, there is no NCD analog to the Gates Foundation from a funding perspective, or to the myriad NGOs and multilaterals that partner and deliver on Gavi and Global Fund grants such as Population Services International (PSI) and the United Nations Development Programme (UNDP). In 2010, PSI served as a Principal Recipient in twelve countries receiving Global Fund grants and, by that time, had done Global Fund–financed work in more than thirty.[15] The UNDP has served as a Principal Recipient for Global Fund grants in close to fifty countries.[16] Currently, no international NGO focused on cancer or heart disease possesses the current breadth of resources, human and otherwise, and geographic scope to PSI. The UNDP manages Global Fund grants in fragile country contexts as well as during emergency situations. From their activities to date, it is unlikely they could play a similar role for NCDs given the greater complexities mentioned earlier, even recognizing the medical, public health, and supply-chain dimensions inherent in managing most Global Fund grants. Additionally, the Gates Foundation has long said that it will not fund NCDs because their efforts focus on diseases that predominantly affect poorer countries (even though NCDs are extracting a tragic toll on countries around the world irrespective of income level).[17] Whether the Bloomberg Family Foundation or another philanthropic funder will emerge and provide a similar and sustained funding boost for NCDs remains to be seen. Similarly, there are no clear signs yet that developing country governments themselves would (or could) increase their own budgetary allocations to NCD prevention and treatment as we have seen happen in relation to HIV/AIDS (and could do so without cutting health funding elsewhere).[18]

Are public-private partnerships such as the Global Fund and Gavi the best models through which to challenge the powerful vested interests that have significant impacts on chronic disease incidence, such as the tobacco industry? Would a cooperative (or even cooptive) model be possible? Richard Horton, the editor in chief of *The Lancet*, has argued that there is much to learn from Gavi for NCDs. In November 2015, he tweeted eight lessons, key among them that such an effort around NCDs needs a clear strategy and set of measurable objectives, a strong group of partners with a shared long-term commitment to combating NCDs, and a high-profile donor to provide substantial funding complemented with a clear long-term plan that ultimately even the poorest countries could sustainably fund their own NCD prevention and treatment work.[19]

Thus far, a measurable results-based focus has been central to new partnership models. However, action on diseases like cancer and diabetes is necessarily complex. For some individuals, risk factors come early in life, as is true of rheumatic heart disease, the most commonly acquired heart disease in children in the developing world. Its origins? An untreated strep infection.[20] Individual-level decisions around tobacco use, diet, physical activity, and alcohol consumption constrained and influenced by environmental factors all correlate to greater NCD risk later in life, and each has a complicated trajectory. Ameliorating those risk factors must involve various combinations of actors working in the public and private sectors as well as across functions as diverse as production, distribution, marketing, and regulation. Achieving results in a short-term timeline amid such a complex playing field may prove to be too formidable a challenge. This raises the following question: Is it possible to reconcile the need to address the deep-rooted, long-tail risk factors for NCDs with the widespread appeal of interventions with clear targets that can be tracked and met within the short-to medium-term? And to do so without sacrificing vital funds targeting infectious diseases? We do not have the answer; we hope our work helps inform those on the frontlines of thinking about these very questions, in developing country governments, in donor governments, in multilateral organizations, in philanthropic institutions, in NGOs, and in private companies.

Universal Health Coverage

Universal health coverage (UHC) presents somewhat similar challenges. On 12 December 2012, UHC received an unequivocal endorsement from the UN General Assembly (including the United States) with the approval of a resolution on UHC that confirmed the "intrinsic role of health in achieving international sustainable development goals."[21] The 2005 World Health Assembly's definition of UHC makes clear what its achievement would look like: "access to key promotive, preventive, curative and rehabilitative health interventions for all at an affordable cost, thereby achieving equity in access,"[22] rather than how it would be achieved. In 2012, a WHO discussion paper on the post-2015 health agenda (what would emerge as the Sustainable Development Goals or SDGs) identified UHC as a "way of bringing all programmatic interests under an inclusive umbrella."[23] Yet despite UHC's growing prominence in the post-2015 agenda, there is not yet any single agreed-upon plan on how institutionally it should be carried forward and financed.[24] This is not particularly surprising. Across countries with UHC, no two versions are alike in their financing, in what they cover, or in how they are structured. Some countries with UHC rely on a public system of coverage while others mandate insurance coverage, requiring individuals to buy health coverage in a regulated private insurance market or from the government, while still others have a mix of the two approaches. Additionally, a further challenge is that the conversations and debates surrounding UHC are rarely tied to those relating to health systems strengthening, community health-worker models, or other health-care delivery priorities. We find this persistent decoupling illogical.

Thus far, neither donors nor developing countries have turned to vertical funds directly to strengthen health systems or to assure health care for all members of society (for example through UHC tied to health systems strengthening).[25] One possible exception to this are the health systems strengthening funds that the Global Fund and Gavi at times have made available; however, these have always remained the significant minority of funds each has disbursed as mentioned in earlier chapters. In addition, to qualify, applicants have had to be clear about how such funds will strengthen health systems with a direct relationship to achieving their respective infectious disease mandates. Not surprisingly then, such funds have not generally supported broader capacity building, despite health-worker shortages across the developing world.[26] In the horizontal-versus-vertical-funding terminology debate we engaged with earlier, this approach is referred to as "diagonal."[27]

For the most part, key donors believe that domestic resources are growing fast enough in most developing countries to enable governments to strengthen their health systems and provide universal health coverage, if that is what they choose as areas of investment.[28] They also worry that governments in developing countries would use any new funds as an excuse to reduce their existing health investments—viewing such aid as a substitute for domestic spending on health, not as an addition to it. Research from the IHME supports these concerns. It also points to this effect only when development assistance flows directly to developing country governments, rather than when it flows to NGOs working within the same country.[29] Arguably, then, this is a valid concern in the context of UHC, as most UHC-targeted development assistance would be expected to flow, at least in significant part, to governments.

Additionally, donors believe that national programs must be country-led (even if donor-influenced) and country-designed because of differences among health systems (such as the presence or absence of a domestic private-care delivery system or preexisting domestic private insurance markets). For some, it is also crucial that such investments be tied to government approaches to fighting disease risk factors (such as tobacco for NCDs). Many donors are also wary of further fragmenting global health governance, cognizant that the aid harmonization efforts of the past decade stretching from Paris to Busan and beyond have largely failed.[30]

Still, Japan plans to make UHC a major priority during its presidency of the 2016 G7. Is UHC a rousing enough topic to get the attention and funding from heads of states and the requisite legitimization from their publics, as happened at the 2000 G7 with what would become the Global Fund?[31] At least at the moment, UHC currently has far from universal donor support. The Gates Foundation has expressed its discomfort with UHC as a unifying post-2015 theme.[32] One strategic idea for raising the profile of UHC is to tie it to health systems strengthening (in a broader context than ever articulated by the Global Fund or Gavi) and to make it a pillar of achieving meaningful global health security.[33] Yet, this strategy is not without possible complications; "global health security" remains a debated term.[34] Since World War II, this concept has become increasingly narrowed to one in which health threats are perceived to be largely related to outbreaks with the potential to affect wealthier and more powerful countries' citizens and interests. Health security became part of national security, instead of its original definition as the health part of human security.[35] In part, this was intentional as seen in UN Resolution 1308, which classified HIV/AIDS as a security threat. At the time, the hope was that such a linkage would increase urgency around the burgeoning epidemic, and that such urgency would be followed with increased political cooperation and funding. On that front, as seen in the advent of the Global Fund and later the US PEPFAR program, it was undeniably successful. Its legacy, however, is one in which it is easy to classify Ebola as a security risk and more challenging to imagine the rising burden of NCDs or persistent lack of UHC as the same in a traditional, or even global health, context.

Pandemic preparedness

It is clear that robust health systems—and ultimately universal health coverage—play a role in combating infectious diseases. Indeed, Ebola's spread across West Africa has shown that health systems must be strengthened not only to provide maternal and child health care and confront NCDs such as cancer and heart ailments but also to fight infectious diseases—to detect and treat them. In our conversations with health ministers from around the world, we have continually heard that developing countries want support from the global community to build an infrastructure capable of both public health activities such as information-gathering and surveillance as well as delivering comprehensive health services to their populations today and in the future.[36] And, understandably, developing countries want those health services to be those anyone would be proud to be a part of or to serve within. We agree that governments should be responsible for leading these efforts, and the goal should be to have domestic sources of revenue fund recurrent expenditures such as health workforce salaries as well as the purchase of commodities. We view such national efforts, with coordination across a regional and global level, supported by donors with an eye toward ultimate self-sustainability, as the best and first-line response to an outbreak and thus the only effective path to pandemic preparedness.

Understandably, health ministers are often wary of new initiatives and plans that jostle them from one disease priority to another. They want to build robust and flexible systems that can deal not only with outbreaks such as Ebola but also with maternal health, respiratory infections, heart disease, diabetes, cancer, and depression—and help prevent outbreaks like Ebola from occurring in the first place. On a basic level, health facilities need to have running water, electricity, laundry facilities, and good sanitation practices, including waste disposal, not to mention a constellation of doctors, nurses, technicians, and community health workers as well as biostatisticians and epidemiologists, among others, to work in and to provide support to health facilities. Rwanda and Ethiopia, for example, established programs to build comprehensive health systems, funded by both increased domestic investment and donor support, in partnership with local and international NGOs under strong country leadership.

Strikingly, even in a moment when vertical funds are delivering on their objectives, and a global pandemic has been called out as the top threat to humankind by Bill Gates, and others,[37] no suggestion has been made for a new vertical outbreak control fund. Instead, the World Bank and WHO have claimed they are the best-positioned to lead in this area, previous failures notwithstanding.[38] The World Bank, through the Pandemic Preparedness Financing Facility, would provide funding during infectious disease emergencies.[39] In theory, WHO could provide more robust convening and coordination functions through a newly created WHO Centre for Emergency Preparedness and Response with a dedicated and protected budget, resourced through a revolving fund. Almost all post-Ebola review efforts (including those we have participated in) have argued that for such a new center to be effective, it must be governed by a separate and independent Board, with control over its agenda, decision-making, and resources.[40] Yet, there is also a broad recognition that a new entity itself is insufficient, and that more attention and resources must concentrate on building resilient health systems around the world. Bill Gates has articulated a clear view that WHO must be the leader in this area, and that health systems strengthening is the best route to achieve global health security.[41] Among bilateral donors, the United States has been a clear leader. In 2014, even before the Ebola outbreak, the United States launched the Global Health Security Agenda to accelerate partner countries' pandemic preparedness. It includes health workforce development support but, as of early 2016, only Jordan and Thailand had received funding in this specific area.[42]

If vertical funds were the global health answer of the late twentieth and early twenty-first century, what is the answer today as broader challenges, such as NCDs, UHC, and pandemic preparedness, claim greater time and attention and, possibly, resources? We believe the answer in part lies in reforming WHO to have a clearer mandate with more focused tools to tackle, for example, coordinating health systems strengthening investments, either through the lens (or excuse) of pandemic preparedness, or through a recommitment to a broader definition of health security than that which prevails today. For certain NCDs, like cancer, the answer may reside in partnerships with advocates for health systems strengthening and in part through NGOs currently working on cancer in wealthier countries looking to build capacity and share their expertise with developing country governments and health professionals. Clearly, the World Bank has a core role to play in each arena as well as in assisting countries that choose to implement UHC and doing so in the most cost-effective—and equitable—means possible. If that proposition is accepted, the financing mechanisms would then need to be determined. Two possible options would be through the Health, Nutrition, and Population division at the World Bank or through a Bank-managed vertical trust fund. Certainly, the governance implications for each would be different.

A third option would be for governments to work with regional development banks, either bilaterally or in regional partnerships with other governments working toward similar ends. There may well be other even more compelling possibilities than those we have imagined. Regardless of the exact financial mechanism, country governments themselves should lead these efforts, supported by expertise and financing from the conventional, "older" multilateral organizations as well as the newer actors on the global health stage.

Notably, during the post-2015 debates leading up to the SDGs, very little attention was given to the questions we address in this book. What are the global governance structures necessary to support the attainment of the new goals? How should such structures be financed? Who should hold them accountable beyond their principals (UN member states), if at all? While it is generally agreed that we need twenty-first-century innovative structures that go beyond WHO's "command and control" model, there is often little detail discussed in such debates on institutional responsibility, monitoring and evaluation, and accountability.[43] We believe such pragmatic thinking is crucial now more than ever given the new challenges—and opportunities—confronting public health in the twenty-first century. We hope those at the UN and elsewhere agree.

CONCLUSION

In 1988, the Global Polio Eradication Initiative (GPEI) was launched at the 41st World Health Assembly. Spearheaded by WHO, Rotary International, the US Centers for Disease Control and Prevention, and UNICEF, the GPEI had a bold ambition from inception: immunize every child at risk with an oral polio vaccine and eradicate polio. In the late 1980s, polio was endemic in more than 125 countries. In 1988, there were an estimated 350,000 polio cases every year, with thousands of those infected suffering long-term effects, including paralysis, with some polio patients dying from the disease. By 2000, polio had been eradicated in the Americas and Europe as well as in parts of Asia and Africa; in 2014, the last polio case on the African continent, in Nigeria, was detected. In 2016, WHO declared that polio could be eradicated within a year, and that WHO and its partners were amplifying their efforts to reach every unvaccinated child in Afghanistan and Pakistan, the two remaining countries that had polio cases in 2015.

If WHO's predictions of a polio-free world in 2017, or earlier, prove correct, it will be a credit to the unparalleled efforts undertaken to vaccinate children around the world, work WHO calls "the largest-ever internationally-coordinated public health effort in history."[44] Since 1988, close to three billion children in two hundred countries have been immunized, in large measure due to the more than twenty million volunteers mobilized to deliver polio vaccines. In addition to the early partners, the Gates Foundation, the World Bank, bilateral donors, development banks, Gavi, developing country governments, NGOs, private companies, and others have all contributed to the GPEI's efforts.[45] Not surprisingly given that list, the initiative considers itself a public-private partnership, and one with clearly designated responsibilities and roles across its four main partners. For example, WHO provides overall strategic planning and technical support, supported by the US Centers for Disease Control; at the same time UNICEF procures and delivers vaccines to still-affected countries, and Rotary International focuses on fund-raising and volunteer recruitment around the world.[46]

Well-funded and coordinated global health efforts can have profound, history-altering effects. We defeated smallpox more than thirty years ago, and we hope soon to see the defeat of polio, possibly even by the time you are reading this book. However, very few major diseases with devastating and deadly consequences are comparable to smallpox and polio. Polio does not have an intermediate host: it does not live in animals, unlike malaria, Dengue, and Zika, which live in and are transmitted by mosquitoes. Polio cannot live long outside a living person, unlike Ebola, which can live for three days and possibly longer in a victim's body, proving deadly even after death. Polio has a vaccine to protect against infection, unlike HIV/AIDS, which currently has no proven vaccine, and polio has an oral vaccine that can be administered by trained volunteers anywhere versus those that require an injection.

Recognizing the unique characteristics of polio does not detract from the incredible efforts mustered to bring the world close to eradicating the disease. Rather, it highlights the reality that to combat other, arguably trickier infectious diseases as well as noncommunicable diseases, we need strong health-care systems and strong public health. This includes curricula in schools that teach children how to protect themselves against infectious diseases, whether washing their hands regularly, wearing bug spray during mosquito seasons, or using a condom during sex (and ensuring equitable access to soap, bug spray, condoms, and other protective measures). It includes public awareness campaigns on airwaves, social media, via SMS (text messaging), and door-to-door efforts by health authorities to help people know how important it is to get rid of stagnant bodies of water in old oil drums, tires, trashcans, or clogged drain pipes, particularly with mosquito-borne Zika, Dengue, and Chikungunya joining old mosquito scourges like malaria. It includes efforts to combat global warming from governments and people alike, around the world, to halt climate change so that places where malaria has been eradicated do not see it return as temperatures rise and mosquitoes carrying malaria once again return. It includes efforts across governments, private companies, NGOs, and philanthropies to make healthy, nutritious food affordable and accessible to families around the world—and to help people understand what nutritious food is, and why diet is so important to preventing and fighting heart disease, cancer, and so many other NCDs. These are only a few illustrative examples.

Governments across the world—supported as needed by international institutions and bilateral aid—must continue to work toward strengthening health systems and broad-based basic health-care coverage. However, this is not sufficient to break the link between sickness and poverty. Commensurate planning, programming, and investments in education, infrastructure, renewable energy, economic empowerment, and more are required. Stronger laws are needed that strengthen protections for women, children, indigenous minorities, workers, and other groups that historically have been disenfranchised, discriminated against, and abused around the world. So too are stronger norms and practices needed that increase opportunities, particularly for women, to be their own economic agents—and the protagonist of their own stories. We recognize that health systems and health insurance alone cannot create or guarantee healthy children, families, or societies.

The institutions we examine in this book and their principals make decisions that meaningfully influence what gets done in global health. We hope our work helps inform those in the UN system, in governments, academia, NGOs, public-private partnerships, philanthropies, and civil society grappling with how best to organize, invest in, and deliver on global health priorities in the twenty-first century. We have made tremendous progress together. We have even more work to do.

NOTES

Preface

1. Shyama Kuruvilla et al., "Success Factors for Reducing Maternal and Child Mortality," *Bulletin of the World Health Organization* 92 (June 2014): 533–44.

Chapter 1

1. "Ebola Situation Reports," WHO, accessed 28 September 2015, http://apps.who.int/ebola/ebola-situation-reports.

2. "Resources for Results III" (report, UN Office of the Special Envoy on Ebola, April 2015), accessed 6 January 2016, https://ebolaresponse.un.org/sites/default/files/rriii_finalf_updated.pdf; "Appeal: Ebola Virus Outbreak—Overview of Needs and Requirements (interagency plan for Guinea, Liberia, Sierra Leone, Region)—October 2014–June 2015," Financial Tracking Service, accessed 28 July 2015, https://fts.unocha.org/reports/daily/ocha_R1_A1060___1511090237.pdf.

3. For more on the history of Zika cases and the 2007 outbreak, please see Mark Duffy et al., "Zika Virus Outbreak on Yap Island, Federated States of Micronesia," *NEJM*, no. 360 (June 2009): 2536–43, http://www.nejm.org/doi/pdf/10.1056/NEJMoa0805715.

4. Sonja Rasmussen, Denise Jamieson, Margaret Honein, and Lyle Petersen, "Zika Virus and Birth Defects—Reviewing the Evidence for Causality," *NEJM*, published online 13 April 2016, accessed 13 April 2016, http://www.nejm.org/doi/full/10.1056/NEJMsr1604338?query=featured_home.

5. Centers for Disease Control and Prevention, "Dengue Homepage," accessed 8 March 2016, http://www.cdc.gov/dengue/epidemiology/.

6. WHO, "WHO Publishes List of Top Emerging Diseases Likely to Cause Major Epidemics," 10 December 2015, accessed 27 March 2016, http://www.who.int/medicines/ebola-treatment/WHO-list-of-top-emerging-diseases/en/.

7. Reference to LSHTM-HSPH Panel *Lancet* paper, David Heymann et al., "Global Health Security: The Wider Lessons from the West African Ebola Virus Disease Epidemic," *Lancet*, no. 385 (May 2015): 1884–1901.

8. "Levels & Trends in Child Mortality: Report 2015," United Nations Interagency Group for Child Mortality Estimation, accessed 6 January 2016, http://www.unicef.org/media/files/IGME_report_2015_child_mortality_final.pdf, 1.

9. "Global Burden of Disease," Institute for Health Metrics and Evaluation, accessed 6 January 2016, http://www.healthdata.org/gbd.

10. "Media Centre: Noncommunicable Diseases," WHO, accessed 6 January 2016, http://www.who.int/mediacentre/factsheets/fs355/en/.

11. Kevin Watkins and Devi Sridhar, "Road Traffic Injuries: The Hidden Development Crisis" (policy briefing, First Global Ministerial Conference on Road Safety, Moscow, Russia, 19–20 November 2009), http://www.fiafoundation.org/media/44127/road-traffic-injuries-kevin-watkins-2009.pdf.

12. WHO, *International Health Regulations (2005):* 2nd ed. (Geneva: WHO Press, 2008), http://www.who.int/ihr/publications/9789241596664/en/.

13. Howard Markel, *When Germs Travel: Six Major Epidemics That Have Invaded America and the Fears They Have Unleashed* (New York: Vintage Books, 2004).

14. Howard Markel, "Worldly Approaches to Global Health: 1851 to the Present," *Public Health*, no. 128 (February 2014): 124–28, http://www.publichealthjrnl.com/article/S0033-3506(13)00265-5/abstract.

15. David Fidler, "The Globalization of Public Health: The First 100 Years of International Health Diplomacy," *Bulletin of the World Health Organization*, no. 79 (2001): 842–49, http://www.who.int/bulletin/archives/79(9)842.pdf.

16. In 1854 Filippo Pacini identified *Vibrio cholerae* in the intestinal walls of people who had died of cholera, publishing extensively on his findings. In recognition of his discovery, in 1965, the organism that causes cholera was renamed *Vibrio cholerae Pacini*.

17. Norman Howard-Jones, "The Scientific Background of the International Sanitary Conferences 1851–1938," *WHO Chronicle*, no. 28 (1974): 159–508, http://apps.who.int/iris/bitstream/10665/62873/1/14549_eng.pdf.

18. David Fidler, *Bulletin of the World Health Organization*, 842–49.

19. In addition to Fidler, for more on the emergence of international health cooperation in the late nineteenth and early twentieth centuries, see Paul

Frederick Basch, "A Historical Perspective on International Health," *Infectious Disease Clinics of North America*, no. 5 (June 1991): 183–96.

20. For a good history of the League of Nations Health Organization, including its work in infectious diseases, health systems, and other areas, see Iris Borowy, *Coming to Terms with World Health: The League of Nations Health Organization 1921–1946* (New York: Peter Lang, 2009).

21. Patrick Meyer, *Succession Between International Organizations* (Geneva: Graduate Institute of International Studies, 2011).

22. Again, see Borowy for more on LNHO throughout the 1930s and early 1940s.

23. Thomas Parran, "The World Health Organization," *Social Security Bulletin* (October 1946): 21.

24. Michael Shimkin, "The World Health Organization," *Science*, no. 104 (September 1946): 281–83.

25. Devi Sridhar, Lawrence Gostin, and Derek Yach, "Healthy Governance: How the WHO Can Regain Its Relevance," *Foreign Affairs*, 24 May 2012, https://www.foreignaffairs.com/articles/2012-05-24/healthy-governance.

26. Public Broadcasting Service, "People and Discoveries: World Health Organization Declares Smallpox Eradicated 1980," accessed 6 January 2016, http://www.pbs.org/wgbh/aso/databank/entries/dm79sp.html.

27. Ibid.

28. For a historical overview of these dynamics, see Kelley Lee, *The World Health Organization (WHO)* (New York: Routledge, 2009).

29. World Health Organization Maximizing Positive Synergies Collaborative Group, "An Assessment of Interactions Between Global Health Initiatives and Country Health Systems," *Lancet*, no. 373 (June 2009): 2137–69, http://www.thelancet.com/journals/lancet/article/PIIS0140-6736(09)60919-3/fulltext.

30. Anne-Emanuelle Birn, "The Stages of International (Global) Health: Histories of Success or Successes of History?," *Global Public Health*, no. 4 (2009): 50–68.

31. Devi Sridhar and Tami Tamashiro, "Vertical Funds in the Health Sector: Lessons for Education from the Global Fund and GAVI" (background paper, UNESCO Education For All Global Monitoring Report 2010).

32. In the late 1970s, "disadvantaged" was a term applied to developing countries. Throughout the book we will use terms that are most favored by specific organizations or were most in favor in specific eras, such as "disadvantaged countries."

33. Gavino Maciocco and Angelo Stefanini, "From Alma-Ata to the Global Fund: The History of International Health Policy," *Revista Brasileira de Saude Materno Infantil*, no. 7 (December 2007): 479–86.

34. Kazuo Takahashi, "Reversing the Decline of ODA: How Effective Is the Current Policy Agenda?" (executive summary, United Nations, Department of Economic and Social Affairs, Division for Sustainable

Development), http://www.un.org/esa/dsd/resources/res_pdfs/
publications/sdt_fin/nairobi_meeting_part2.pdf.

35. Julia Walsh and Kenneth Warren, "Selective Primary Health Care—An
Interim Strategy for Disease Control in Developing Countries," *NEJM*,
no. 301 (November 1979): 967–74, http://www.nejm.org/doi/pdf/10.1056/
NEJM197911013011804.

36. Rifat Atun, Sara Bennett, and Antonio Duran, "When Do Vertical
(Stand-alone) Programmes Have a Place in Health Systems?" (policy
brief, WHO European Ministerial Conference on Health Systems:
"Health Systems, Health and Wealth," Tallinn, Estonia, 25–27 June
2008).

37. Anne-Emanuelle Birn, "Gates's Grandest Challenge: Transcending
Technology as Public Health Ideology," *Lancet*, no. 366 (August 2005):
514–19; Devi Sridhar and Karen Grepin, "Population: Better Lives, Not
Just Contraceptives," *Nature*, no. 488 (August 2012), http://www.nature
.com/nature/journal/v488/n7409/full/488032c.html.

38. Devi Sridhar and Rajaie Batniji, "Misfinancing Global Health: A Case for
Transparency in Disbursements and Decision Making," *Lancet*, no. 372
(September 2008): 1185–91.

39. UNHCR, UNICEF, WFP, UNDP, UNFPA, UNODC, ILO, UNESCO,
UNWOMEN, WHO, World Bank.

40. UNAIDS, "Final Report of Five-Year Evaluation of UNAIDS" (report,
13th meeting of the Programme Coordinating Board, Lisbon, Portugal,
11–12 December 2002).

41. Michael Merson, Jeffrey O'Malley, David Serwadda, and Chantawipa
Apisuk, "The History and Challenge of HIV Prevention," *Lancet*, no. 372
(August 2008): 475–88.

42. Steven Hoffman, Clarke Cole, and Mark Pearcey, "Mapping Global
Health Architecture to Inform the Future" (research paper, Centre on
Global Health Security, Chatham House, January 2015), accessed 14
April 2016, 7, https://www.chathamhouse.org/sites/files/chathamhouse/
field/field_document/20150120GlobalHealthArchitectureHoffmanColePe
arceyUpdate.pdf.

43. Sonja Bartsch, "Global Public-Private Partnerships in Health: A Question
of Accountability and Legitimacy," (paper prepared for the 2007 Wall
Summer Institute for Research, Vancouver, 25–28 June 2007).

44. W. H. Reinicke et al., *Critical Choices: The United Nations, Networks, and
the Future of Global Governance.* (International Development Research
Centre: Canada, 2000).

45. Kent Buse and Gill Walt, "Global Public–Private Health Partnerships:
II: What Are the Issues for Global Governance?" *Bulletin of the World
Health Organization*, 2000, 78; Roy Widdus, "Public-Private Partnerships
for Health: Their Main Targets, Their Diversity, and Their Future
Directions," *Bulletin of the World Health Organization*, no. 79 (2001):

713–20, http://www.scielosp.org/scielo.php?script=sci_arttext&pid=S0042
-96862001000800006.

46. Marissa Miley, "Public-Private Partnerships: A 'Win-Win' for Global
Health?," *Global Post*, 8 July 2014, accessed 6 January 2016, http://www
.globalpost.com/dispatch/news/health/can-PPPs-improve-global-health.

47. Joint United Nations Programme on HIV/AIDS and the World Health
Organization, "AIDS epidemic update" (document, Geneva, December
2001), accessed 6 January 2016, http://data.unaids.org/Publications/
IRC-pub06/epiupdate01_en.pdf.

48. "Home," United Nations Population Fund, accessed 6 January 2016,
http://www.unfpa.org/.

49. Joint United Nations Programme on HIV/AIDS, "Report on the Global
HIV/AIDS Epidemic" (document, Geneva, July 2002), accessed 6
January 2016, http://data.unaids.org/pub/Report/2002/brglobal_aids_
report_en_pdf_red_en.pdf, p. 147.

50. Kent Buse, Nick Drager, Suzanne Fustukian, and Kelley Lee,
"Globalisation and Health Policy: Trends and Opportunities," in *Health
Policy in a Globalising World*, ed. Kelley Lee, Kent Buse, and Suzanne
Fustukian (Cambridge: Cambridge University Press, 2002), 251–80.

51. Benedicte Bull and Desmond McNeill, *Development Issues in Global
Governance: Public-Private Partnerships and Market Multilateralism* (New
York: Routledge, 2007).

52. Mark Dybul, executive director of the Global Fund (interview by authors,
3 June 2015).

53. Kenneth Abbott and Duncan Snidal, "The Governance Triangle:
Regulatory Standards Institutions and the Shadow of the State" (paper
prepared for the Global Governance Project, Oxford University, October
2006).

54. General Assembly, "Role of the United Nations in Promoting
Development in the Context of Globalization and Interdependence:
Report of the Secretary-General" (agenda item 104, 54th sess., 15
September 1999), accessed 6 January 2016, http://www.un.org/
documents/ga/docs/54/plenary/a54-358.htm.

55. Karl-Oskar Lindgren and Thomas Persson, "Input and Output
Legitimacy: Synergy or Trade-off? Empirical Evidence from an EU
Survey," *Journal of European Public Policy*, no. 17 (May 2010): 449–67,
http://www.tandfonline.com/doi/abs/10.1080/13501761003673591#.
VmSed2BHW4Q.

56. Studies such as Bartsch provide a useful framework in terms of evaluating
PPPs, but much more evidence needs to be gathered.

57. Mark Zacher and Tania Keefe, "The Transformation of Global Health
Governance: Utilization and Expansion of Control Strategies Since the
1990s" (paper presented at Wall Summer Institute for Research [WSIR]
2007: Civil Society Organizations and Global Health Governance); Kent

Buse and Andrew Harmer, "Seven Habits of Highly Effective Public-Private Partnerships: Practice and Potential," *Social Science and Medicine*, no. 64 (2007): 259–71.

58. Buse and Harmer, 2007.

59. Thomas Pogge, *World Poverty and Human Rights* (Cambridge: Polity, 2008), 255.

60. Ibid.

61. Richard Feachem (personal interview, conducted by phone, 16 December 2011).

62. Ruairi Brugha, "The Global Fund at Three Years—Flying in Crowded Air Space," *Tropical Medicine and International Health*, no. 10 (July 2005): 625.

63. In Pogge's reasoning, while these companies may not have the business acumen in place for delivery of health solutions, this can be developed from their experience in marketing other consumables. Thomas Pogge (presentation, Trinity College, Dublin, Ireland, 12 September 2007).

64. As one such example, see "Project Last Mile," USAID, accessed 10 April 2016, https://www.usaid.gov/cii/project-last-mile.

65. Author's own assessment. GEF has received attention from international relations scholars, including Robert Keohane, and has been the subject of book-length work, see Zoe Young, *A New Green Order?: The World Bank and the Politics of the Global Environmental Facility* (London: Pluto Press, 2002).

66. For US-based examples, see Roger Bate, "Transparency and the Global Fund's Healthy Crisis" (congressional staff foreign policy brief, American Enterprise Institute for Public Policy Research, 3 February 2011), https://www.aei.org/publication/transparency-and-the-global-funds-healthy-crisis; Michael Gerson, "Putting Fraud Into Context," *Washington Post*, 4 February 2011, http://www.washingtonpost.com/wp-dyn/content/article/2011/02/03/AR2011020305176.html; regarding the US Congress's simultaneous critiques and more positive recognition, see Tiaji Salaam-Blyther and Alexandra Kendall, "The Global Fund to Fight AIDS, Tuberculosis and Malaria: Issues for Congress and US Contributions from FY2001 to FY2013" (report for Congress, Congressional Research Service, 15 May 2012), 13–14. As Europe-based examples, see praise of the Fund in European Commission, "2012 Annual Report on the European Union's Development and External Assistance Policies and Their Implementation in 2011" (Brussels, Belgium, September 2012), 15–120, https://ec.europa.eu/europeaid/sites/devco/files/annual-report-2012-eu-development-external-assistance-policies-implementation-in-2011_en.pdf; for the European Commission's strong criticism of the Fund's governance during the same year, see Ann Danaiya Usher, "Donors Continue to Hold Back Support from Global Fund," *Lancet*, no. 378 (August 2011): 471–72.

67. Beatrice Bernescut, Ian Grubb, Ralf Jurgens, and Paula Hacopian, "The Global Fund Annual Report 2010" (report, Global Fund to Fight AIDS,

Tuberculosis and Malaria, Geneva, May 2011). See also "PEPFAR Blueprint: Creating an AIDS-free Generation" (report, The Office of the Global AIDS Coordinator, Washington, DC, November 2012).

68. "Celebrating Life: The U.S. President's Emergency Plan for AIDS Relief" (Annual Report to Congress, Washington, DC, 2009), and "The Global Fund Annual Report 2009" (report, Global Fund to Fight AIDS, Tuberculosis and Malaria, Geneva May 2010).

69. For an overview of principal-agent theory and its application to international organizations, see Darren Hawkins, David Lake, Daniel Nielson, and Michael Tierney, "Delegation under Anarchy: States, International Organizations, and Principal-agent Theory," in *Delegation and Agency in International Organizations*, ed. Darren Hawkins, David Lake, Daniel Nielson, and Michael Tierney (Cambridge: Cambridge University Press, 2006), 3–38.

Chapter 2

1. Robert Keohane and Joseph Nye, *Power and Interdependence: World Politics in Transition* (Boston: Little, Brown, 1977).

2. This is discussed in regards to environmental cooperation by Oran Young and Gail Osherenko, "Testing Theories of Regime Formation: Findings from a Large Collaborative Research Project," in *Regime Theory and International Relations*, ed. Volker Rittberger and Peter Mayer (New York: Oxford University Press, 1993).

3. See Chelsea Clinton, "The Global Fund to Fight AIDS, TB and Malaria: A Response to Global Threats. A Part of a Global Future" (MPhil thesis, University of Oxford, 2003), 11–38.

4. Although Mearsheimer argues that this overstates the role of institutions. See John Mearsheimer, "The False Promise of International Institutions," *International Security*, no. 19 (Winter 1994): 5–49.

5. Martha Finnemore and Kathryn Sikkink, "International Norm Dynamics and Political Change," *International Organization*, no. 52 (Autumn 1998): 887–917.

6. Lawrence O. Gostin and Devi Sridhar, "Global Health Law," *NEJM*, no. 370 (May 2014): 1732–40.

7. Kenneth Abbott and Duncan Snidal, "Why States Act Through Formal International Organizations," *Journal of Conflict Resolution*, no. 42 (Winter 1998): 3–32.

8. Joseph Jupille and Duncan Snidal, "The Choice of International Institutions: Cooperation, Alternatives and Strategies" (annual meeting, American Political Science Association, Washington, DC, 2005).

9. Michael Barnett and Martha Finnemore, "The Politics, Power, and Pathologies of International Organizations," *International Organization*, no. 53 (Autumn 1999): 699–732.

10. Robert Keohane, *After Hegemony: Cooperation and Discord in the World Political Economy* (Princeton, NJ: Princeton University Press, 1984).

11. Institute for Health Metrics and Evaluation (IHME), "Financing Global Health 2014: Shifts in Funding as the MDG Era Closes," accessed 16 January 2016, http://www.healthdata.org/policy-report/financing-global-health-2014-shifts-funding-mdg-era-closes; Organization for Economic Cooperation and Development (OECD), "2012 DAC Report on Multilateral Aid," accessed 15 January 2016, http://www.oecd.org/dac/aid-architecture/DCD_DAC(2012)33_FINAL.pdf.

12. Authors' calculation using Institute for Health Metrics and Evaluation (IHME) raw data: IHME, "DAH by Sources of Funding, 1990–2014," accessed 2 August 2015, http://www.healthdata.org/sites/default/files/files/policy_report/2015/FGH2014/IHME_PolicyReport_FGH_2014_0.pdf, p. 18.

13. OECD, "2011 DAC Report on Multilateral Aid," accessed 15 January 2016, http://www.oecd.org/dac/aid-architecture/49014277.pdf, 5.

14. Ibid., 7–20.

15. See Roland Vaubel, "Principal-Agent Problems in International Organizations," Review International Organization, no. 1 (2006): 125–38.

16. See Darren Hawkins, David Lake, Daniel Nielson, and Michael Tierney, eds., Delegation and Agency in International Organizations (Cambridge: Cambridge University Press, 2006), 3–38.

17. As an example, Daniel Nielson and Michael Tierney, "Principals and Interests: Common Agency and Multilateral Development Bank Lending" (working paper, November 2006), http://ncgg.princeton.edu/IPES/2006/papers/nielson_tierney_F2006_1.pdf.

18. See Hawkins et al., Delegation and Agency, 3–38, for an overview of principal-agent theory and its application to international organizations.

19. Ibid.

20. According to Lyne et al. 2006, collective principals are "overwhelmingly the most common type we observe when analyzing IOs." See Mona Lyne, Daniel Nelson, and Michael Tierney, "Who Delegates? Alternative Models of Principals in Development Aid," in Hawkins, Delegation and Agency, 44.

21. Hawkins et al., Delegation and Agency, 4.

22. See Mark Pollack, "Principal-Agent Analysis and International Delegation: Red Herrings, Theoretical Clarifications, and Empirical Disputes" (paper, Workshop on Delegating Sovereignty, Duke University, 3–4 March 2006), http://papers.ssrn.com/sol3/papers.cfm?abstract_id=1011324.

23. Hawkins et al., Delegation and Agency, 8.

24. Mark Copelovitch, The International Monetary Fund in the Global Economy: Banks, Bonds, and Bailouts (Cambridge: Cambridge University Press, 2010), 44.

25. World Bank, "The World Bank Annual Report 2014," accessed 15 January 2016, https://openknowledge.worldbank.org/handle/10986/20093, 21.

26. Ibid., 59.

27. Authors' calculations based on "Disbursements," Global Fund, accessed 30 September 2015, http://www.theglobalfund.org/en/financials/.

28. Authors' calculations based on "Disbursements," Gavi, accessed 27 February 2016, http://www.gavi.org/results/disbursements/.

29. For example, relating to WHO: "Evaluation of WHO's Contribution to '3 by 5'" (main report, Geneva, 2006); relating to the World Bank: World Bank Independent Evaluation Group, "Improving Effectiveness and Outcomes for the Poor in Health, Nutrition and Population: An Evaluation of World Bank Group Support since 1997" (report, World Bank, Washington, DC, 2009); relating to the Global Fund: Chunling Lu, Catherine Michaud, Kashif Khan, and Christopher Murray, "Absorptive Capacity and Disbursements by the Global Fund to Fight AIDS, Tuberculosis and Malaria: Analysis of Grant Implementation," *Lancet*, no. 368 (August 2006): 483–88; relating to Gavi: Joseph Naimoli, "Global Health Partnerships in Practice: Taking Stock of the GAVI Alliance's New Investment in Health Systems Strengthening," *International Journal of Health Planning and Management*, no. 24 (Winter 2009): 3–25.

30. Niyi Awofeso, "Re-defining 'Health,'" *Bulletin of the World Health Organization*, no. 83 (2005): 802, accessed 15 January 2016, http://www.who.int/bulletin/bulletin_board/83/ustun11051/en.

31. Ibid.

32. "Declaration of Alma-Ata" (declaration, International Conference on Primary Health Care, Alma-Ata, USSR, 6–12 September 1978), accessed 21 January 2011, http://www.who.int/publications/almaata_declaration_en.pdf.

33. WHO and World Bank Group, "Tracking Universal Health Coverage: First Global Monitoring Report" (report, Geneva, June 2015), accessed 2 July 2015, http://www.who.int/healthinfo/universal_health_coverage/report/2015/en/; WHO, "Research for Universal Health Coverage: World Health Report 2013" (report, Geneva, August 2013), accessed 3 October 2015, http://www.who.int/whr/2013/report/en/.

34. Most recent search conducted 12 October 2015. Search terms included: World Health Organization Annual Report; WHO Annual Report; Links to two results referenced in n33: Lymphatic filariasis Annual reports, found at: "Lymphatic filariasis/Annual reports," WHO, accessed 12 October 2015, http://www.who.int/lymphatic_filariasis/resources/annual_reports/en/; World Cancer Report, found at: WHO, *World Cancer Report 2014* (Lyon: International Agency for Research on Cancer, 2014), http://www.iarc.fr/en/publications/books/wcr/.

35. WHO Executive Board, "Resolutions and Decisions" (136th session proceedings, Geneva, 26 January–3 February 2015), accessed 15 January 2016, http://apps.who.int/gb/ebwha/pdf_files/EB136-REC1/B136_REC1.pdf#page=21, 1–4.

36. See http://www.rollbackmalaria.org/, accessed 28 August 2015.

37. "Health: Overview," World Bank, accessed 30 September 2015, http://www.worldbank.org/en/topic/health/overview#3.

38. "Multi-Country HIV/AIDS Program for Africa (MAP)," World Bank, accessed 12 March 2012, http://web.worldbank.org/WBSITE/EXTERNAL/COUNTRIES/AFRICAEXT/EXTAFRHEANUTPOP/EXTAFRREGTOPHIVAIDS/0,,contentMDK:20415735~menuPK:1001234~pagePK:34004173~piPK:34003707~theSitePK:717148,00.html; "Meeting the Challenge: The World Bank and HIV/AIDS," World Bank, 3 April 2013, accessed 2 October 2015, http://www.worldbank.org/en/results/2013/04/03/hivaids-sector-results-profile.

39. See Desmond McNeill and Kristin Ingstad Sandberg, "Trust in Global Health Governance: The GAVI Experience," *Global Governance: A Review of Multilateralism and International Organizations*, no. 20 (Spring 2014): 325–43.

40. Thomas Weiss and Rorden Wilkinson, *International Organization and Global Governance* (New York: Routledge, 2014), 378 claim that Gavi and the Global Fund have in common the following features with traditional international organizations: "large staff, secretariat, and regionally based offices."

41. Gavi, "Disbursements."

42. Sarah Dykstra, Amanda Glassman, Charles Kenny, and Justin Sandefur, "Refocusing Gavi for Greater Impact" (brief, Center for Global Development, 9 September 2015), accessed 15 January 2016, http://www.cgdev.org/publication/ft/refocusing-Gavi-greater-impact.

43. "History of Gavi," Gavi, accessed 15 January 2016, http://www.Gavi.org/about/mission/history/.

44. "Global and Regional Immunization Profile," WHO, 18 December 2015, accessed 27 March 2016, http://www.who.int/immunization/monitoring_surveillance/data/gs_gloprofile.pdf?ua=1.

45. See "Board Composition," Gavi, accessed 15 January 2016, http://www.gavi.org/about/governance/gavi-board/composition/.

46. "New coverage figures show more children than ever being reached with immunization in poorest countries," Gavi, 17 July 2015, accessed 15 January 2016, http://www.gavi.org/Library/News/GAVI-features/2015/New-coverage-figures-show-more-children-than-ever-being-reached-with-immunisation-in-poorest-countries/.

47. "Home," Gavi, accessed 2 August 2014, http://www.gavi.org/.

48. Sarah Dykstra, Amanda Glassman, Charles Kenny, and Justin Sandefur, "Understanding Gavi's Impact on Vaccination Rates" (global health policy blog, Center for Global Development, 9 February 2015), accessed 15 January 2016, http://www.cgdev.org/blog/understanding-gavis-impact-vaccination-rates.

49. "Vaccines Boost Economic Growth in Poorest Countries," Gavi, accessed 15 January 2016, http://www.Gavi.org/library/news/roi/2010/vaccines-boost-economic-growth-in-poorest-countries/.

50. For example see, "Public Health's 'Best Buy,'" Gavi, accessed 2 May 2015, http://www.Gavi.org/about/value/cost-effective/.

51. Ibid.

52. "GAVI Impact on Vaccine Market Behind Price Drop," Gavi, accessed 15 January 2016, http://www.Gavi.org/library/news/roi/2010/Gavi-impact-on-vaccine-market-behind-price-drop/.

53. In disclosure, the Clinton Health Access Initiative (CHAI) has participated in multiple vaccine negotiations, including around the pentavalent and rotavirus vaccines. For more on CHAI's vaccine work, please visit http://www.clintonhealthaccess.org/history/initial-vaccines-work/.

54. Gavi, "2013–2014 Business Plan and Budget" (report to the Gavi Alliance Board, Geneva, 4–5 December 2012), 2.

55. Global Fund funding model evolved over time (see chapter 6). For more on the current (as of early 2016) funding model, please visit "Funding Model," Global Fund to Fight AIDS, Tuberculosis and Malaria, accessed 15 January 2016, http://www.theglobalfund.org/en/fundingmodel/.

56. "About WHO," WHO, accessed 15 January 2016, http://www.who.int/about/en/ and "How UNICEF works," UNICEF, accessed 15 January 2016, http://www.unicef.org/about/structure/index_structure.html.

57. The Fund uses "implementing" to describe countries and constituencies that receive its grants, rather than developing country or recipient.

58. "Financials," Global Fund to Fight AIDS, Tuberculosis and Malaria, accessed 1 October 2015, http://www.theglobalfund.org/en/financials/.

59. Global Fund to Fight AIDS, Tuberculosis and Malaria, "Results Report 2015" (report, Geneva, 2015).

60. Global Fund, "Annual Report 2010" (report, Geneva, May 2011). See also PEPFAR, "Blueprint for Creating an AIDS-free Generation" (Washington, DC: The Office of the Global AIDS Coordinator, 2012).

61. Department for International Development, "Multilateral Aid Review: Ensuring Maximum Value for Money for UK Aid Through Multilateral Organizations" (review, London, UK, March 2011), 187.

62. Global Fund, "Annual Report 2010," 4.

63. Authors' calculations: "The President's Emergency Plan for AIDS Relief (PEPFAR)," Henry J. Kaiser Family Foundation, 5 November 2015, accessed 5 December 2015, http://kff.org/global-health-policy/fact-sheet/the-u-s-presidents-emergency-plan-for/.

64. We principally rely on publicly available sources, including those from our selected case study institutions. These include, from each organization, selected Annual Reports; Board documents; Budgets; databases relating to

pledge and contribution amounts (particularly for WHO, Global Fund, Gavi); transparency policies; formal efforts to engage civil society; other pertinent information discoverable on their websites; databases relating to grants (particularly for the Global Fund and Gavi); documents relating to key performance indicators; and, independent evaluations, some done at the request of the institutions themselves (e.g., for the Global Fund, the independent High-Level Review Panel in 2011, and for the World Bank, reports from the Bank's Independent Evaluation Group). Additional key data sources include data compiled by IHME, as well as raw data from both the DAC statistics database and the activity-specific Creditor Reporting System (CRS), each as reported to the OECD. We also draw on, as relevant, Annual Reports and additional relevant publications from the Gates Foundation and PEPFAR, as well as extensive scholarly literature, particularly as relates to the Bank and WHO.

Chapter 3

1. Lawrence Gostin and Devi Sridhar, "Global Health Law," *NEJM*, no. 370 (May 2014): 1732–40.
2. Dr. Mark Dybul, Executive Director of the Global Fund, interview by authors, 3 June 2015.
3. Authors' assessment based on a review of all publicly available documents from the Transitional Working Group, June–December 2001. As of March 2016, most are accessible online: http://www.theglobalfund.org/en/archive/twg/.
4. "Board composition," Gavi, accessed 14 December 2015, http://www.Gavi.org/about/governance/Gavi-board/composition/.
5. "Top 100 U.S. Foundations by Asset Size," Foundation Center, accessed 21 September 2015, http://foundationcenter.org/findfunders/topfunders/top100assets.html.
6. Chevron, "Chevron Increases Total Investment to $55 Million in the Global Fund to Fight AIDS, Tuberculosis and Malaria: New Investment of $25 million Makes Chevron the Single Largest Private Sector Partner" (press release, 5 October 2010), accessed 25 February 2013, http://www.chevron.com/chevron/pressreleases/article/10052010_chevronincreasestotalinvestmentto55millionintheglobalfund.news.
7. "Funding Model—Eligibility," Global Fund, accessed 14 December 2015, http://www.theglobalfund.org/en/fundingmodel/process/eligibility/.
8. "Funding Model–Allocations," Global Fund, accessed 14 December 2015, http://www.theglobalfund.org/en/fundingmodel/process/allocations/.
9. Authors' count based on information available at: http://www.theglobalfund.org/en/fundingmodel/process/eligibility/. The Russian Federation is an example of a transition country, as it is receiving HIV/AIDS grant funding under the Global Fund's NGO Rule. Russia is not eligible to apply for new Global Fund grants.

10. Gavi, "Gavi Independent Review Committee Report New Proposals March 2015," accessed 3 February 2016, www.**gavi**.org/library/**gavi**-documents/irc-reports/final-report-for-irc-march-2015/.

11. Gavi, "Countries Eligible for Support," accessed 15 June 2015, http://www.gavi.org/support/apply/countries-eligible-for-support/.

12. Devi Sridhar and Ngaire Woods, "Trojan Multilateralism: Global Cooperation in Health," *Global Policy* 4, no. 4 (November 2013): 325–35.

13. Ibid.

14. Michael H. Merson, "The HIV-AIDS Pandemic at 25—The Global Response," *NEJM*, no. 354 (June 2006): 2414–17, http://www.nejm.org/doi/full/10.1056/NEJMp068074#t=article.

15. GPA Management Committee, "Report of the Ad Hoc Working Group of the GPA Management Committee" (report, WHO, Geneva, 1992).

16. Ruth Levine, Ngaire Woods, Danielle Kuczynski, and Devi Sridhar, "UNAIDS: Preparing for the Future" (report, UNAIDS Leadership Transition Working Group, Center for Global Development, Washington, DC, 2009).

17. "Composition of the Programme Coordinating Board (PCB) 1 January to 31 December 2015," UNAIDS, accessed 14 December 2015, http://www.unaids.org/sites/default/files/sub_landing/PCB_Members_1January2015_en.pdf.

18. Levine et al., "UNAIDS: Preparing for the Future," 2009.

19. Transitional Working Group, "First Meeting of the Transitional Working Group to Establish a Global Fund to Fight AIDS, Tuberculosis, and Malaria, Brussels, 11–12 October 2001" (report, Brussels, Belgium, 2001).

20. It is clear from the Transitional Working Group documents that its members, including donors, never considered the Bank as a potential home for what emerged as the Global Fund. Certain unnamed Working Group members even expressed skepticism about the Bank's ability to act as the Fund's fiduciary agent and wanted a stronger separation between the Fund and the Bank. For more, see the Transitional Working Group documents available at http://www.theglobalfund.org/en/archive/twg/ (accessed 28 June 2016).

21. United Nations, "Secretary-General Proposes Global Fund for Fight Against HIV/AIDS and Other Infectious Diseases at African Leaders Summit" (press release, Secretary-General Kofi Annan, 26 April 2001), accessed 15 January 2016, http://www.un.org/press/en/2001/SGSM7779R1.doc.htm.

22. Ruairi Brugha et al., "The Global Fund: Managing Great Expectations," *Lancet*, no. 364 (July 2004): 95–100.

23. DFID, "Multilateral Aid Review: Ensuring Maximum Value for Money for UK Aid Through Multilateral Organisations," March 2011.

24. Ibid.

25. DFID, "Multilateral Aid Review: Taking Forward the Findings of the UK Multilateral Aid Review" (report, London, March 2011), accessed 15 January 2016, https://www.gov.uk/government/uploads/system/uploads/attachment_data/file/224993/MAR-taking-forward.pdf.

26. Ibid., 15.

27. Darren Hawkins, David Lake, Daniel Nielson, and Michael Tierney, "Delegation under Anarchy: States, International Organizations, and Principal-agent Theory," in *Delegation and Agency in International Organizations*, ed. Darren Hawkins, David Lake, Daniel Nielson, and Michael Tierney (Cambridge: Cambridge University Press, 2006), 3–38.

28. DFID, "Multilateral Aid Review: Taking Forward the Findings," 15.

29. Patrick Goodenough, "U.K. Becomes Latest Donor Country to Withdraw from U.N. Development Agency," *CNSNews.com*, http://www.cnsnews.com/news/article/uk-becomes-latest-donor-country-withdraw-un-development-agency 2 March 2011, accessed 15 January 2016, http://www.cnsnews.com/news/article/uk-becomes-latest-donor-country-withdraw-un-development-agency.

30. WHO, "The Future of Financing for WHO: Report of an Informal Consultation Convened by the Director-General" (report, Geneva, 2010), accessed 15 January 2016, http://www.who.int/dg/future_financing/who_dgo_2010_1/en/index.html.

31. Piera Tortora and Suzanne Steensen, "Making Earmarked Funding More Effective: Current Practices and a Way Forward" (report, OECD Development Co-operation Directorate, 2014), 8, accessed 14 December 2015, http://www.oecd.org/dac/aid-architecture/Multilateral%20Report%20N%201_2014.pdf.

32. International Development Association, "Additions to IDA: Thirteenth Replenishment" (report, Washington, DC, September 2002), 77, accessed 10 January 2016, http://www.worldbank.org/ida/papers/IDA13_Replenishment/FinaltextIDA13Report.pdf; International Development Association, "Table 1: Contributions to the Sixteenth Replenishment" (report, Washington, DC, March 2011), accessed 10 January 2016, http://www.worldbank.org/ida/papers/IDA16_Donor_Contributions_Table_1.pdf.

33. Catherine Gwin, "U.S. Relations with the World Bank, 1945–1992," in *The World Bank: Its First Half Century*, ed. Devesh Kapur, John Lewis, and Richard Webb (Washington, DC: Brookings Institution, 1997), 1150.

34. "Gavi Pledging Conference June 2011," Gavi, accessed 14 December 2015, http://www.gavi.org/funding/how-gavi-is-funded/resource-mobilisation-process/gavi-pledging-conference-june-2011/.

35. Gavi, "Immunisation's Vital Role in UN Health Strategy" (press release, 6 October 2010), accessed 15 January 2016, http://www.gavi.org/Library/News/Press-releases/2010/Immunisation-s-vital-role-in-UN-health-strategy/.

36. Global Fund, "Resource Mobilization," accessed 11 June 2016, http://www.theglobalfund.org/en/replenishment/.

37. Aidspan, "Global Fund Inspector General," *Global Fund Observer Newsletter*, no. 43 (24 April 2005).

38. Sarah Boseley, "Can the Global Fund Weather the Corruption Storm?," *Guardian,* 28 January 2011, accessed 15 January 2016, http://www.theguardian.com/society/sarah-boseley-global-health/2011/jan/28/aids-infectiousdiseases.

39. Sridhar and Woods, "Trojan Multilateralism", 325–35.

40. "Expert Advisory Panels and Committees," World Health Organization, accessed 15 January 2016, http://www.who.int/rpc/expert_panels/Factsheet_EAP2010.pdf.

41. Author's own calculation based on TRP reports through 2014 alongside the relevant Global Fund Board minutes. TRP reports available at http://www.theglobalfund.org/en/trp/.

42. Steven Radelet and Bilal Siddiqi, "Global Fund Grant Programmes: An Analysis of Evaluation Scores," *Lancet*, no. 369 (26 May–1 June 2007): 1807–13 as well as author's own literature review through December 2015.

43. "Technical Review Panel–Members," Global Fund, accessed 28 November 2015, http://www.theglobalfund.org/en/trp/members/.

44. Author's own calculations based on the IRC reports through 2014 alongside the relevant Gavi Board (legacy and consolidated Gavi) minutes. IRC reports available at http://www.gavi.org/support/apply/independent-review-committee/.

45. Sridhar and Woods, "Trojan Multilateralism," 325–35.

46. Jonathan Bendor, Amihai Glazer, and Thomas Hammond, "Theories of Delegation," *Annual Review of Political Science*, no. 4 (June 2001): 235–69.

47. DFID, "Multilateral Aid Review: Ensuring Maximum Value for Money," 54.

48. GAO, "Global Fund to Fight AIDS, TB and Malaria Has Improved Its Documentation of Funding Decisions but Needs Standardized Oversight Expectations and Assessments" (report to Congressional Committees, Washington, DC, May 2007), accessed 15 January 2016, http://www.gao.gov/products/GAO-07-627.

49. Authors' review of all WHO Executive Board participants' lists, conducted on 29 June 2016, available at http://apps.who.int/gb/gov/.

50. This challenge has been in existence since the creation of WHO. See Charles Ascher, "Current Problems in the World Health Organization's Program," *International Organization*, no. 6 (February 1952): 27–50.

51. Gavin Yamey, "Have the Latest Reforms Reversed WHO's Decline?" *BMJ*, no. 325 (November 2002): 1107.

52. Ngaire Woods, *The Globalizers: The IMF, the World Bank, and Their Borrowers* (Ithaca, NY: Cornell University Press, 2006).

53. Ibid.

54. Daniel Nelson and Michael Tierney, "Delegation to International Organizations: Agency Theory and World Bank Environmental Reform," *International Organization*, no. 57 (Spring 2003): 243. For a full treatment of the politics of the Inspection Panel, see Theresa Bridgeman, "Accountable to Whom? The World Bank and Its Inspection Panel 1994–2004" (DPhil thesis, University of Oxford, 2011).

55. DFID, "Multilateral Aid Review: Ensuring Maximum Value for Money," 55.

56. Ibid., 175.

57. Ibid., 177.

58. Ibid., 206.

59. Gates Foundation, "2013 Annual Report," accessed 1 May 2015, http://www.gatesfoundation.org/Who-We-Are/Resources-and-Media/Annual-Reports/Annual-Report-2013; this definition excludes other programs impacting on health delivered by the Gates Foundation Global Development Team.

60. UNAIDS, "Health 8 Group Meet to Discuss Maximizing Health Outcomes With Available Resources and Getting 'More Health for the Money'" (feature story, 23 February 2011), accessed 7 August 2015, http://www.unaids.org/en/resources/presscentre/featurestories/2011/february/20110223bh8.

61. Dybul, interview, 3 June 2015.

62. Gates Foundation, "The Bill & Melinda Gates Foundation Announces New $776 Million Investment in Nutrition to Tackle Child Mortality and Help All Women and Children Survive and Thrive" (press release and statement, Brussels, Belgium, 3 June 2015), accessed 1 August 2015, http://www.gatesfoundation.org/Media-Center/Press-Releases/2015/06/Nutrition-Strategy-Launch.

63. Susan Okie, "Global Health—The Gates-Buffett Effect," *NEJM*, no. 355 (September 2006): 1084–88.

64. "What We Do–Integrated Delivery: Strategy Overview," Gates Foundation, accessed 5 July 2015, http://www.gatesfoundation.org/What-We-Do/Global-Development/Integrated-Delivery.

65. David McCoy, Gayatri Kembhavi, Jinesh Patel, and Akish Luintel, "The Bill & Melinda Gates Foundation's Grant-Making Programme for Global Health," *Lancet*, no. 373 (May 2009): 1645–53.

66. Devi Sridhar and Rajaie Batniji, "Misfinancing Global Health: A Case for Transparency in Disbursements and Decision Making," *Lancet*, no. 372 (September 2008): 1185–91.

67. Aside from McCoy et al., "Gates Foundation's Grant-Making Programme for Global Health," and Sridhar and Batniji, "Misfinancing Global Health."

68. Anne-Emanuelle Birn, "Gates's Grandest Challenge: Transcending Technology as Public Health Ideology," *Lancet*, no. 366 (March 2005):

515–19; Katerini Storeng, "The GAVI Alliance and the 'Gates Approach' to Health System Strengthening," *Global Public Health*, no. 9 (August 2014): 865–79.

69. Tamara Hafner and Jeremy Shiffman, "The Emergence of Global Attention to Health Systems Strengthening," *Health Policy and Planning*, no. 28 (2013): 41–50.

70. Marine Kiromera, "Investigating the Bill and Melinda Gates Foundation's Funding Policies for Child Health Research from 2005–2014" (MPH diss., University of Edinburgh, 2015); Gabrielle Geonnotti, "Investigating how the Bill and Melinda Gates Foundation Has Invested in Global Child Health Research from 2005–2014" (MPH diss., University of Edinburgh, 2015). See also fig. 3.10.

71. Robert Black, Maharaj Bhan, Mickey Chopra, Igor Rudan, and Cesar Victoria, "Accelerating the Health Impact of the Gates Foundation," *Lancet*, no. 373 (2009): 1584–85.

72. Kiromera, "Investigating...Funding Policies for Child Health Research" and Geonnotti, "Investigating...Global Child Health Research."

73. Jef Leroy, Jean-Pierre Habicht, Gretel Pelto, and Stefano Bertozzi, "Current Priorities in Health Research Funding and Lack of Impact on the Number of Child Deaths per Year," *American Journal of Public Health*, no. 97 (February 2007): 219–23.

74. Ibid.

75. Black et al., "Accelerating the Health Impact."

76. "What We Do—Integrated Delivery: Strategy Overview," Gates Foundation.

77. Storeng, "The GAVI Alliance," *Global Public Health*, 865–79.

Chapter 4

1. IHME, "Financing Global Health 2014: Shifts in Funding as the MDG Era Closes" (report, Seattle, 2015), 81 and 97.

2. World Bank Group, "Aid Architecture: An Overview of the Main Trends in Official Development Assistance Flows," in "Brief History of Aid Institutions" (paper, Washington, DC, 2007), 2–3.

3. Authors' calculations using raw data available from OECD, "Compare Your country: Official Development Assistance 1960–2014," accessed 30 September 2015, http://www.compareyourcountry.org/oda?cr=20001&cr1=oecd&lg=en&page=1.

4. IHME, "Financing Global Health 2014," 9.

5. Christopher Murray, "Shifting to Sustainable Development Goals— Implications for Global Health," *NEJM*, no. 373 (2015): 1393.

6. See discussion of WHO's budget cycle in Kelley Lee, *The World Health Organization (WHO)*, Global Institutions (London: Routledge, 2008), 41–42.

7. IDA and the Global Fund hold replenishments every three years, Gavi every four years.

8. IHME, "Financing Global Health 2012: The End of the Golden Age?" (report, Seattle, 2012).

9. Chelsea Clinton, "The Global Fund to Fight AIDS, TB and Malaria: A Response to Global Threats. A Part of a Global Future" (MPhil thesis, University of Oxford, 2003); Seth Berkley, CEO of Gavi (phone interview, 13 March 2015).

10. Global Fund to Fight AIDS, Tuberculosis and Malaria, "The Framework Document of the Global Fund to Fight AIDS, Tuberculosis and Malaria: Title, Purpose, Principles, and Scope of the Fund" (Geneva, 2002).

11. See Howard Friedman, "Casual Inference and the Millennium Development Goals (MDGs): Assessing Whether There Was an Acceleration in MDG Development Indicators Following the MDG Declaration" (working paper, Munich Personal RePEc Archive, August 2013), https://mpra.ub.uni-muenchen.de/48793/1/MPRA_paper_48793.pdf.

12. For one example of such influence, see Kirstin Matthews and Vivian Ho, "The Grand Impact of the Gates Foundation. Sixty Billion Dollars and One Famous Person Can Affect the Spending and Research Focus of Public Agencies," *EMBO Reports*, no. 9 (May 2008): 409–12, http://www.ncbi.nlm.nih.gov/pmc/articles/PMC2373372/.

13. "Source and Distribution of Funds Available/Contributors/Bill & Melinda Gates Foundation," WHO, accessed 2 October 2015, http://extranet.who.int/programmebudget/Biennium2014/Contributor.

14. "Assessed Contribution Status Report, as of 31 December 2015," WHO, accessed 16 June 2016, http://www.who.int/about/resources_planning/AC_Status_Report_2015.pdf?ua=1. and "Assessed Contribution Status Report, as of 31 December 2014," WHO, accessed 16 June 2016,http://www.who.int/about/resources_planning/AC_Status_Report_2014.pdf?ua=1.

15. WHO membership as of 27 October 2015. Please see http://www.who.int/countries/en/.

16. Fiona Godlee, "WHO in Retreat: Is It losing Its Influence?" *BMJ* (December 1994): 1491, accessed 27 October 2014, http://www.bmj.com/content/309/6967/1491; the WHO secretariat has, over the years, made multiple proposals to the WHA that all, or at least half, of membership dues be assessed in Swiss Francs given that a significant portion of WHO's costs are in Swiss Francs given the location of its headquarters in Geneva. As of early 2016, a portion of certain assessments are denominated in Swiss Francs. As one such example of proposals for the greater adoption of Swiss Francs as a core currency for WHO membership assessments, see the World Health Organization, "Scale of assessments for 2014–2015: Foreign exchange risk management" (report by the Secretariat, 66th World Health Assembly, 22 March 2013), http://apps.who.int/gb/ebwha/pdf_files/WHA66/A66_32-en.pdf.

17. Timothy Mackey and Thomas Novotny, "Improving United Nations Funding to Strengthen Global Health Governance: Amending the

Helms—Biden Agreement," *Global Health Governance*, no. 6 (Autumn 2012), accessed 13 January 2016, http://blogs.shu.edu/ghg/files/2012/12/GHGJ-VOLUME-VI-ISSUE-1-FALL-2012-Improving-United-Nations-Funding-to-Strengthen-Global-Health-Governance-Amending-the-Helms-Biden-Agreement.pdf, http://blogs.shu.edu/ghg/files/2012/12/GHGJ-VOLUME-VI-ISSUE-1-FALL-2012-Improving-United-Nations-Funding-to-Strengthen-Global-Health-Governance-Amending-the-Helms—-Biden-Agreement.pdf.

18. For a discussion of what motivated the US position on freezing real budget funds (RBFs) throughout the UN system, such as concerns over bloated budgets, see Brett Schaefer, "The History of the Bloated UN Budget: How the U.S. Can Rein It In" (report, Heritage Foundation, 2 April 2012), http://www.heritage.org/research/reports/2012/04/the-history-of-the-bloated-un-budget-how-the-us-can-rein-it-in.

19. Lester Brown, Michael Renner, and Christopher Flavin, *Vital Signs 1998: The Environmental Trends That Are Shaping Our Future* (New York: W. W. Norton, 1998), 82.

20. HIV/AIDS was first clinically observed in 1981.

21. WHO's essential medicines list includes those that WHO determines "satisfy the priority health care needs" of a country's population and "are intended to be available within the context of functioning health systems at all times…at a price the individual and community can afford." Although WHO has long positioned the essential medicines list as a "guide" and not a global standard, it is often viewed as such. For more information, see "Essential Medicines and Health Products," WHO, accessed 28 October 2015, http://www.who.int/medicines/services/essmedicines_def/en/.

22. Godlee, "WHO in Retreat," 1492.

23. Halfdan Mahler, Director-General of WHO, "World Health For All" (speech, 40th World Health Assembly, 5 May 1987), as quoted in Nitsan Chorev, *The World Health Organization: Between North and South* (Ithaca, NY: Cornell University Press, 2012), 144–45.

24. Yves Beigbeder, Mahyar Nashat, Marie-Antoinette Orsini, and Jean-Francois Tiercy, *The World Health Organization* (Boston: Martinus Nijhoff Publishers, 1998), 163.

25. Theodore Brown, Marcos Cueto, and Elizabeth Fee, "The World Health Organization and the Transition from 'International' to 'Global' Public Health," *American Journal of Public Health*, no. 96 (January 2006): 62–72, accessed 17 July 2015, http://www.ncbi.nlm.nih.gov/pmc/articles/PMC1470434/#r36.

26. Beigbeder et al., *World Health Organization*, 163, and WHO, "Proposed Programme Budget for the Financial Period 1996–1997: Cost Increases" (report by the Director-General, Executive Board, 95th sess., 14 December 1994), accessed 13 January 2016, http://apps.who.int/iris/bitstream/10665/172125/1/EB95_21_eng.pdf.

27. "Annex 1, Figure 1. Rate of collection of contributions, Percentage collected as of 31 December, from 1991 to 2000" in WHO, "Status of Collection of Assessed Contributions, Including Members in Arrears to an Extent Which Would Justify Invoking Article 7 of the Constitution" (report by the Director-General, 107th sess., Geneva, 11 January 2001), http://apps.who.int/gb/archive/pdf_files/EB107/ee10.pdf.

28. WHO, "Status of Collection of Assessed Contributions, Including Members in Arrears to an Extent Which Would Justify Invoking Article 7 of the Constitution" (report of the Administration, Budget, and Finance Committee of the Executive Board, 52nd World Health Assembly, 18 May 1999), http://apps.who.int/gb/archive/pdf_files/WHA52/ew27.pdf.

29. Elizabeth Olson, "Other Nations Balk at Picking Up Tab: UN Health Agency Reduces U.S. Dues," *New York Times*, 23 May 2001, accessed 7 July 2015, http://www.nytimes.com/2001/05/23/news/23iht-who_ed3_.html.

30. WHO, "Status of Collection of Assessed Contributions, Including Members in Arrears in the Payment of Their Contributions to an Extent Which Would Justify Invoking Article 7 of the Constitution" (report by the Secretariat, 21st meeting of the Administration, Budget, and Finance Committee of the Executive Board, 7 May 2004), http://www.who.int/governance/eb/committees/EBABFC21_2-en.pdf.

31. WHO, "Status of Collection of Assessed Contributions, Including Members in Arrears in the Payment of Their Contributions to an Extent Which Would Justify Invoking Article 7 of the Constitution" (report by the Secretariat, 68th World Health Assembly, 10 April 2015), http://apps.who.int/gb/ebwha/pdf_files/WHA68/A68_39-en.pdf.

32. Dr. Gro Harlem Brundtland, Director-General elect, "Speech to the 51st World Health Assembly" (speech, Geneva, 13 May 1998), http://apps.who.int/gb/archive/pdf_files/WHA51/eadiv6.pdf.

33. As cited in Kelley Lee, *World Health Organization*, 40.

34. Ibid., 40 (through 2007) and then authors' analyses of WHO's budgets and audited financial statements through December 2014.

35. Authors' calculations based on raw data available in: World Health Organization, "Annex to the Financial Report for the year ended 31 December 2014, Voluntary contributions by fund and by contributor" (document, 68th World Health Assembly, 1 May 2015) and World Health Organization, "Financial Report and Audited Financial Statements for the year ended 31 December 2014" (provisional agenda item, 68th World Health Assembly, 24 April 2015).

36. United Nations, "Funding for United Nations Development Cooperation: Challenges and Options," 13, accessed 4 December 2015, http://www.un.org/esa/coordination/Funding_for_United_Nations_Development_Cooperation.pdf.

37. As noted in "The World Health Organization (WHO): Budget Challenges and the 2014 Ebola Outbreak," Council on Foreign Relations, accessed 2 January 2015, http://www.cfr.org/public-health-threats-and-pandemics/world-health-organization-/p20003.

38. Fiona Godlee, "The World Health Organisation: WHO in Crisis," *BMJ*, no. 309 (November 1994): 1424, accessed 27 October 2014, http://www.bmj.com/content/309/6966/1424.

39. Laurie Garrett, "Ebola's Lessons: How the WHO Mishandled the Crisis," *Foreign Affairs*, September/October 2015, accessed 20 August 2015, https://www.foreignaffairs.com/articles/west-africa/2015-08-18/ebolas-lessons?campaign=Garrett.

40. WHO, "Programme Budget 2012–2013: Performance Assessment Report" (document, Geneva, October 2014), 10–11, http://www.who.int/about/resources_planning/HQPRP14.1_PBPA2012-2013.pdf.

41. In the 2012–2013 Programme Budget and associated Performance Assessment Report, noncommunicable diseases are combined with injuries (strategic objective 3). As a result, we have grouped them together in the description of percentages of assessed and voluntary contributions.

    (SO1 + SO2)=Infectious diseases
    (SO3)=Noncommunicable diseases and injuries
    (SO = WHO Strategic Objective 1, 2, 3)

42. WHO, "Programme Budget 2012–2013: Performance Assessment Report," accessed 13 January 2016, http://www.who.int/about/resources_planning/HQPRP14.1_PBPA2012-2013.pdf.

43. As one example, see Muhammad Yussuf, Juan Luis Larrabure, and Cihan Terzi, "Voluntary Contributions in United Nations System Organizations: Impact on Programme Delivery and Resource Mobilization Strategies" (report, United Nations Joint Inspection Unit, Geneva, 2007), 13, accessed 2 October 2015, https://www.unjiu.org/en/reports-notes/archive/JIU_REP_2007_1_English.pdf.

44. According to WHO, "just 7% of all voluntary contributions from the 2014–2015 biennium have been made to the Core Voluntary Contributions Account." Cited from "Voluntary Contributions," WHO, accessed 2 October 2015, http://www.who.int/about/finances-accountability/funding/voluntary-contributions/en/.

45. According to WHO Budget and Contribution data from 2000 to 2015 available through: "Funding WHO," WHO, accessed 30 October 2015, http://www.who.int/about/finances-accountability/funding/en/. As one example, see WHO, "Annex to the Financial Report and Audited Financial Statements for the year end 31 December 2013" (document, 67th World Health Assembly, 17 April 2014).

46. Peter Piot, *No Time to Lose: A Life in Pursuit of Deadly Viruses* (New York: W. W. Norton, 2013).

47. Most recent biennial for which we have complete contribution data (versus only budget predictions).

48. "The World Health Organization," Gavi, accessed 9 April 2016, http://www.gavi.org/about/partners/who/.

49. "Financing WHO's Programme Budget," WHO, accessed 2 December 2014, http://www.who.int/about/funding/financing_the_pb/en/.

50. Authors' calculation using a basic CAGR formula and the WHO 2014–2015 Approved Budget.

51. See United Nations, "Resolution No. 67/238" (agenda item, 67th sess., General Assembly of the United Nations, 24 December 2012), accessed 13 January 2016, http://www.un.org/en/ga/67/resolutions.shtml. In accordance with Resolution No. 55/235, peacekeeping assessments are largely based on the relative scale of assessments for member states as relates to the UN's general budget.

52. Cristian Baeza, director, Health, Nutrition and Population, World Bank, "The World Bank in Health 2012: Challenges, Priorities, and Role in the Global Health Aid Architecture" (presentation, 31 January 2012), 5; IHME, "Financing Global Health 2014," 122.

53. When these efforts were unsuccessful, China announced a new Asian Development Bank in which it would have a significantly greater stake (and voting power).

54. World Bank, "Annual Report 2013," 48, accessed 13 January 2016, http://siteresources.worldbank.org/EXTANNREP2013/ Resources/9304887-1377201212378/9305896-1377544753431/1_ AnnualReport2013_EN.pdf.

55. As of October 2015, there are eighty-five countries that qualify for IBRD loans. For the most recent list, see: "Country and Lending Groups," World Bank, accessed 13 January 2016, http://data.worldbank.org/about/ country-and-lending-groups#IBRD.

56. As of October 2015, there are seventy-seven countries that qualify for IDA grants, credits, and loans. For the most recent list, see "Country and Lending Groups," The World Bank, accessed 13 January 2016, http://data.worldbank.org/about/country-and-lending-groups#IDA.

57. Sarah Tenney and Anne Salda, *Historical Dictionary of the World Bank* (Lanham, MD: Scarecrow Press, 2014), 149.

58. Independent Evaluation Group, "World Bank Group Support to Health Financing" (report, World Bank, Washington, DC, July 2014), 24, accessed 14 January 2016, http://ieg.worldbank.org/Data/reports/chapters/ health_fin_app_all1.pdf.

59. World Bank Fiscal Years run from 1 July of the previous year (2013 in this instance) to 30 June of the following year (2014).

60. Authors' calculations drawn from lending data by sector included in World Bank, "Annual Report 2014," 59, accessed 13 January 2016, https://openknowledge.worldbank.org/handle/10986/2127.

61. See comparisons of FY2010–FY2014 in World Bank, "Annual Report 2014," 59.

62. Kelley Lee and Jennifer Fang, *Historical Dictionary of the World Health Organization* (Lanham, MD: Scarecrow Press, 2013), 24.

63. Ibid., 25.

64. World Bank, "Annual Report 2000: Annual review and summary financial information," 33, accessed 13 January 2016, http://www-wds .worldbank.org/external/default/WDSContentServer/WDSP/IB/2001/03/ 07/000094946_01021605430221/Rendered/PDF/multi_page.pdf.

65. Baeza, "The World Bank in Health 2012," 6.

66. Ibid., 5.

67. World Bank, "Healthy Development: The World Bank Strategy for Health, Nutrition, and Population Results" (document, Washington, DC, 24 April 2007), accessed 13 January 2016, http://siteresources. worldbank.org/HEALTHNUTRITIONANDPOPULATION/ Resources/281627-1154048816360/HNPStrategyFINALApril302007.pdf.

68. As one example, see World Bank, "Financing Health Services in Developing Countries: An Agenda for Reform" (policy study, Washington, DC, 1987).

69. WHO, "Macroeconomics and Health: Investing in Health for Economic Development" (report of the Commission on Macroeconomics and Health, Geneva, 2001).

70. See new HNP thematic lending by theme and region at "World Bank HNP Lending," World Bank, accessed 13 January 2016, http://datatopics .worldbank.org/hnp/worldbanklending.

71. Independent Evaluation Group, "Results and Performance of the World Bank Group 2014: An Independent Evaluation, Appendixes," 11 February 2015, 28.

72. Evidence to Policy Initiative, "PROFILE: The World Bank," February 2013, 5.

73. In 2013, administrative fees and expenses related to trust funds amounted to $218 million. See World Bank Group, "2013 Trust Fund Annual Report" (report, Washington, DC, 4 April 2015), 56, accessed 13 January 2016, http://siteresources.worldbank.org/CFPEXT/ Resources/299947-1274110249410/CFP_TFAR_AR13_High.pdf.

74. Jeff Tyson, "The World Bank's New Approach to Trust Funds," *Devex*, 12 February 2015, https://www.devex.com/news/the-world-bank-s-new- approach-to-trust-funds-85477.

75. World Bank Group, "2013 Trust Fund Annual Report," 25.

76. Ibid., 65.

77. Bretton Woods Project, "World Bank Trust Funds," 31 March 2015, accessed 18 April 2016, http://www.brettonwoodsproject.org/2015/03/ world-bank-trust-funds/.

78. World Bank Group, "2013 Trust Fund Annual Report," 30.

79. Funded by Norway and the UK, the HRITF is financed at an expected level of $575 million from inception in 2007 through 2022.

80. World Bank Group, "2013 Trust Fund Annual Report," 30.

81. Total commitments were yielded from the addition of World Bank "New IBRD/IDA HNP Thematic Commitments" and "Summary of Contributions to Financial Intermediary Funds" (finances section). The

calculation of trust fund contributions to health commitments relied solely on financial intermediary funds (FIFs). In an attempt to develop a more holistic picture of trust fund commitments, we examined the World Bank's website, annual report, and annual trust fund report. The only fund for which we found quantifiable health data was the FIF; "World Bank HNP Lending," World Bank, accessed 13 January 2016, http://datatopics.worldbank.org/hnp/worldbanklending; "Summary of Contributions to Financial Intermediary Funds," World Bank, accessed 13 January 2016, http://data.worldbank.org/topic/health.

82. See the finances section of: "Finances," World Bank, accessed 13 January 2016, http://data.worldbank.org/topic/health.

83. Piera Tortora and Suzanne Steensen, "Making Earmarked Funding More Effective: Current Practices and a Way Forward" (report, OECD, 2014), accessed 4 January 2016, https://www.oecd.org/dac/aid-architecture/Multilateral%20Report%20N%201_2014.pdf.

84. For example, through Debt2Health, a Fund program in which creditor countries, like Germany, "swap" the debt principal and interest of a debtor country, like Tanzania, for domestic investment in HIV/AIDS, TB, malaria, or health systems strengthening.

85. Authors' calculations based on raw Global Fund contribution data 2000–2014: "Financials," Global Fund, accessed 2 December 2014, http://www.theglobalfund.org/en/financials/.

86. Chelsea Clinton, "The Global Fund: An Experiment in Global Governance" (DPhil diss., University of Oxford, 2014), 46–48.

87. Authors' calculations.

88. The British prime minister Gordon Brown initially proposed an international financing facility for the Fund, not Gavi. Although Aidspan reported some donor support and the idea was discussed by the Board in 2005, the Board never formally voted on it. For more on Brown's original conceptualization, see Bernard Rivers, "Brown and Chirac Propose New Ideas to Finance the Global Fund," *Global Fund Observer Newsletter* (February 2005).

89. This tension was subsequently addressed early in its second decade.

90. Global Fund to Fight AIDS, Tuberculosis and Malaria, "Turning the Page from Emergency to Sustainability: Final Report of the High-Level Independent Review Panel on Fiduciary Controls and Oversight Mechanisms of the Global Fund to Fight AIDS, Tuberculosis and Malaria" (report, Washington, DC, 19 September 2011), 9.

91. "Private & NGO Partners, (RED)," Global Fund, accessed 8 March 2016, http://www.theglobalfund.org/en/privatengo/red/.

92. As one example, see Juan Manuel Suarez del Toro, then-president of the International Federation of Red Cross and Red Crescent Societies (speech to United Nations General Assembly, 2003), accessed 8 July 2012, http://www.ifrc.org/en/news-and-media/press-releases/general/federation-

president-calls-for-equitable-contributions-framework-to-sustain-global-fund-for-hivaids/. This concept first found formal expression in a 1970 UN Resolution. Similar to the Fund's focus on aid effectiveness, much of the dialogue in the 2000s centered on effectiveness, as seen in the 2005 Paris Declaration on Aid Effectiveness and subsequent High-Level Forums in Accra (2008) and Busan (2011).

93. At least not one reflected in the Board record. The clearest example of this is what the Secretariat published on the Fund's website in advance of the 2005 Rome replenishment meeting, accessed 2 January 2011, http://www.theglobalfund.org/en/about/replenishment/rome.

94. Authors' analysis of all Global Fund Board minutes through the first twenty-eight Board meetings.

95. For a good history of Gavi and UNITAID's bilateral origins and then more inclusive and staff-driven evolution, see Philippe Douste-Blazy, coordinator, "Innovative Financing For Development: The I-8 Group Leading Innovative Financing for Equity (LIFE)" (report, United Nations, New York, 2009).

96. Authors' calculations based on Global Fund raw pledges and contributions data, through 2013, accessed 24 May 2015, http://www.theglobalfund.org/en/donors/.

97. In 2014, 28 percent of its funding came from philanthropic foundations and private individuals. See International AIDS Vaccine Initiative, "Annual Report 2014," accessed 5 September 2015, https://www.iavi.org/annual_reports/2014.

98. Dr. Mark Dybul, Executive Director of the Global Fund (interview by authors, 3 June 2015).

99. Ibid.

100. Clinton, "The Global Fund: An Experiment," 318–19.

101. All based on authors' calculations, using "Annual Donor Contributions to Gavi, 2000-2033, as of 31 March 2014," Gavi, The Vaccine Alliance, accessed 12 September 2014, http://www.gavi.org/funding/donor-contributions-pledges/.

102. Gavi raw data, cash contributions 2000–2013, authors' calculations.

103. Authors' calculations of Gavi raw data, cash contributions 2000–2013, and Gavi, The Vaccine Alliance, "GAVI Alliance Annual Financial Report 2013" (report, Geneva, September 2014), 12–13.

104. Gavi, "GAVI Alliance Annual Financial Report 2013." and "Funding and finance," Gavi, accessed 7 July 2012, http://www.gavialliance.org/funding/; Gavi, The Vaccine Alliance, "Cash received by GAVI 2000–2010," 31 December 2010, accessed 3 May 2013, http://www.gavialliance.org/funding/donor-contributions-pledges/.

105. HIV Vaccines and Microbicides Resource Tracking Working Group, "Investing to End the AIDS Epidemic: A New Era for HIV Prevention Research & Development" (report, July 2012), 4.

106. Desmond McNeill and Kristin Sandberg, "Trust in Global Health Governance: The GAVI Experience," *Global Governance: A Review of Multilateralism and International Organizations*, no. 20 (Spring/Summer 2014): 325–43.

107. Sheri Fink, "Cuts at W.H.O. Hurt Response to Ebola Crisis," *New York Times*, 3 September 2014, accessed 3 September 2014, http://www .nytimes.com/2014/09/04/world/africa/cuts-at-who-hurt-response-to-ebola-crisis.html.

Chapter 5

1. As one example, see Robert Keohane, "Global Governance and Democratic Accountability," in *Taming Globalization: Frontiers of Governance*, ed. David Held and Mathias Koenig-Archibugi (Cambridge: Polity Press, 2003).

2. As one example, see WHO, "Report of the Review Committee on the Functioning of the International Health Regulations (2005) in relation to Pandemic (H1N1) 2009" (agenda item, 64th World Health Assembly, 5 May 2011), 10, accessed 3 September 2015, http://apps.who.int/gb/ ebwha/pdf_files/WHA64/A64_10-en.pdf.

3. For a discussion on the perception of membership enlargement and diversity as normatively positive, see Julia Gray, René Lindstädt, and Jonathan Slapin, "The Dynamics of Enlargement in International Organizations," *International Studies Quarterly* (February 2015): 1–40.

4. As one example, see "Statement of PHM at the Consultation of WHO's Engagement with Non-state Actors," People's Health Movement, 18 October 2013, accessed 4 December 2015, http://www.phmovement. org/en/node/8123.

5. "Democracy Index 2014," Economist Intelligence Unit, accessed 2 September 2015, http://www.eiu.com/public/topical_report.aspx?campaig nid=Democracy0115.

6. For a discussion of the democratic deficit in international organizations, see Andrew Moravcsik, "Is there a 'Democratic Deficit' in World Politics? A Framework for Analysis," *Government and Opposition*, no. 39 (Spring 2004): 336–63.

7. WHO, "Report of the Review Committee on the Functioning of the International Health Regulations (2005) in relation to Pandemic (H1N1) 2009," 5 May 2011.

8. WHO, "Financial Report and Audited Financial Statements for the Year Ended 31 December 2014" (document, 68th World Health Assembly, 24 April 2015).

9. WHO, "Principles Governing Relations Between the World Health Organization and Nongovernmental Organizations" (text, 40th World Health Assembly, Resolution WHA40.25), accessed 25 September 2015, http://apps.who.int/gb/bd/PDF/bd47/EN/principles-governing-rela-en .pdf?ua=1.

10. WHO, "English/French List of 202 Nongovernmental Organizations in Official Relations with WHO Reflecting Decisions of EB136, January 2015," accessed 30 October 2015, http://www.who.int/civilsociety/relations/NGOs-in-Official-Relations-with-WHO.pdf?ua=1.

11. WHO, "Principles," 86; although the Gates Foundation is not on the official NGO list, Bill Gates has addressed the World Health Assembly twice, in 2005 and 2011.

12. For more information on RBM and UNITAID, please visit "Home," Roll Back Malaria Partnership, http://www.rollbackmalaria.org/. and "Home," UNITAID, http://www.unitaid.eu/en/.

13. WHO, "Guidelines on Working with the Private Sector to Achieve Health Outcomes: Report by the Secretariat" (provisional agenda item 8.3, Executive Board, 107th sess., 30 November 2000), accessed 2 November 2015, http://apps.who.int/iris/bitstream/10665/78660/1/ee20.pdf.

14. WHO, "Mapping of WHO's Engagement with Non-State Actors" (background paper, Executive Board, 134th sess., January 2014), 1–2, accessed 2 November 2015, http://www.who.int/about/who_reform/governance/mapping-of-WHO-engagement-with-non-State-actors.pdf?ua=1.

15. WHO, "Principles."

16. As one example, see the 133rd meeting: "Documentation: EB133," World Health Organization, accessed 18 April 2016, http://apps.who.int/gb/e/e_eb133.html.

17. See resolution: WHO, "Framework of Engagement with Non-State Actors" (draft resolution, 68th World Health Assembly, 26 May 2015), accessed 2 September 2015, http://apps.who.int/gb/ebwha/pdf_files/WHA68/A68_ACONF3Rev1-en.pdf.

18. As one example, see Catherine Saez and William New, "WHO Engagement With Non-State Actors: No Deal This Year, Work To Continue," *Intellectual Property Watch*, 26 May 2015, accessed 28 May 2015, http://www.ip-watch.org/2015/05/26/who-engagement-with-non-state-actors-no-deal-this-year-work-to-continue/.

19. Global Policy Forum, "WHO: Work on Non-State Actors Engagement Policy Continues," 28 May 2015, accessed 15 January 2016, https://www.globalpolicy.org/component/content/article/270-general/52767-who-work-on-non-state-actors-engagement-framework-to-continue.html.

20. This argument is fleshed out in Lawrence Gostin, Devi Sridhar, and Daniel Hougendobler, "The Normative Authority of the World Health Organization," *Public Health*, no. 129 (July 2015): 854–63, accessed 18 November 2015, http://scholarship.law.georgetown.edu/cgi/viewcontent.cgi?article=2510&context=facpub.

21. WHO, "Report of the Ebola Interim Assessment Panel" (report, Geneva, July 2015), accessed 8 July 2015, http://www.who.int/csr/resources/publications/ebola/ebola-panel-report/en/.

22. WHO, "Report of the Ebola Interim Assessment Panel," 21.

23. As only one example, see Human Rights Watch, "At Your Own Risk: Reprisals Against Critics of World Bank Group Projects," 22 June 2015, accessed 20 November 2015, https://www.hrw.org/report/2015/06/22/your-own-risk/reprisals-against-critics-world-bank-group-projects.

24. World Bank, "Civil Society Organizations," accessed 23 November 2015, http://web.worldbank.org/WBSITE/EXTERNAL/TOPICS/CSO/0,,contentMDK:20127718~menuPK:288622~pagePK:220503~piPK:220476~theSitePK:228717,00.html.

25. For a full list of World Bank Consultations with CSOs from 2010 to 2012 (the most recent data available at the time of writing), please see World Bank, "World Bank-Civil Society Engagement: Review of Fiscal Years 2010–2012" (report, Washington, DC, 2013), 13. For the HNP portfolio, also see 31.

26. "Archives: 'Firsts' in World Bank History," World Bank, accessed 23 November 2015, http://web.worldbank.org/WBSITE/EXTERNAL/EXTABOUTUS/EXTARCHIVES/0,,contentMDK:20080767~pagePK:36726~menuPK:214047~piPK:36092~theSitePK:29506,00.html.

27. "The World Bank," MIT, accessed 23 November 2015, http://web.mit.edu/urbanupgrading/upgrading/resources/organizations/world-bank.html.

28. As one example, see The World Bank Operations Evaluation Department, "Lessons and Practices No. 18: Non-Governmental Organizations and Civil Society Engagement in World Bank Supported Projects—Lessons from OED Evaluations," 28 August 2002, 1–2, accessed 24 September 2015, http://lnweb90.worldbank.org/oed/oeddoclib.nsf/DocUNIDViewForJavaSearch/851D373F39609C0B85256C230057A3E3/$file/LP18.pdf.

29. World Bank, "World Bank-Civil Society Engagement: Review," 21.

30. "The World Bank and Civil Society Engagement: How the Bank Engages," World Bank, accessed 25 September 2015, http://web.worldbank.org/WBSITE/EXTERNAL/TOPICS/CSO/0,,contentMDK:20092185~menuPK:220422~pagePK:220503~piPK:220476~theSitePK:228717,00.html.

31. "Search," WHO, accessed 30 September 2015, http://www.who.int/en/.

32. Ibid.

33. "Grantee Projects," Global Partnership for Social Accountability, accessed 25 September 2015, http://www.thegpsa.org/sa/project.

34. "The Little Data Book on Private Sector Development 2015," World Bank, accessed 23 November 2015, http://data.worldbank.org/products/data-books/little-data-book-on-private-sector-dvlpmnt.

35. According to a 2005 World Bank study, more than 90 percent of the hospitals and more than 80 percent of the doctors in India are in the private sector. See Ismail Radwan, "India—Private Health Services for the Poor" (discussion paper, World Bank Group, Washington, DC, 2005).

36. We do not address the International Finance Corporation (IFC), which is part of the World Bank Group and has an explicit charge to work with and through the private sector and private-public partnerships in the developing world.

37. "CSO Constituency: Steering Committee," Gavi CSO Constituency for Immunisation and Stronger Health Systems, accessed 25 September 2015, http://www.gavi-cso.org/home-1/steering-committee.

38. "Civil Society Organisation Support: Improved Health Outcomes and Equity," Gavi, accessed 25 September 2015, http://www.gavi.org/support/cso/.

39. "Civil Society Access to Gavi Vaccine Prices: Frequently Asked Questions August 2015," Gavi, accessed 25 September 2015, http://www.gavi.org/support/cso/.

40. Authors' calculation based on information as of 23 November 2015; "Civil Society Organisation Support," Gavi, accessed 23 November 2015, http://www.gavi.org/support/cso/.

41. "Civil Society Organisation Support: Past Response," Gavi, accessed 25 September 2015, http://www.gavi.org/support/cso/.

42. "GAVI Programmatic Support to Civil Society Organisations Implementation Framework," Gavi (CSO Implementation and Results Framework, March 2013), 1, accessed 25 September 2015, http://www.gavi.org/support/cso/.

43. "GAVI Programmatic Support to Civil Society Organisations Implementation Framework," 2.

44. "Civil Society Organisation Support: Current Response," Gavi, accessed 25 September 2015, http://www.gavi.org/support/cso/.

45. For example, in 2011 the Gates Foundation and other donors offered to match newly pledged funds. In late 2012/early 2013, three partners collectively pledged $12.5 mm, less than .5 percent of what Gates contributed to Gavi in 2012. See "GAVI Alliance Significantly Expands Private Sector Involvement in Saving Lives," Gavi, accessed 23 November 2015, http://www.gavi.org/library/news/press-releases/2013/gavi-alliance-significantly-expands-private-sector-involvement-in-saving-lives/. Authors' calculations based on raw Gavi contribution data 2000–2003, as of 31 March 2014.

46. The World Bank encourages countries to engage with the private sector at the national level, but it has not built institutional relationships with the private sector in the ways Gavi, for example, has. As one example, see The International Finance Corporation, "Healthy Partnerships: How Governments Can Engage the Private Sector to Improve Health in Africa" (report, Washington, DC, 2011), accessed 15 January 2016, https://openknowledge.worldbank.org/handle/10986/2304.

47. Andrew Jack, "Conflict of Interest Fears Over Vaccine Group," *Financial Times*, 27 May 2011, accessed 23 November 2015, http://www.ft.com/intl/

cms/s/0/484e8ada-87c2-11e0-a6de-00144feabdc0.html?siteedition=uk#axz
z3sSONjbat.

48. CEPA LLP, Applied Strategies, and Ulla Griffiths, "Gavi Second Evaluation Report" (evaluation, 13 September 2010), 70.

49. UNICEF, "Pentavalent Vaccine: Market & Supply Update" (report, New York, July 2015), 2, accessed 2 October 2015, http://www.unicef .org/supply/files/Pentavalent_Vaccine_Market_and_Supply_Update_ July_2015.pdf.

50. As one example, see Laurie Garrett, "The Challenge of Global Health," *Foreign Affairs*, no. 86 (Winter 2007): 14–38.

51. For example, see coverage of such critiques in Devi Sridhar and Tami Tamashiro, "Vertical Funds in the Health Sector: Lessons for Education from the Global Fund and Gavi" (background paper, Education for All Global Monitoring Report 2010, 2009), 30, accessed 24 November 2015, http://unesdoc.unesco.org/images/0018/001865/186565e.pdf.

52. See Katerini Storeng, "The Gavi Alliance and the 'Gates Approach' to Health Systems Strengthening," *Global Public Health*, no. 9 (2014): 865–79, accessed November 2015, http://www.tandfonline.com/doi/pdf/1 0.1080/17441692.2014.940362.

53. Authors' calculation using Gavi raw disbursement data, accessed 14 June 2016, http://www.gavi.org/results/disbursements/.

54. Authors' calculation using Global Fund raw disbursement data, accessed 14 June 2016, http://www.theglobalfund.org/en/portfolio/.

55. Gavi, "New Private Sector Partners Bring Technical Expertise and Innovative Finance to Help Save Children's Lives" (press release, Geneva, 21 January 2015), accessed 22 January 2015, http://www.gavi .org/Library/News/Press-releases/2015/New-private-sector-partners- bring-technical-expertise-and-innovative-finance-to-help-save- children-s-lives/.

56. Authors' evaluation of all Global Fund Board Members, from 2001 through 2013.

57. See Global Fund, "Report of the Eighth Board Meeting," accessed 8 December 2015, http://www.theglobalfund.org/en/board/meetings/09/; and the "Report of the 18th Board Meeting," accessed 8 December 2015, http://www.theglobalfund.org/en/board/meetings/19/.

58. Global Fund, "Final Report of the 8th Board Meeting."

59. Global Fund Working Group, "Challenges and Opportunities for the New Executive Director of the Global Fund: Seven Essential Tasks" (report, Center for Global Development, Washington, DC, 26 October 2006), 22, http://www.cgdev.org/publication/challenges-and- opportunities-new-executive-director-global-fund-seven-essential-tasks.

60. As one example, see "Analysis of Private Sector Contributions in Round 8 and 9: Opportunities for Co-Investment," Global Fund, 2010, accessed 2 July 2012, http://www.theglobalfund.org/en/civilsociety/reports.

61. "The Office of the Inspector General Progress Report for March–October 2010 and 2011 Audit Plan and Budget," Global Fund (report, 22nd Board meeting, Sofia, Bulgaria, 13–15 December 2010).

62. "Turning the Page from Emergency to Sustainability: The Final Report of the High-Level Independent Review Panel on Fiduciary Controls and Oversight Mechanisms of the Global Fund to Fight AIDS, Tuberculosis and Malaria," High-Level Independent Panel (report, Geneva, 19 September 2011).

63. "Procurement for Impact," Global Fund, accessed 2 January 2014, http://www.theglobalfund.org/en/blog/2013-11-07_Global_Fund_News_Flash_Issue_29.

64. "Sourcing and Procurement—Overview," Global Fund, accessed 12 November 2015, http://www.theglobalfund.org/en/sourcingprocurement/.

65. As an example, see Global Fund, "Report of the 21st Board Meeting."

66. Authors' assessment of all Board documentation through 2012, 1st–25th Meetings. "Board: Board Meetings & Calendar," Global Fund, accessed 18 April 2016, http://theglobalfund.org/en/board/meetings/.

67. Authors' review of all published "US Government Positions on Decision Points from Global Fund Board Meetings" documents through 2014, all available at pepfar.gov.

68. Different translations exist for the original quotation from Juvenal's *Satires of Juvenal* 6.347–48. It is often misattributed to Plato and his *Republic*.

69. One arena where this is particularly clear is in the corporate sector. For example, countries from the United States and Denmark to Brazil and India have introduced reporting requirements for companies intended to provide greater transparency into how their businesses impact the societies in which they operate, the environment, and human rights. For more, please visit: UN Global Compact, "Nowhere to Hide: Transparency is Becoming the New Norm," accessed 12 August 2015, http://globalcompact15.org/report/findings-level-1/6transparency-is-becoming-the-new-norm.

70. As one example, see Ivan Krastev, *In Mistrust We Trust: Can Democracy Survive When We Don't Trust Our Leaders?* TED Books (New York: Simon & Schuster, 2012).

71. Robert Keohane and Joseph Nye, "Power and Interdependence in the Information Age," *Foreign Affairs* (September/October 1998): 89.

72. As one example, see Thomas Blanton, "The Struggle for Openness in the International Financial Institutions," in *The Right to Know: Transparency for an Open World*, ed. Ann Florini (New York: Columbia University Press, 2007), 243–78.

73. Joseph Nye, *Power in the Global Information Age: From Realism to Globalization* (New York: Routledge, 2004), 89.

74. See Barbara Koremenos, "Open Covenants, Clandestinely Arrived At" (working paper, *International Theory*), available at https://www.researchgate.net/publication/251781284_Open_Covenants_Clandestinely_Arrived_At.

75. We will point, as have other scholars, to Hans Morgenthau's *Politics Among Nations: The Struggle for Power and Peace* (New York: Alfred A. Knopf, 1950) for a robust argument in favor of providing confidential spaces for nations (and other powers) to discuss in the shadows.

76. "WHO Open-access Policy: Frequently Asked Questions for Recipients of WHO Funding," WHO, accessed 18 January 2016, http://www.who.int/about/open-access-faq/en/index1.html.

77. "Executive Board Webcasts," WHO, accessed 18 January 2016, http://www.who.int/mediacentre/executive-board-live/en/.

78. "Alert, Response, and Capacity Building Under the International Health Regulations (IHR): IHR Procedures Concerning Public Health Emergencies of International Concern (PHEIC)," World Health Organization, accessed 18 January 2016, http://www.who.int/ihr/procedures/pheic/en/.

79. "Media Centre: WHO Statement on the First Meeting of the International Health Regulations (2005) (IHR 2005) Emergency Committee on Zika Virus and Observed Increase in Neurological Disorders and Neonatal Malformations," WHO, accessed 1 February 2016, http://www.who.int/mediacentre/news/statements/2016/1st-emergency-committee-zika/en/.

80. "Media Centre: Statement on the First Meeting of the IHR Emergency Committee on the 2014 Ebola Outbreak in West Africa," WHO, accessed 10 August 2014, http://www.who.int/mediacentre/news/statements/2014/ebola-20140808/en/.

81. Nicole Winfield, "WHO Chief Promises Transparency in Ebola Review," *Yahoo News*, 19 November 2014, accessed 19 November 2014, http://news.yahoo.com/chief-promises-transparency-ebola-response-161135028.html.

82. "Media Centre: WHO Calls for Increased Transparency in Medical Research," WHO, accessed 2 August 2015, http://www.who.int/mediacentre/news/notes/2015/medical-research-transparency/en/.

83. Suerie Moon et al., "Will Ebola Change the Game? Ten Essential Reforms before the Next Pandemic: The Report of the Harvard-LSHTM Independent Panel on the Global Response to Ebola," *Lancet*, no. 386 (November 2015): 2204–21.

84. Department for International Development(DFID), "Multilateral Aid Review Update: Driving Reform to Achieve Multilateral Effectiveness" (report, UKAID, London, England, December 2013), accessed 9 January 2014, https://www.gov.uk/government/uploads/system/uploads/attachment_data/file/297523/MAR-review-dec13.pdf.

85. DFID, "Multilateral Aid Review: Ensuring Maximum Value for Money for UK Aid Through Multilateral Organisations."

86. Barry Bloom, "WHO Needs Change," *Nature*, no. 473 (May 2011): 143–45, accessed 2 June 2015, http://www.nature.com/nature/journal/v473/n7346/full/473143a.html.

87. "About IATI," International Aid Transparency Initiative, accessed 2 August 2015, http://www.aidtransparency.net/about.

88. "IATI DATA: Publishers," International Aid Transparency Initiative, accessed 18 January 2016, http://www.iatiregistry.org/publisher and "Results," Publish What You Fund, accessed 18 January 2016, http://ati.publishwhatyoufund.org/index-2014/results.

89. Authors' assessment as of 9 December 2015.

90. Authors' assessment as of 9 December 2015, "Violence and Injury Prevention: Road Traffic Injuries," WHO, accessed 18 January 2016, http://www.who.int/violence_injury_prevention/road_traffic/en/.

91. Authors' assessment as of 9 December 2015, "Global Health Observatory (GHO) Data: The Data Repository," WHO, accessed 18 January 2016, http://www.who.int/gho/database/en/.

92. Andrea Bianchi and Anne Peters, eds., *Transparency in International Law* (New York: Cambridge University Press, 2013), 289.

93. For example, Devi Sridhar and Lawrence Gostin, "Reforming the World Health Organization," *JAMA*, 29 March 2011, accessed 18 January 2016, http://scholarship.law.georgetown.edu/cgi/viewcontent.cgi?article=1622&context=facpub.

94. Davesh Kapur, John Lewis, and Richard Webb, *World Bank: Its First Half Century*, vol. 1 (Washington, DC: Brookings Institution Press, 1997), 222.

95. Robert Wade, "Greening the Bank: The Struggle over the Environment, 1970–1995," in *The World Bank: Its First Half Century*, ed. Davesh Kapur, John Lewis, and Richard Webb, 2:611–72 (Washington, DC: Brookings Institution Press, 1997).

96. As one example, see "Extractive Industries Transparency Initiative: Results Profile," World Bank, 15 April 2013, accessed 2 June 2015, http://www.worldbank.org/en/results/2013/04/15/extractive-industries-transparency-initiative-results-profile.

97. "Overview," World Bank, accessed 5 May 2015, http://www.worldbank.org/en/access-to-information/overview, and World Bank, "Policy on Access to Information" (brochure, Washington, DC, 2015), accessed 2 December 2015, http://pubdocs.worldbank.org/pubdocs/publicdoc/2015/7/740621437416268169/AI-Brochure-2015.pdf.

98. "Open Learning Campus," World Bank Group, accessed 18 April 2016, http://wbi.worldbank.org/wbi/webinar/open-contracting-principles-practice.

99. "Projects & Operations," World Bank, accessed 8 December 2015, http://web.worldbank.org/WBSITE/EXTERNAL/PROJECTS/0,,menuPK:41389~pagePK:95863~piPK:95983~targetDetMenuPK:228424~targetProjDetPK:73230~targetProjResPK:95917~targetResMenuPK:232168~theSitePK:40941,00.html#Documents.

100. "World Bank HNP Lending," World Bank, accessed 8 December 2015, http://datatopics.worldbank.org/hnp/worldbanklending.

101. "Projects & Operations: Health System Improvement Project," World Bank, accessed 8 December 2015, http://www.worldbank.org/projects/P113349/health-system-improvement-project?lang=en.

102. Independent Evaluation Group, "Improving Effectiveness & Outcomes for the Poor in Health, Nutrition & Population: An Evaluation of World Bank Group Support since 1997" (report, Washington, DC, 2009).

103. Independent Evaluation Group, "Implementation of the World Bank's Strategy for Health, Nutrition, and Population Results: Achievements, Challenges, and the Way Forward" (progress report, Washington, DC, 19 March 2009).

104. Parliament, House of Commons, International Development Committee, "The World Bank: Report, together with formal minutes, oral and written evidence" (4th report of session 2010–2011, London, England), 41.

105. Douglas Gillison, "Freedom of Information: World Bank Lags Behind Many Member States," 100Reporters, 11 March 2015, accessed 2 August 2015, https://100r.org/2015/03/freedom-of-information-the-world-bank-lags-behind-many-member-states.

106. World Bank is a leader with its open access information policy and open data platforms (as recognized by the OECD), *Aid Effectiveness in the Health Sector: Progress and Lessons* (Paris: OECD Publishing, 2012), 52.

107. "World Bank—International Development Association," Publish What You Fund, accessed 2 January 2015, http://ati.publishwhatyoufund.org/donor/world-bank-ida.

108. "Are We There Yet? The World Bank's Anti-Corruption Record," Transparency International, 28 June 2012, accessed 2 August 2015, http://www.transparency.org/news/feature/are_we_there_yet_the_world_banks_anti_corruption_record.

109. Benno Torgler, "Trust in International Organizations: An Empirical Investigation Focusing on the United Nations," *Review of International Organizations*, no. 3 (March 2008): 65–93; Martin Edwards, "Public Support for the International Economic Organizations: Evidence from Developing Countries," *Review of International Organizations*, no. 4 (June 2009): 185–209; Roderick Kramer and Karen Cook, *Trust and Distrust in Organizations: Dilemmas and Approaches* (New York: Russell Sage Foundation, 2004).

110. Desmond McNeill and Kristin Ingstad Sandberg, "Trust in Global Health Governance: The GAVI Experience," *Global Governance: A Review of Multilateralism and International Organizations*, no. 20 (Spring 2014): 325–43.

111. "Transparency and Accountability Policy," Gavi, accessed 2 August 2015, http://www.gavi.org/about/governance/programme-policies/tap/.

112. As an example, see Afghanistan, the first country listed alphabetically in Gavi's vaccine hub: "Country Hub: Afghanistan," Gavi, accessed 23 November 2015, http://www.gavi.org/country/afghanistan/.

113. "Disbursements and Commitments," Gavi, accessed 23 November 2015, http://www.gavi.org/results/disbursements/.

114. "Full Country Evaluations," Gavi, accessed 23 November 2015, http://www.gavi.org/results/evaluations/full-country-evaluations/.

115. As one example, see the Health System Strenghening (HSS) platform list of current participating countries, available: "The Gavi CSO Constituency CSO Platforms Project," Gavi CSO Constituency for Immunisation and Stronger Health Systems, accessed 25 September 2015, http://www.gavi-cso.org/cso-hss-platforms.

116. "Results & Evidence: Full Country Evaluations," Gavi, accessed 18 January 2016, http://www.gavi.org/Results/Evaluations/Full-country-evaluations/.

117. "Results," Publish What You Fund, accessed 18 January 2016, http://ati.publishwhatyoufund.org/index-2014/results/.

118. Kevin Klock, former Head of Governance and Assistant Secretary for Gavi (phone interview, 17 June 2015).

119. Authors' analysis of shared documentation from Board meetings and sessions from 2013 to 2015: "Gavi Board Minutes 2015," Gavi, accessed 15 January 2016, http://www.gavi.org/about/governance/gavi-board/minutes/2015/.

120. "GAVI: Overview," Publish What You Fund, accessed 15 January 2016, http://ati.publishwhatyoufund.org/donor/gavi.

121. "Goal-level Indicators," Gavi, accessed 30 December 2015, http://www.gavi.org/results/goal-level-indicators/.

122. United Nations, "Secretary-General Proposes Global Fund for Fight Against HIV/AIDS and Other Infectious Diseases at African Leaders Summit" (press release, 26 April 2001), accessed 18 January 2016, http://www.un.org/press/en/2001/SGSM7779R1.doc.htm. Secretary-General Kofi Annan called these the "diseases of the poor."

123. "LFAs in Countries," Global Fund, accessed 4 December 2015, http://www.theglobalfund.org/en/lfa/.

124. For example, referred to as such in Todd Summers, "The Global Fund to Fight AIDS, Tuberculosis and Malaria: A Progress Report" (document, CSIS HIV/AIDS Task Force, March 2003), accessed 18 January 2016, http://csis.org/files/media/csis/pubs/030103_global_fund_progress_report_.pdf.

125. As one example, see the Global Fund Office of the Inspector General, "Follow-Up Review of the Global Fund Grants to Uganda" (audit report, Geneva, 9 September 2009), accessed 2 July 2011, http://www.theglobalfund.org/en/oig/reports/.

126. For example, "Nigeria: Overview," Global Fund, accessed 24 December 2015, http://www.theglobalfund.org/en/portfolio/country/?loc=NGA.

127. "Bill & Melinda Gates Foundation Open Access Policy," Gates Foundation, accessed 2 November 2015, http://www.gatesfoundation.org/How-We-Work/General-Information/Open-Access-Policy.

128. Richard Van Noorden, "Gates Foundation Announces World's Strongest Policy on Open Access Research" (blog, *Nature*, 21 November 2014), accessed 22 November 2014, http://blogs.nature.com/news/2014/11/gates-foundation-announces-worlds-strongest-policy-on-open-access-research.html.

129. "Report of the Finance and Audit Committee," Global Fund (report, 16th Board meeting, Kunming, China, 12–13 November 2007).

130. Robert Bourgoing, "The Global Fund and the Fears of Transparency" (commentary, AIDSPAN, 4 March 2014), accessed 24 August 2015, http://www.aidspan.org/gfo_article/global-fund-and-fears-transparency.

131. At least in the Board meetings in which Board members and observers are identified by name, as mentioned earlier.

132. Kevin Klock (phone interview, 17 June 2015).

133. The Global Fund, "Report of the 20th Board Meeting" (21st Board meeting, Geneva, 28–30 April 2010), 11.

134. Garrett Wallace Brown, "Safeguarding Deliberative Global Governance: The Case of the Global Fund to Fight AIDS, Tuberculosis and Malaria," *Review of International Studies*, no. 36 (2010): 522–23.

135. Samantha Custer, Zachary Rice, Takaaki Masaki, Rebecca Latourell, and Bradley Parks, "Listening to Leaders: Which Development Partners Do They Prefer and Why?" (report, AidData, Williamsburg, VA, 2015), http://aiddata.org/sites/default/files/publication_full_2.pdf, 48.

136. Ibid.

Chapter 6

1. Devi Sridhar and Ngaire Woods, "Trojan Multilateralism: Global Cooperation in Health," *Global Policy*, no. 4 (October 2013): 325–35.

2. Ibid.

3. Charles Allen, "World Health and World Politics," *International Organization*, no. 4 (February 1950): 27–43.

4. "Home," FCTC WHO Framework Convention on Tobacco Control, accessed 6 January 2016, http://www.who.int/fctc/en/.

5. Sridhar and Woods, "Trojan Multilateralism," 325–35.

6. Barbara Koremenos, Charles Lipson, and Duncan Snidal, "The Rational Design of International Institutions," *International Organization*, no. 55 (Autumn 2001): 761–99.

7. Suerie Moon et al., "Will Ebola Change the Game? Ten Essential Reforms before the Next Pandemic. The Report of the Harvard-LSHTM Independent Panel on the Global Response to Ebola," *Lancet*, no. 386 (November 2015): 2204–21; "The Politics Behind the Ebola Crisis

Report," http://www.crisisgroup.org/~/media/Files/africa/west-africa/232-the-politics-behind-the-ebola-crisis.pdf.

8. Endang Sedyaningsih, Siti Isfandari, Triono Soendoro, and Siti Supari, "Towards Mutual Trust, Transparency and Equity in Virus Sharing Mechanism: The Avian Influenza Case of Indonesia," *Annals, Academy of Medicine*, no. 37 (June 2008): 482–88.

9. Seth Berkley (phone interview, 13 March 2015).

10. Ruairi Brugha, "The Global Fund at Three Years—Flying in Crowded Air Space," *Tropical Medicine & International Health*, no. 10 (June 2005): 625.

11. Gates Foundation, "Bill & Melinda Gates Foundation Announces $750 Million Gift to Speed Delivery of Life-Saving Vaccines" (press release, November 1999), accessed 2 July 2015, http://www.gatesfoundation.org/Media-Center/Press-Releases/1999/11/Global-Alliance-for-Vaccines-and-Immunization.

12. Seth Berkley (phone interview, 13 March 2015).

13. Agbakwuru Chinedu and Joanne Beswick, "A Comparison of The Global Fund and The GAVI Alliance with Emphasis on Health System Strengthening" (draft, May 2009), 37, accessed 27 May 2012, sihp.brandeis.edu/ighud/PDFs/GF-GAVI-Comparison-May-2009.pdf.; in November 2011, the Gavi Board formally approved the introduction of PBF, tied to immunization coverage and equity. As 2013 is the earliest Gavi recipient countries would receive a portion of their funds under Gavi's PBF scheme, it is too soon to assess Gavi's implementation of PBF at a country or global level.

14. As one example, in 2011, the Gavi Board approved introducing performance-based funding for Gavi's health systems strengthening funding. Gavi Alliance, "Gavi Alliance Board Meeting" (final minutes, Dhaka, Bangladesh, 16–17 November 2011), accessed 11 January 2016, http://www.gavi.org/about/governance/gavi-board/minutes/2011/16-november/.

15. Institute of Medicine (US) Committee on the Children's Vaccine Initiative: Planning Alternative Strategies, *The Children's Vaccine Initiative: Achieving the Vision*, ed. Violaine Mitchell, Nalini Philipose, and Jay Sanford (Washington, DC: National Academies Press, 1993), accessed 2 December 2015, http://www.ncbi.nlm.nih.gov/books/NBK236423/.

16. WHO, UNICEF, and World Bank, *State of the World's Vaccines and Immunization*, 3rd ed. (Geneva: WHO Press, 2009), 43.

17. Seth Berkley (phone interview, 13 March 2015).

18. Gavi, "Interview with Bill Gates," YouTube, March 2015, accessed 13 January 2016, http://www.gavi.org/Library/Audio-visual/Videos/Interview-with-Bill-Gates/.

19. "Market-shaping Goal Indicators," Gavi, The Vaccine Alliance, accessed 2 March 2015, http://www.gavi.org/results/goal-level-indicators/market-shaping-goal-indicators/.

20. Gavi, "The Vaccine Alliance Progress Report 2014: Summary," accessed 2 August 2015, http://www.gavi.org/progress-report/.

21. Gavi, "'Deliver, Deliver, Deliver'—Dagfinn Høybråten reflects on five years as Gavi Board Chair," accessed 11 January 2016, http://www.gavi.org/Library/News/GAVI-features/2015/Deliver-deliver-deliver-Dagfinn-Hoybraten-reflects-on-five-years-as-Gavi-Board-Chair/.

22. Gavi, "Gavi, The Vaccine Alliance 2014 Annual Financial Report" (report, Geneva, August 2015), 8.

23. United Nations Children's Fund, "UNICEF Annual Report 2000" (report, New York, NY, 2000), 27–32, accessed 2 October 2015, http://www.unicef.org/publications/files/pub_ar00_en.pdf.

24. Kevin Klock (phone interview, 10 June 2015).

25. Independent Evaluation Group (IEG), "The World Bank's Partnership with the GAVI Alliance" (report, Washington, DC, 2014), 1, accessed 12 December 2015, http://ieg.worldbank.org/Data/reports/chapters/wbp_gavi_alliance_chap1.pdf.

26. Gavi, "2002 Annual Report" (report, Washington, DC, 2002), 34.

27. Deloitte, "The GAVI Fund: Consolidated Financial Statements as of and for the Years Ended December 31, 2007 and 2006 (As restated), and Independent Auditors' Report" (document, Washington, DC, 2008).

28. Independent Evaluation Group, "The World Bank's Partnership with the Gavi Alliance," 2.

29. George Wellde (personal interview, 23 September 2015).

30. Kevin Klock (10 June 2015) and George Wellde (23 September 2015) interviews.

31. Gavi, "Gavi Alliance Progress Report 2007" (document, Washington, DC, 2007), 5.

32. For a detailed assessment of the Fund's performance against these early ambitions, see Chelsea Clinton, "The Global Fund: An Experiment in Global Governance" (DPhil diss., University of Oxford, 2014).

33. Institute of Medicine, *Evaluation of PEPFAR* (Washington, DC: The National Academies Press, 2013); World Bank/IEG, "The Global Fund to Fight AIDS, Tuberculosis and Malaria, and the World Bank's Engagement with the Global Fund" (main report, vol. 1, Washington, DC, 8 February 2011); David McCoy and Kelvin Kinyua, "Allocating Scarce Resources Strategically—An Evaluation and Discussion of the Global Fund's Pattern of Disbursements," *PLoS ONE*, no. 7 (May 2012), accessed 8 January 2016, http://www.plosone.org/article/fetchObject.action?uri=info:doi/10.1371/journal.pone.0034749&representation=PDF.

34. Author's own calculations based on raw Global Fund contribution data 2000–2014: "Financials," Global Fund, accessed 2 December 2014, http://www.theglobalfund.org/en/financials/.

35. Global Fund, Framework Document, 2001, 91–92.

36. When the Global Fund employed a rounds-based financing approach, it would issue calls for proposals from applicant country-coordinating

mechanisms and then review the applications as a group, approving in whole or part applications its TRP and then its Board judged as technically sound. In general, during the Fund's first decade there was approximately one funding round per year.

37. As one example, in 2010, the Secretariat recommended to the Global Fund Board that it waive all conditions it had previously imposed on two round 5 grants (NGR-506-G04-M & NGR-506-G05-T) to Niger because of the then on-going civil war. See Global Fund, "Electronic Decision Points" (submitted to the 22nd Board Meeting, 2011), 10.

38. As one example, Macro International, "The Five-Year Evaluation of the Global Fund to Fight AIDS, Tuberculosis and Malaria: Synthesis of Study Areas 1, 2 and 3," 2009, 31.

39. Australian Aid, "Australian Multilateral Assessment March 2012: Global Fund to Fight AIDS, Tuberculosis and Malaria (The Global Fund)," document, Australian Government, 2012, 3, accessed 2 November 2012, https://dfat.gov.au/about-us/publications/Documents/global-fund-assessment.pdf.

40. At least one academic paper (from 2002 through 12) argued that while the Fund continued to rely on process, input, and output measurements, in successive rounds, it looked to incorporate more outcome-based measurements, at least in malaria. See Jinkou Zhao, Marcel Lama, Swarup Sarkar, and Rifat Atun, "Indicators Measuring the Performance of Malaria Programs Supported by the Global Fund in Asia, Progress and the Way Forward," *PLoS ONE*, no. 6 (December 2011), accessed 3 March 2012, http://journals.plos.org/plosone/article?id=10.1371/journal.pone.0028932.

41. Clinton, "The Global Fund: An Experiment," 319.

42. See Chelsea Clinton, "The Global Fund to Fight AIDS, TB and Malaria: A Response to Global Threats. A Part of a Global Future" (MPhil thesis, University of Oxford, 2003).

43. Xavier Bosch, "Europe Refuses to Match US Cash for Ailing Global Fund," *Lancet*, no. 362 (July 2003): 299.

44. See Clinton, "The Global Fund: An Experiment," 9–10. As one example, "Can the Global Fund to Fight Aids, Tuberculosis and Malaria Restore Its Reputation as the Best and Cleanest in the Aid Business?" *Economist*, 17 February 2011, http://www.economist.com/node/18176062.

45. For example, UNICEF and UNDP only release aggregate fraud numbers, none of which is ever above 1 percent and none of which is ever tied to specific programs.

46. Global Fund, *Results with Integrity: The Global Fund's Response to Fraud* (Geneva: Global Fund, 2011), 5.

47. Most notably in Secretary of State Hillary Clinton, "Creating an Aids-Free Generation" (speech, the National Institutes of Health, Bethesda, Maryland, 8 November 2011), http://www.state.gov/secretary/20092013clinton/rm/2011/11/176810.htm.

48. Global Fund, "Board Retreat Progress Report" (document, submitted by General Manager Jaramillo to the 26th Board meeting, 2012).

49. High-Level Independent Review Panel, "Turning the Page from Emergency to Sustainability: The Final Report of the High-Level Independent Review Panel on Fiduciary Controls and Oversight Mechanisms of the Global Fund to Fight AIDS, Tuberculosis and Malaria" (report, Geneva, 19 September 2011), 31.

50. See Amanda Glassman, "Why a Banker Is Good for the Global Fund" (global health policy blog, Center for Global Development, 30 January 2012), accessed 30 January 2012, http://www.cgdev.org/blog/why-banker-good-global-fund; Laurie Garrett, "Global Health Hits Crisis Point," *Nature*, no. 482 (February 2012), accessed 1 February 2012, http://www.nature.com/news/global-health-hits-crisis-point-1.9951.

51. Betsy McKay, "New Chief Unveils Plan to Revive Disease-Fighting Fund," *Wall Street Journal*, 30 January 2012, http://online.wsj.com/article/SB10001424052970203363504577187224148489882.html.

52. Clinton "The Global Fund: An Experiment," 325.

53. Authors' assessment of all documents related to the Fourth Replenishment: The Global Fund, "Fourth Replenishment," 28 December 2013, http://www.theglobalfund.org/en/replenishment/.

54. High-Level Independent Review Panel, "Turning the Page from Emergency to Sustainability," 9.

55. Lawrence Gostin, Devi Sridhar, and Daniel Hougendobler, "The Normative Authority of the World Health Organization," *Public Health*, no. 129 (July 2015): 854–63; Lawrence Gostin, *Global Health Law* (Cambridge, MA: Harvard University Press, 2014).

56. Gavi, "Gavi Alliance Board Meeting" (board and committee minutes, Geneva, 2–3 December 2015), 31, accessed 17 December 2015, http://www.gavi.org/about/governance/gavi-board/minutes/2015/2-dec/.

57. WHO, "World Health Forum" (concept paper, Geneva, 22 June 2011), accessed 12 January 2016, http://www.who.int/dg/reform/en_who_reform_world_health_forum.pdf.

58. WHO Committee of Experts on Tobacco Industry Documents, "Tobacco Company Strategies to Undermine Tobacco Control Activities at the World Health Organization" (report, Geneva, July 2000), accessed 12 January 2016, http://apps.who.int/iris/handle/10665/67429.

59. WHO, "WHO Reforms for a Healthy Future: An Overview" (paper, Geneva, 20 July 2011), accessed 12 January 2016, http://www.who.int/dg/reform/en_who_reform_overview.pdf; WHO, "WHO Reforms for a Healthy Future: Report by the Director-General" (provisional agenda item, executive board, special session on WHO reforms, Geneva, 15 October 2011), accessed 12 January 2016, http://apps.who.int/gb/ebwha/pdf_files/EBSS/EBSS2_2-en.pdf.

60. Lawrence Gostin, "A Framework Convention on Global Health: Health for All, Justice for All," *Journal of the American Medical Association*, no. 307 (May 2012): 2087–92.

61. Gaudenz Silberschmidt, Don Matheson, and Ilona Kickbusch, "Creating a Committee C of the World Health Assembly," *Lancet*, no. 371 (2008): 1483–86.

62. WHO, "Principles Governing Relations Between the World Health Organization and Nongovernmental Organizations" (document, 40th World Health Assembly), accessed 23 March 2015, http://apps.who.int/ gb/gov/assets/ngo-principles-governing-rela-en.pdf.

63. Christophe Lanord, "A Study of WHO's Official Relations System with Nongovernmental Organizations" (document, WHO Civil Society Initiative, June 2002), accessed 12 January 2016, http://www.who.int/ civilsociety/documents/en/study.pdf; Thomas Schwarz, "A Stronger Voice for Civil Society at the World Health Assembly?"; see web page, Medicus Mundi International Network, June 2010, accessed 23 March 2015, http:// www.medicusmundi.org/en/contributions/reports/2010/a-stronger-voice-of-civil-society-at-the-world-health-assembly.

64. Kevin Klock, "The Soft Law Alternative to the WHO's Treaty Powers," *Georgetown Journal of International Law*, no. 44 (2013), http://www.law .georgetown.edu/academics/law-journals/gjil/recent/upload/ zsx00213000821.PDF.

65. In 2009, the Global Fund Board approved financial support for facilitating implementing countries' convenings and communications between Board meetings. See Global Fund, "Report of the Twentieth Board Meeting," Annex 3. At least by 2009, Gavi had introduced a similar program for its developing-country Board members. See also Kevin Klock (phone interview, 10 June 2015).

66. WHO, "Policy for Relations with Nongovernmental Organizations: Note by the Director-General" (provisional agenda item, 57th World Health Assembly, Geneva, 1 April 2004); WHO, "Status of Proposal for a New Policy to Guide WHO's Relations with NGOs," accessed 23 March 2015, http://apps.who.int/iris/handle/10665/20112

67. Moon et al., "Will Ebola Change the Game?," *Lancet*, no. 386 (November 2015).

68. David Stuckler, Sanjay Basu, and Martin McKee, "Global Health Philanthropy and Institutional Relationships: How Should Conflicts of Interest Be Addressed?" *PLoS Medicine*, no. 8 (April 2011).

69. Linsey McGoey, *No Such Thing as a Free Gift: The Gates Foundation and the Price of Philanthropy* (New York: Verso, 2015).

70. Donald McNeil, "Gates Foundation's Influence Criticized," *New York Times*, 16 February 2008, http://www.nytimes.com/2008/02/16/ science/16malaria.html?_r=0.

71. Gostin, Sridhar, and Hougendobler, "Normative Authority," *Public Health*; Gostin, *Global Health Law*, 2014.

72. WHO, "Proposed Programme Budget 2016–2017" (provisional agenda item, 68th World Health Assembly, Geneva, 30 April 2015).

73. WHO, "Implementation of the International Health Regulations (2005): Report of the Review Committee on the Functioning of the International

Health Regulations (2005) in relation to Pandemic (H1N1) 2009"
(provisional agenda item, 64th World Health Assembly, 5 May 2011).

74. United Kingdom Department for International Development,
"Multilateral Aid Review: Ensuring Maximum Value for Money for
UK Aid through Multilateral Organisations" (document, London,
March 2011), accessed 12 January 2016, https://www.gov.uk/government/
uploads/system/uploads/attachment_data/file/67583/multilateral_
aid:review.pdf.

75. WHO, "Independent Formative Evaluation of the World Health
Organization" (concept paper, Geneva, 22 June 2011), accessed
12 January 2016, http://www.who.int/dg/reform/en_who_reform_
evaluation.pdf.

76. While often not a challenge explicitly discussed, it is one often hinted at
and addressed through other areas at WHO. As one example, see WHO,
"Human Resources: Report by the Secretariat" (provisional agenda item
23.1, 68th World Health Assembly, Geneva, 12 May 2015), accessed 14 April
2016, http://apps.who.int/gb/ebwha/pdf_files/WHA68/A68_44-en.
pdf?ua=1.

77. WHO, "Report of the Ebola Interim Assessment Panel" (report, Geneva,
July 2015), accessed 12 January 2016, http://www.who.int/csr/resources/
publications/ebola/ebola-panel-report/en/.

78. Laurie Garrett, "Garrett on Global Health," *Council on Foreign Relations
Newsletter*, 25 January 2016, http://www.cfr.org/about/newsletters/
onthefly.php?id=3493.

79. WHO, "WHO Reforms for a Healthy Future: Report by the Director-
General" (provisional agenda item, special session on WHO reform,
Executive Board, Geneva, 15 October 2011).

80. WHO, "Proposed Programme Budget 2016–2017" (provisional agenda
item, 68th World Health Assembly, Geneva, 30 April 2015).

81. Sheri Fink, "Cuts at WHO Hurt Response to Ebola Crisis," *New York
Times*, 3 September 2014, http://www.nytimes.com/2014/09/04/world/
africa/cuts-at-who-hurt-response-to-ebola-crisis.html?_r=0.

82. WHO, "Medium-term Strategic Plan 2008–2013" (document, 9th
plenary meeting, Geneva, 21 May 2007); WHO, "Proposed Programme
Budget 2014–2015" (provisional agenda item, 66th World Health
Assembly, Geneva, 19 April 2013); Sridhar and Woods, "Trojan
Multilateralism," 325–35.

83. PricewaterhouseCoopers, "WHO Financing Dialogue Evaluation: Final
report" (report, Geneva, 17 April 2014), accessed 12 January 2016, http://
www.who.int/about/resources_planning/financing_dialogue/FD_
EvaluationFinalReport.pdf.

84. Lawrence Gostin and Devi Sridhar, "Global Health and the Law," *New
England Journal of Medicine*, no. 370 (May 2014): 1732–40.

85. International Conference on Primary Health Care, "Declaration of
Alma-Ata" (document, Alma-Ata, USSR, 6–12 September 1978), accessed

12 January 2015, http://www.who.int/publications/almaata_declaration_en.pdf.

86. US Government, "Observations by the United States of America on 'The Right to Health, Fact Sheet No. 31,'" accessed 12 January 2016, http://www.state.gov/documents/organization/138850.pdf.

87. Lawrence Gostin, John Monahan, Mary DeBartolo, and Richard Horton, "Law's Power to Safeguard Global Health: A Lancet-O'Neill Institute, Georgetown University Commission on Global Health and the Law," *Lancet*, no. 385 (April 2015): 1603–4.

88. Gostin and Sridhar, "Global Health and the Law."

89. David Fidler and Lawrence Gostin, "The WHO Pandemic Influenza Preparedness Framework: A Milestone in Global Governance for Health," *Journal of the American Medical Association*, no. 306 (July 2011): 200–201.

90. Gostin, Sridhar, and Hougendobler, "Normative Authority," *Public Health*; Gostin, *Global Health Law*, 2014.

91. Ngaire Woods, "How to Save the World Bank," Project Syndicate, 12 January 2016, accessed 13 January 2016, https://www.project-syndicate.org/commentary/saving-the-world-bank-by-ngaire-woods-2016-01.

92. See Anne Krueger, "Whither the World Bank and the IMF?" *Journal of Economic Literature*, no. 36 (December 1998): 1983–2020.

93. Robert Wade, "Greening the Bank: The Struggle Over the Environment, 1975–1995," in *The World Bank: Its First Half Century*, vol. 1, ed. Devesh Kapur, John Prior Lewis, Richard Charles (New York: Oxford University Press, 1997), 611–734; https://books.google.co.uk/books?id=bNBmKae6n UcC&pg=PA611&lpg=PA611&dq=robert+wade+greening+the+bank+stru ggle+over+environment&source=bl&ots=D8K6O4kbwm&sig=B88HVoI M3AQTW7nI9ny2rrXl-3c&hl=en&sa=X&ved=0ahUKEwiYp8iop8 DNAhVGJcAKHfLHB9QQ6AEIHDAA#v=onepage&q=robert%20 wade%20greening%20the%20bank%20struggle%20over%20 environment&f=false.

94. Woods, "How to Save the World Bank."

95. Robert Zoellick, "Why We Still Need the World Bank: Looking Beyond Aid," *Foreign Affairs*, March/April 2012, accessed 12 January 2016, https://www.foreignaffairs.com/articles/2012-02-16/why-we-still-need-world-bank; Nancy Birdsall, "A New Mission for the World Bank," Project Syndicate, 30 June 2015, accessed 12 January 2016, http://www.project-syndicate.org/commentary/world-bank-global-public-goods-cgiar-by-nancy-birdsall-2015-06.

96. Devi Sridhar, "Addressing Under-nutrition in India: Do 'Rational' Approaches Work?" in *Paradoxes of Modernization: Unintended Consequences of Public Policy Reform*, ed. Helen Margetts and Christopher Hood, 134 (Oxford: Oxford University Press, 2010).

97. William Ascher, "New Development Approaches and the Adaptability of International Agencies: The Case of the World Bank," *International Organization*, no. 37 (Summer 1983): 430.

98. Taken from transcript of Bank meeting, cited in Devi Sridhar, *The Battle Against Hunger: Choice, Circumstance, and the World Bank* (New York: Oxford University Press, 2008).

99. Ngaire Woods, "How to Save the World Bank."

100. As one example, draft Project Preparation Mission aide-mémoire prepared for Bangladesh states: Given the fact that (1) the support for HNPSP [HNP Sector Programme] needs to be approved by the World Bank and DP [Development Partners] by December 2004, and (2) a HNP Strategic Investment Plan for the period 2005–2010 (or further) is in an early stage of development, the timeline for project preparation (see Annex 1) is constrained. However, project approval by the Executive Board of the World Bank could be achieved by December 2004, if good use is made of existing policy papers—including the Conceptual Framework and Policy Options paper come to mind—and PIP 2003–2006. Government and DPs have developed numerous papers dealing with subsectoral or multisectoral HNP issues. Bangladesh is also developing a National Strategy for Economic Growth and Poverty Reduction (PRSP). Therefore, the development of a six-year Strategic Investment Plan 2005–2010 (SIP) for the HNP sector should heavily rely on these documents. The SIP would only need to be detailed only for the first few years of the program, both in terms of interventions and in financial plans.

101. Ngaire Woods, *The Globalizers: The IMF, the World Bank, and Their Borrowers* (Ithaca, NY: Cornell University Press, 2006), 63 and 55 respectively.

102. Sridhar, *Battle Against Hunger*.

103. Woods, *Globalizers*.

104. Ibid.

105. Ngaire Woods, "The US, the World Bank and the IMF," in *US Hegemony and International Organizations*, ed. Rosemary Foot, Neil MacFralane, and MichaelMastanduno (New York: Oxford University Press, 2003), http://www.oxfordscholarship.com/view/10.1093/0199261431.001.0001/acprof-9780199261437-chapter-5

106. Philip Musgrove, "Idea Versus Money: A Conversation with Jean-Louis Sarbib," *Health Affairs* (August 2005), accessed 12 January 2016, http://content.healthaffairs.org/content/early/2005/08/02/hlthaff.w5.341.full.pdf.

107. Jeff Tyson, "Jim Kim Reflects on World Bank Reforms," Devex, 23 April 2015, accessed 12 January 2016, https://www.devex.com/news/jim-kim-reflects-on-world-bank-reforms-85974.

108. Jim Kim, "On Universal Health Coverage in Emerging Economies" (speech, World Bank, Washington, DC, 14 January 2014), accessed 12 January 2016, http://www.worldbank.org/en/news/speech/2014/01/14/speech-world-bank-group-president-jim-yong-kim-health-emerging-economies.

109. Ngaire Woods, "How to Save the World Bank."

110. "Home," Global Health Watch 2, 17 August 2009, accessed 12 January 2016, https://www.ghwatch.org/ghw2; Anne-Emanuelle Birn and Klaudia Dmitrienko, "The World Bank: Global Health or Global Harm?" *American Journal of Public Health*, no. 95 (July 2005): 1091–92.

111. Sridhar, *Battle Against Hunger*.

112. World Bank, "Lending Data: Fiscal 2011–2015," accessed 1 April 2016, http://pubdocs.worldbank.org/pubdocs/publicdoc/2015/11/804131447347453530/WBAR15-LendingData-rev.pdf.

113. See diversity and lack of agreement in list of health systems metrics in Soumya Alva, Eckhard Kleinau, Amanda Pomeroy, and Kathy Rowan, "Measuring the Impact of Health Systems Strengthening: A Review of the Literature" (report, USAID, Washington, DC, November 2009), 13–14, accessed 12 January 2016, https://www.k4health.org/sites/default/files/measuring%20reform%20hss.pdf.

114. Global Economic Governance Program, "High-Level Working Group of Developing Country Health Ministers" (meeting report, 2008).

115. Charles Clift, "WHO, the World Bank and Universal Health Coverage," *Chatham House*, 28 May 2013, accessed 12 January 2016, https://www.chathamhouse.org/media/comment/view/191697.

116. International Bank for Reconstruction and Development, "IBRD Articles of Agreement: Article IV, Section 10" (provisions, World Bank, February 1989), accessed 12 January 2016, http://siteresources.worldbank.org/EXTABOUTUS/Resources/ibrd-articlesofagreement.pdf.

117. Clyde Farnsworth, "Diplomatic World Bank Chief," *New York Times*, 12 April 1982, accessed 16 January 2016, http://www.nytimes.com/1982/04/12/business/diplomatic-world-bank-chief.html?pagewanted=all.

118. Sam Jones, "Senior UN Official Castigates World Bank Over Its Approach to Human Rights," *Guardian*, 22 October 2015, accessed 12 January 2016, http://www.theguardian.com/global-development/2015/oct/22/world-bank-human-rights-un-special-rapporteur-philip-alston; Sridhar, *Battle Against Hunger*.

119. Sridhar, *Battle Against Hunger*.

120. Robert Wade, "The Rising Inequality of World Income Distribution," *Finance & Development*, no. 38 (December 2001).

121. Philip Musgrove, "Idea Versus Money: A Conversation with Jean-Louis Sarbib," *Health Affairs* (August 2005), accessed 12 January 2016, http://content.healthaffairs.org/content/early/2005/08/02/hlthaff.w5.341.full.pdf.

122. Sudhir Anand, Fabienne Peter, and Amartya Sen, eds., *Public Health, Ethics, and Equity* (New York: Oxford University Press, 2004).

123. Devi Sridhar et al., "Universal Health Coverage and the Right to Health: From Legal Principle to Post-2015 Indicators," *International Journal of Health Services*, no. 45 (July 2015): 495–506.

124. With major funding from the Wellcome Trust, we will be leading a new project titled "The Economic Gaze: the World Bank's Influence in Global

Public Health" in a robust, independent, and detailed way from 2016 to 2020.

Chapter 7

1. Chris Murray, "Shifting to Sustainable Development Goals— Implications for Global Health," *NEJM*, no. 373 (October 2015): 1393.
2. Richard Horton, "GBD 2010: Understanding Disease, Injury, and Risk," *Lancet*, no. 380 (December 2012): 2053–54.
3. "Health Statistics and Information Systems/Estimates for 2000–2012/ Disease Burden/Global Summary Estimates," WHO, accessed 17 January 2016, http://www.who.int/healthinfo/global_burden_disease/estimates/ en/index2.html.
4. Commission on Social Determinants of Health, "Closing the Gap in a Generation: Health Equity Through Action on the Social Determinants of Health" (final report, WHO, Geneva, 2008).
5. Devi Sridhar et al., "Recent Shifts in Global Governance: Implications for the Response to Non-communicable Diseases," *PLoS Medicine*, no. 10 (July 2013).
6. IHME, "Financing Global Health 2012: The End of the Golden Age?" (report, Seattle, WA, 2012).
7. David Stuckler, Lawrence King, Helen Robinson, and Martin McKee, "WHO's Budgetary Allocations and Burden of Disease: A Comparative Analysis," *Lancet*, no. 372 (November 2008): 1563–69.
8. WHO, "Programme Budget 2008–2009 Performance Assessment Report," (WHO, Geneva, 2010), vii, accessed 13 July 2016, http://www .who.int/about/resources_planning/PBPA-1.pdf.
9. Rachel Nugent and Andrea B. Feigl, "Where Have All the Donors Gone? Scarce Donor Funding for Non-Communicable Diseases," (Center for Global Development Working Paper 228, November 2010), accessed 13 July 2016, http://www.cgdev.org/publication/where-have-all-donors-gone-scarce-donor-funding-non-communicable-diseases-working-paper.
10. Thomas Bollyky, "Developing Symptoms: Noncommunicable Diseases Go Global," *Foreign Affairs* (May/June 2012), accessed 15 January 2016, https://www.foreignaffairs.com/articles/2012-05-01/developing-symptoms.
11. Dawn Primarolo, Mark Malloch-Brown, and Ivan Lewis, "Health is Global: A UK Government Strategy for 2008–13," *Lancet*, no. 373 (February 2009): 443–45; Tone Torgersen, Oyvind Giaever, and Ole Stigen, "Developing an Intersectoral National Strategy to Reduce Social Inequities in Health: The Norwegian Case" (document, Intersectoral Action Project, WHO Commission on the Social Determinants of Health, Oslo, Norway, August 2007); Government of Canada, "The Federal Initiative to Address HIV/AIDS in Canada: Strengthening Federal Action in the Canadian Response to HIV/AIDS" (document, Minister of Public Works and Government Services Canada, Ontario,

Canada, 2004), accessed 16 January 2016, http://www.cpha.ca/uploads/portals/hiv/federal_initiative_e.pdf.

12. Derek Yach and Yasmin von Schirnding, "Public Health Lives: Gro Harlem Brundtland," *Public Health*, no. 128 (February 2014): 148–50.

13. Lawrence Gostin and Devi Sridhar, "Global Health and the Law," *NEJM*, no. 370 (2014): 1732–40.

14. David Stuckler and Marion Nestle, "Big Food, Food Systems, and Global Health," *PLoS Medicine*, no. 9 (6): e1001242 (June 2012), http://journals.plos.org/plosmedicine/article?id=10.1371/journal.pmed.1001242.

15. Global Fund to Fight AIDS, Tuberculosis and Malaria, Office of the Inspector General, "Audit of Global Fund Grants Managed by Population Services International" (executive summary, Geneva, 31 October 2011).

16. "About the UN Global Fund Partnership," UNDP, accessed 11 January 2016, http://www.undp-globalfund-capacitydevelopment.org/home/service/about-us.aspx.

17. Devi Sridhar and Rajaie Batniji, "Misfinancing Global Health: A Case for Transparency in Disbursements and Decision Making," *Lancet*, no. 372 (September 2008): 1185–91.

18. Devi Sridhar and Eduardo Gomez, "Health Financing in Brazil, Russia and India: What Role Does the International Community Play?" *Health Policy and Planning*, no. 26 (2011): 12–24.

19. Richard Horton, Twitter Feed, accessed 16 January 2016, https://twitter.com/richardhorton1?lang=en.

20. World Heart Federation, "Rheumatic Heart Disease," accessed 17 June 2016, http://www.world-heart-federation.org/press/fact-sheets/rheumatic-heart-disease/.

21. United Nations, "Adopting Consensus Text, General Assembly Encourages Member States to Plan, Pursue Transition of National Health Care Systems Towards Universal Coverage" (meeting coverage, 67th General Assembly, Geneva, Switzerland, 12 December 2012), accessed 16 January 2016, http://www.un.org/press/en/2012/ga11326.doc.htm.

22. WHO, "Sustainable Health Financing, Universal Coverage and Social Health Insurance" (resolution, 58th World Health Assembly, Geneva, April 2005), accessed 16 January 2016, http://www.who.int/health_financing/documents/cov-wharesolution5833/en/.

23. WHO, "Positioning Health in the Post-2015 Development Agenda" (discussion paper, Geneva, October 2012).

24. Thomas O'Connell, Kumanan Rasanathan, and Mickey Chopra, "What Does Universal Health Coverage Mean?" *Lancet*, no. 383 (January 2014): 277–79.

25. Devi Sridhar and Chelsea Clinton, "Overseeing Global Health," *Finance & Development*, no. 51 (December 2014), accessed 15 January 2016, http://www.imf.org/external/pubs/ft/fandd/2014/12/sridhar.htm.

26. Marko Vujicic, Stephanie E. Weber, Irina A. Nicolic, Rifat Atun, and Ranjana Kumar, "An Analysis of Gavi, the Global Fund and World Bank Support for Human Resources for Health in Developing Countries," *Health Policy and Planning*, published online 13 February 2012, accessed 17 March 2016, http://heapol.oxfordjournals.org/content/ early/2012/02/13/heapol.czs012.full.pdf+html.

27. Gorik Ooms, Wim Van Damme, Brook Baker, Paul Zeitz, and Ted Schrecker, "The 'Diagonal' Approach to Global Fund Financing: A Cure for the Broader Malaise of Health Systems?" *Globalization and Health*, no. 4 (March 2008).

28. John-Arne Rottingen et al., *Shared Responsibilities for Health: A Coherent Global Framework for Health Financing* (London: Chatham House, The Royal Institute of International Affairs, 2014).

29. Chunling Lu et al., "Public Financing of Health in Developing Countries: A Cross-National Systematic Analysis," *Lancet*, no. 375 (April 2010): 1375–87, accessed July 2015, http://www.ncbi.nlm.nih.gov/ pubmed/20381856.

30. Devi Sridhar, "Post-Accra: Is There Space for Country Ownership in Global Health?" *Third World Quarterly*, no. 30 (October 2009): 1363–77, accessed 15 January 2016, http://www.tandfonline.com/doi/ abs/10.1080/01436590903134981.

31. Gavin Yamey, "Can Japan Rouse the G7 Nations to Action on Universal Health Coverage?" *BMJ*, 22 December 2015, accessed 15 January 2016, http://blogs.bmj.com/bmj/2015/12/22/gavin-yamey-can-japan-rouse-the-g7-nations-to-action-on-universal-health-coverage/.

32. Carol Welch and Clint Pecenka, "Health in the Post-2015 Development Agenda" (document, Gates Foundation, 2013).

33. Save the Children, "A WAKE-UP CALL: Lessons from Ebola for the World's Health Systems" (report, London, 2015); editorial, "Health Security: The Defining Challenge of 2016," *Lancet*, no. 386 (December 2015): 2445.

34. David Heymann et al., "Global Health Security: The Wider Lessons from the West African Ebola Virus Disease Epidemic," *Lancet*, no. 385 (May 2015): 1884–1901.

35. Ibid.

36. Chelsea Clinton and Devi Sridhar, "Ebola Shows How Our Global Health Priorities Need to be Shaken Up," *Guardian*, 6 May 2015, accessed 15 January 2016, http://www.theguardian.com/commentisfree/2015/ may/06/ebola-global-health-priorities-chelsea-clinton.

37. Ezra Klein, "The Most Predictable Disaster in the History of the Human Race," Vox.com, 27 May 2015, accessed 16 January 2016, http://www.vox .com/2015/5/27/8660249/gates-flu-pandemic.

38. See http://www.worldbank.org/en/news/press-release/2016/05/21/ world-bank-group-launches-groundbreaking-financing-facility-to-protect-

poorest-countries-against-pandemics; http://www.who.int/dg/
speeches/2016/ebola-road-to-recovery/en/.

39. "Pandemic Emergency Facility: Frequently Asked Questions," World
Bank, accessed 16 January 2016, http://www.worldbank.org/en/topic/
pandemics/brief/pandemic-emergency-facility-frequently-asked-
questions; Suerie Moon et al., "Will Ebola Change the Game? Ten
Essential Reforms Before the Next Pandemic. The Report of the Harvard-
LSHTM Independent Panel on the Global Response to Ebola," *Lancet*,
no. 386 (November 2015): 2204–21; Institute of Medicine, *Global Health
Risk Framework, Governance for Global Health: Workshop Summary*
(Washington, DC: The National Academies Press, 2016).

40. Suerie Moon et al., "Will Ebola Change the Game?".

41. Bill Gates, "The Next Epidemic—Lessons from Ebola," *NEJM*, no. 372
(April 2015): 1381–84.

42. "Home," Global Health Security Agenda, accessed 11 January 2016,
https://ghsagenda.org/packages/d5-workforce-development.html.

43. Ole Ottersen, Julio Frenk, and Richard Horton, "The *Lancet*—University
of Oslo Commission on Global Governance for Health, in Collaboration
with the Harvard Global Health Institute," *Lancet*, no. 378 (November
2011): 1612–13.

44. "10 Facts on Polio Eradication," WHO, October 2015, accessed 14 April
2016, http://www.who.int/features/factfiles/polio/en/.

45. UNICEF, "UNICEF's Engagement in the Global Polio Eradication
Initiative," 2012, accessed 14 April 2016, http://www.unicef.org/partners/
files/Partnership_profile_2012_Polio_revised.pdf, 2.

46. "About Us," GPEI, accessed 14 April 2016, http://www.polioeradication
.org/aboutus.aspx.

INDEX

———◦◦———

Note: Page numbers in *italics* indicate charts and tables.

Abbott, Kenneth, 16, 25
Additional Financing for the
    Health System
    Improvement Project, 149
agency slack, 31–32, 71–72
Aidspan, 68, 111
Aid Transparency Index, 145,
    151–52, 159
Alma-Ata Conference, 9, 187
Angola, 53
Annan, Kofi, 16, 62
antiretroviral drugs, 14, 19, 45
Asian Infrastructure
    Investment Bank, 190
assessed contributions
    and DAH funding, 89
    and incentive structures, 65
    and shifts in governance
        structures, 53
    and WHO funding, 91,
        94–95, *95*, 97
    and WHO reforms, 185
asymmetries of information,
    69–72
Australia, *51*, 95, *95*, 206
    AusAid, 172
Austria, 5

autoimmune diseases, 2.
    See also HIV/AIDS crisis
Avian and Human Influenza
    Facility, 106

Bangladesh, 151
Bartsch, Sonja, 13
bed nets, 9, 18–20, 45–46,
    133–34, 172, 202
Belgium, *51*
Berkley, Seth, 165
bilateral aid agencies, 26–27,
    61, 75, 86, 109–10, 117
Bill & Melinda Gates
    Foundation
    and alignment of global
        health objectives, 60
    and background of global
        health cooperation, 10
    child health-related
        programs, 78–79, *105*
    and consequences of new
        institutional models, 165
    and critiques of the
        WHO, 36
    and DAH funding, 84, 88–89
    and data sources, 228

    and Gavi funding, 113–17,
        114, 116
    and Gavi governance, 130
    and Gavi's impact on aid
        landscape, 167–69
    and Gavi's mission, 41, 42
    and Global Fund funding,
        108–9, 112
    and Global Fund's impact
        on aid landscape, 171, 177
    and global institution
        governance structures,
        138–39
    and growth of public-
        private partnerships,
        15–16
    influence on global aid
        system, 203
    and legitimacy of
        public-private
        partnerships, 17
    and mechanics of
        international
        cooperation, 23, 27–28
    and noncommunicable
        disease efforts, 205, 207–8
    open access research, 153–54

Bill & Melinda Gates
    Foundation (*continued*)
    origin and influence
        of, 76–82
    and polio eradication
        efforts, 215
    principal-agent perspective
        on, 32
    and purpose of study, 22
    and rise of public-private
        partnerships, 13
    scope of global health
        aid, 28–29
    and shifts in governance
        structures, 48, 50–53,
        51, 52
    and source vs. channel
        funding, 86
    and transparency, 153
    and universal health
        coverage efforts, 211
    and WHO funding, 94,
        96, 119
    and WHO governance,
        123, 126
    and WHO reforms, 178,
        181, 184
    and World Bank's
        comparative
        advantage, 197
Birdsall, Nancy, 190
birth attendants, ix
Bloomberg, Michael, 181
Bloomberg Family
    Foundation, 205, 208
Bono, 110
Brazil, 2, 189
breastfeeding, 78
British Medical Journal, 93–94
Brundtland, Gro Harlem, 35,
        73–74, 91–92, 207
bubonic plague (Black
        Death), 5
Buffett, Warren, 52, 76–77
Bull, Benedict, 15
Buse, Kent, 13, 17
Bush, George W., 62

Canada
    bilateral vs. multilateral aid,
        27, *28*
    and Gavi funding, *114*, 115,
        116

and IDA funding, *101, 102*
and noncommunicable
    disease efforts, 206
and shifts in governance
    structures, *51*
and WHO funding, 95, *95*
cancer, 211–13
cause-specific funding, 78–79
Chan, Margaret, 2, 120,
        122, 144
channel funding
    and alignment of global
        health objectives, 61
    bilateral vs. multilateral
        aid, *28*
    and Global Fund's impact
        on aid landscape, 173–74
    and Global Fund's
        mission, 45
    and importance of
        governance, 4
    and incentive structures, 66
    and mechanics of
        international
        cooperation, 26–27
    and revolutionizing global
        aid, 18
    source funding contrasted
        with, 86–87
    and WHO funding, 93
    and World Bank funding,
        101, 103
Chevron, 53
Chikungunya, 216
child mortality, ix, 3, 107,
        167–68
Children's Vaccine Initiative
    (CVI), 166–67
China
    and early global health
        cooperation efforts, 5–6
    and Global Fund funding,
        108
    and Global Fund
        governance, 140
    and Global Fund's impact
        on aid landscape, 177
    voting power of, *194*
    and WHO funding, 95, *95*
    and World Bank funding, 99
    and World Bank reforms,
        189–90, 193
cholera, 4–6, 24, 39, 218n16

civil society, 178–79
Civil Society Organizations
    (CSOs)
    and accountability, 119–20
    and composition of Gavi
        board, *58*
    and Gavi governance,
        129–30, 132
    and Gavi's impact on aid
        landscape, 168
    and Gavi's mission, 42
    and Global Fund
        governance, 133, 134–35
    and global institution
        governance structures,
        137–39, 138–39
    and growth of public-
        private partnerships, 16
    and history of global health
        cooperation, 5
    and membership standards
        for multilaterals, 121–22
    and monitoring of global
        agencies, 72
    principal-agent perspective
        on, 29
    and rise of public-private
        partnerships, 13
    and shifts in governance
        structures, 50, 52, *52*
    and transparency, 141–42,
        144, 147, 151, 153
    and WHO practices, 38
    and WHO reforms,
        178–80, 187, 188
    and World Bank
        governance, 126–29
    and World Bank
        practices, 39
    and World Bank reforms,
        200
    and World Bank's
        comparative advantage,
        199
    See also nongovernmental
        organizations (NGOs);
        nonstate actors
Clausen, Alden "Tom,"
        198–99
Climate Investment Fund, 106
Clinton Foundation, x
Clinton Health Access
    Initiative, x

Cold War, 26, 119
collective action, x, 23–24,
    31, 81
compromise, 143, 144
conditional authority, 30
cooperation in global health,
    3–12. *See also* collective
    action
corruption, 140–41
Country Assistance Strategies
    (CASs), 137
country-coordinating
    mechanisms (CCMs)
    and Global Fund
        governance, 134, *138*
    and Global Fund grants,
        54
    and Global Fund's impact
        on aid landscape, 171–74,
        176–77
    and Global Fund's mission,
        44–45
    and monitoring of global
        agencies, 73, 75
    and Rounds-based
        financing, 254n36
Creditor Reporting System
    (CRS), *101*, 228n64
Crucell, 131

democratic deficit, 122, 162
Dengue fever, 2, 215–16
Denmark, *51*
depression, 212
developing countries, 41, 159,
    188
Development Assistance
    Committee (DAC), 30,
    228n64
development assistance for
    health (DAH), 26–28, *29*,
    83–86, *84*, 88, 205
diabetes, 212
diphtheria, 41, 167
Disability Adjusted Life Years
    (DALYs), 10
discretionary funding
    and consequences of new
        institutional models,
        162–63
    and critiques of the
        WHO, 37
    and DAH funding, 82

and incentive structures, 66,
    68–69
and trend toward vertical
    initiatives, 56
and WHO governance, 122
and WHO reforms, 185
disease risk factors, 210–11
Djibouti, 68
DPT$_3$ vaccine, 41–42, 55,
    152, 167
Dybul, Mark, 16, 112

Ebola crisis
    and the case for good
        governance, 202
    and case study overviews, 35
    and consequences of new
        institutional models, 164
    and critiques of the World
        Bank, 126
    and importance of
        governance, 1–4
    and ODA trends, 200
    and pandemic preparedness,
        204, 211–13
    and polio eradication
        efforts, 215
    and stakeholder
        engagement, 160
    and transparency, 144–45
    and WHO budget, 87
    and WHO funding, 93
    and WHO governance,
        125
    and WHO reforms, 180,
        182, 184, 187–88
    and World Bank's
        comparative advantage,
        198
The Economist, 174
Emanuel, Ezekiel J., 67–68
epidemic diseases
    and alignment of global
        health objectives, 61
    and background of global
        health cooperation,
        6–7, 10
    and case study overviews, 35
    and consequences of new
        institutional models,
        163–64
    and importance of
        governance, 3

and information
    asymmetries, 71
and noncommunicable
    disease efforts, 206
and purpose of study, 20
and transparency, 146
and universal health
    coverage efforts, 211
and WHO reforms, 182, 184
See also specific diseases
Ethiopia, 212
European Commission, 19, *51*,
    65, 96, 174
European Union, 14, 31,
    114, 122
Evans, Tim, 198
extrabudgetary funding
    and alignment of global
        health objectives, 61
    disbursements over
        time, *104*
    and Gavi funding, 116–17
    and incentive structures,
        64–65
    and monitoring of global
        agencies, 73–74
    and noncommunicable
        disease efforts, 205
    and WHO funding, 90,
        92–94, *93*, 96–97
    and WHO governance, *136*
    and WHO reforms, 181

Feachem, Richard, 18, 68, 165
financial crisis (1980s), 9
Financial Intermediary Funds
    (FIFs), 240n81
Financial Times, 131
Five-Year Evaluations, 172
Food and Agricultural
    Organization (FAO), 75
Ford Foundation, 77
Foreign Affairs, 94
France
    bilateral vs. multilateral aid,
        27, 28
    and Gavi funding, *114*, 115
    and Global Fund funding,
        112
    and IDA funding, *101, 102*
    and mechanics of
        international
        cooperation, 27

France (*continued*)
  and shifts in governance
    structures, *51*
  and WHO funding, *95*
  and World Bank
    reforms, 193
fraud, 174, *175*
funding, 81–86
  and Gavi, 113–18
  and the Global Fund,
    107–13
  "Golden Age" of DAH
    funding, 88–89
  membership due vs/
    voluntary contributions,
    87–88
  and the World Bank,
    97–107
  and the World Health
    Organization, 89–97
  See also channel funding

G7 countries, 10, *27*, *28*, 62,
  119, 211
Garrett, Laurie, 94
Gates, Bill and Melinda
  and DAH funding, 89
  and Gavi funding, 117
  and Gavi governance, 130
  and influence of the Gates
    Foundation, 78–81
  and origin of the Gates
    Foundation, 76
  and pandemic preparedness,
    212–13
  principal-agent perspective
    on, 29
  and WHO reforms, 181
Gates Foundation. *See* Bill &
  Melinda Gates
  Foundation
generic pharmaceuticals, 16
Germany
  bilateral vs. multilateral aid,
    27, *28*
  and debt swap programs,
    240n84
  and development assistance
    for health funding, *29*
  and Global Fund
    funding, 112
  and IDA funding, *101*, *102*
  and incentive structures, 68

and shifts in governance
  structures, *51*
voting power of, *194*
and WHO funding, *95*
and World Bank
  reforms, 193
GlaxoSmithKline, 15
Global Alliance for Improved
  Nutrition (GAIN), 12,
  26, *55*
Global Alliance for Vaccines
  and Immunization (Gavi)
  and advanced market
    commitment donors, 115,
    116, *139*
  and alignment of global
    health objectives, 60, 63
  and background of global
    health cooperation, 10, 12
  and the case for good
    governance, 202–4
  and case study methods, 40,
    46–47
  and changing accountability
    standards, 120–21
  composition of governing
    board, *58*
  and consequences of new
    institutional models,
    162, 165
  contrasted with "old"
    institutions, 107–8
  cooperation with nonstate
    actors, 129–32
  and critiques of the WHO,
    35, 36, 37
  and DAH funding, 86,
    88–89
  donors to, *114*
  and dues vs. voluntary
    contributions, 87–88
  and funding for global
    health initiatives,
    113–18
  and funding shifts, *33*
  fundraising efforts, 169
  and Gates Foundation aid,
    28–29
  and Gavi funding,
    115–16, *116*
  and Gavi's mission, 41–44
  and Global Fund funding,
    110, 111–12

and Global Fund
  governance, 133–35, *138*
and Global Fund's impact
  on aid landscape, 173
and Global Fund's mission,
  44–45
governance structure of, *139*
and growth of public-private
  partnerships, 14, 16
impact on aid landscape,
  166–70
and incentive structures, 65,
  67–68
Independent Review
  Committee (IRC), 71, 75
and influence of the Gates
  Foundation, 76–77, 81
and information
  asymmetries, 69, 70–71
and legitimacy of
  public-private
  partnerships, 17
and mechanics of
  international
  cooperation, 23, 25–27
and monitoring of global
  agencies, 74–75
and noncommunicable
  disease efforts, 207–8
and polio eradication
  efforts, 215
principal-agent perspective
  on, 30, 32–33
and purpose of study, 20,
  21–22
and revolutionizing global
  aid, 18–19
and rise of public-private
  partnerships, 12–13
and shifts in governance
  structures, 48,
  50–56, *52*
and stakeholder
  engagement, 159–60
and transparency, 142, 144,
  145–46, 150–52, 153–54,
  158, 159
and trend toward vertical
  initiatives, *55*
and universal health
  coverage efforts, 210–11
and WHO funding, 91, 94,
  96–97

and WHO governance,
123–25
and WHO reforms, 178,
180–81, 183
and World Bank funding,
101, 104–5
and World Bank reforms,
200
and World Bank's
comparative advantage,
197
Global Environmental Facility,
106
Global Fund Observer, 74–75
Global Fund to Fight AIDS,
Tuberculosis and Malaria
and Affected Communities,
134–35
and alignment of global
health objectives, 60,
62–63
and background of global
health cooperation, 10, 12
and the case for good
governance, 202–4
and case study methods, 40,
44–46, 46–47
and changing accountability
standards, 119–21
composition of governing
board, *58*
and composition of
governing boards, 59
and consequences of new
institutional models,
162, 165
contrasted with "old"
institutions, 107–13
cooperation with nonstate
actors, 129
and critiques of the WHO,
35–37
and DAH funding,
88–89
debt swaps, 108, 240n84
and dues vs. voluntary
contributions, 87–88
and faith-based
organizations, 127
Framework Document, 88
fraud in grants, *175*
and funding sources, 107–13,
115

fundraising, 108–9, 111–12,
133–34
and Gates Foundation aid,
28–29
Gavi contrasted with, 166
and Gavi governance, 130,
132
and Gavi's impact on aid
landscape, 168–70
and Global Fund's impact
on aid landscape, 170–77
governance structure of,
133–40, *138*
and growth of public-
private partnerships,
14–15, 16
High-Level Panel, 110, 134,
175, 177
and importance of
governance, 3
and incentive structures, 65,
67–68
and influence of the Gates
Foundation, 76, 81
and information
asymmetries, 69–71
Inspector General, 68, 154
and legitimacy of
public-private
partnerships, 17
Local Fund Agents (LFAs),
153
and mechanics of
international
cooperation, 23
membership policy,
133–40
and monitoring of global
agencies, 72, 74–75
New Funding Model, 172,
176
and noncommunicable
disease efforts, 207–8
Partnership Forums, 135
Portfolio and
Implementation
Committee, 70
principal-agent perspective
on, 30, 32–33
and purpose of study, 20,
21–22
and revolutionizing global
aid, 18–19

and rise of public-private
partnerships, 12–13
Rounds-based approach, 171
and shifts in governance
structures, 48, 50, *51*,
51–54
and source vs. channel
funding, 86–87
and stakeholder
engagement, 159–60
Technical Review Panel
(TRP), 70–71, 74, 153,
171–72, 176
top donors, *109*
and transparency, 142,
144–46, 149–50, 152–59,
157
and trend toward vertical
initiatives, *55*, 56
and universal health
coverage efforts, 210, 211
WHO contrasted with,
117–18
and WHO funding, 91–92,
94, 97
and WHO governance, 125
and WHO reforms, 178,
180, 183, 184–85
and World Bank funding,
101, 104–7
and World Bank reforms,
200
and World Bank's
comparative advantage,
197
See also principal recipients
(PRs) of Global Fund
grants
global governance, x–xi, 81
Global Health Security
Agenda, 213
globalization, x
Global Partnership for Social
Accountability (GPSA),
128
Global Partnership for TB
Control, 106
Global Partnership to Eradicate
Poliomyelitis, 128
Global Polio Eradication
Initiative, 17
Godlee, Fiona, 93–94
good governance, 22

Gostin, Larry, 179
gross national income (GNI),
    54–55
growth monitoring, oral
    rehydration,
    breastfeeding, and
    immunization
    (GOBI), 10
Guinea, 163, 198
Guinea Worm Eradication
    Partnership, 17

H₁N₁ pandemic, 69
H₁N₁ Review Committee, 182
H8, 76
Harmer, Andrew, 17
Harvard School of Public
    Health (HSPH), 3
Hawkins, Darren, 30–32
Health, Nutrition, and
    Population (HNP)
    (World Bank)
    composition of
        commitments, 105
    and funding shifts, 33
    and pandemic preparedness,
        213–14
    and transparency, 148, 156
    and World Bank funding,
        97, 101, 104–6
    and World Bank reforms,
        191, 192
Health for All by 2000 initiative, 10
Health Results Innovation
    Trust Fund (HRITF), 107
health-worker shortages, 210
heart disease, 212
Hepatitis B, 43
HIV/AIDS crisis
    and alignment of global
        health objectives, 60–62
    and background of global
        health cooperation, 10–11
    and changing WHO
        priorities, 35
    and consequences of new
        institutional models, 162
    and critiques of "old
        actors," 40
    and DAH funding, 88–89
    and Gates Foundation, 28
    and Gavi funding, 115–16
    and Gavi governance, 132

and the Global Fund,
    45–46, 53–54, 110
and Global Fund
    governance, 135, 138
and Global Fund's impact
    on aid landscape, 170–71
and growth of public-private
    partnerships, 14–15
and importance of
    governance, 3–4
and influence of the Gates
    Foundation, 77
and information
    asymmetries, 70
and legitimacy of
    public-private
    partnerships, 17
and mechanics of
    international
    cooperation, 24–25
and noncommunicable
    disease efforts, 205–6, 208
and polio eradication
    efforts, 215
principal-agent perspective
    on, 30
and purpose of study,
    20, 21
and source vs. channel
    funding, 87
and transparency, 152–53
and universal health
    coverage efforts, 211
and WHO funding, 91
and WHO governance, 125
and WHO strategies, 49
and World Bank funding,
    97, 105–6
and World Bank practices, 39
See also Global Fund to
    Fight AIDS, Tuberculosis
    and Malaria
horizontal approach to
    health-care challenges
    and background of global
        health cooperation, 8–12
    and Gavi governance, 132
    and Global Fund's impact
        on aid landscape, 176
    and influence of the Gates
        Foundation, 78–79, 81
    and trend toward vertical
        initiatives, 55, 56

and universal health
    coverage efforts, 210
and World Bank's comparative
    advantage, 197–98
See also vertical approach to
    health-care challenges
Horton, Richard, 208
Høybråten, Dagfinn, 168

incentive structures, 63–69
Independent Evaluation
    Group (IEG), 105,
    148–49, 170, 228n64
Independent Panel on the
    Global Response to
    Ebola, 3
India, 147, 189, 196, 206
Indonesia, 53
infectious disease, 3, 5–9, 12,
    211–14. See also pandemics
    and pandemic
    preparedness; specific
    diseases
Influenza A (H₁N₁) pandemic,
    182
in-kind contributions
    and DAH funding, 26,
        83, 85
    and Gavi governance, 132
    and the Global Fund, 110,
        112, 133–35
    and global institution
        governance structures,
        138–39
    and rise of public-private
        partnerships, 13
    and transparency, 150–51
    and WHO governance,
        123–24
    and the World Bank, 97
input legitimacy, 17
Institute for Health Metrics
    and Evaluation (IHME)
    on annual disbursements
        over time, 104
    and critiques of the
        WHO, 36
    and DAH funding,
        84, 88
    and data sources, 228n64
    and noncommunicable
        disease efforts, 205
    and transparency, 151, 158

and universal health
    coverage efforts, 210
and World Bank funding, 97
Internal Revenue Service
    (IRS), 77
International AIDS Vaccine
    Initiative (IAVI), 112, 115,
    241n97
International Aid Transparency
    Initiative (IATI), 145, 149,
    150, 155
International Bank for
    Reconstruction and
    Development
    (IBRD), 194
and alignment of global
    health objectives, 63
annual disbursements over
    time, 104
and dues vs. voluntary
    contributions, 87
funding for global health
    efforts, 98
and Gavi grants, 55
Global Fund funding
    contrasted with, 110
and incentive structures, 66
origin of, 38
and shifts in governance
    structures, 49–50
and transparency, 150
and trend toward vertical
    initiatives, 55
and World Bank funding,
    99, 101, 107
and World Bank
    governance, 137
and World Bank Group
    structure, 99
and World Bank reforms,
    189, 190, 193
and World Bank's
    comparative advantage, 196
See also World Bank
International Centre for
    Settlement of Investment
    Disputes (ICSID) (World
    Bank), 38, 99, 193
International Conference on
    Primary Health Care, 9
International Congress of
    Charities, Corrections,
    and Philanthropy, 5

International Development
    Association (IDA)
    (World Bank)
and alignment of global
    health objectives, 63
annual disbursements over
    time, 104
donor contributions over
    time, 101
and dues vs. voluntary
    contributions, 87–88
funding for global health
    efforts, 98
and Gavi funding, 44, 113
and Gavi grants, 55
and Gavi's mission, 41
and IDA funding, 102
and incentive structures,
    65–67
and replenishment funding,
    100, 108
and shifts in governance
    structures, 49–50
and transparency, 150, 151,
    159, 203
and trend toward vertical
    initiatives, 55
and World Bank funding,
    99–101, 107
and World Bank
    governance, 137
and World Bank Group
    structure, 99
and World Bank practices,
    38–39
and World Bank reforms,
    189, 193
and World Bank's
    comparative advantage,
    196, 198–99
International Development
    Committee (UK
    Parliament), 149
International Drug Purchasing
    Facility (UNITAID), 111,
    123
International Federation of
    Pharmaceutical
    Wholesalers, 132
International Finance
    Corporation (IFC)
    (World Bank), 38,
    99, 137

International Financing
    Facility for Innovation
    Mechanism (IFFIm), 115,
    139, 168
International Health
    Boards (Rockefeller
    Foundation), 6
International Health
    Regulations (IHR)
and alignment of global
    health objectives, 60
and background of global
    health cooperation, 5
and changing WHO
    priorities, 35–36
and consequences of new
    institutional models,
    163–64
and importance of
    governance, 4
and WHO reforms, 182,
    184, 187
International Labor
    Organization (ILO), 6,
    26, 40, 65
International Monetary Fund
    (IMF), 30, 32, 49, 126,
    142–43, 193
International Red Cross,
    5, 6
International Sanitary
    Conference, 5, 7, 24
Investing in Health (World
    Bank), 10
Ireland, 51, 95
Italy
and background of global
    health cooperation, 5
bilateral vs. multilateral aid,
    27, 28
and Gavi funding, 114, 115,
    116
and Global Fund funding,
    109
and IDA funding, 102
and shifts in governance
    structures, 51
and WHO funding, 96

Jacques-François, Martin, 169
Japan
and background of global
    health cooperation, 5

Japan (*continued*)
   bilateral vs. multilateral aid,
      27, 28
   and Global Fund funding,
      109, 112
   and IDA funding, *101, 102*
   and shifts in governance
      structures, *51*
   and transparency, *156*
   and universal health
      coverage efforts, 211
   voting power of, *194*
   and WHO funding, 95, *95*
   and World Bank
      reforms, 193
Japanese encephalitis, 42
Jaramillo, Gabriel, 174–75

Keefe, Tania, 17
Keohane, Robert, 26, 142
Kim, Jim, 129, 195, 198
knowledge mobilization, 15

Lagarde, Christine, 193
The Lancet, 208
languages used by global
      institutions, 144, 151,
      155–58, 159
League of Nations, 6
League of Nations Health
      Organization (LNHO),
      6–8
League of Nations Health
      Section, 7
Liberia, 198
Lob-Levyt, Julian, 169
London School of Hygiene
      and Tropical Medicine
      (LSHTM), 3
Luxembourg, *51*

Mahler, Halfdan, 91
malaria
   and alignment of global
      health objectives, 60, 62
   and background of global
      health cooperation, 8, 11
   and changing WHO
      priorities, 35
   and critiques of "old
      actors," 40
   and critiques of the
      WHO, 37

and DAH funding, 88
and Gavi governance, 132
and the Global Fund,
   44–46, 53–54, 110
and Global Fund
   governance, 135, *138*
and Global Fund's impact
   on aid landscape,
   170, 172
and information
   asymmetries, 70
and noncommunicable
   disease efforts, 205
and polio eradication
   efforts, 215–16
and purpose of study, 20
and transparency, 153
and WHO funding, 92
and World Bank funding,
   106
See also Global Fund to
   Fight AIDS, Tuberculosis
   and Malaria
Mali, 68, 134
malnutrition, 39, 78
Mandela, Nelson, 169
Mann, Jonathan, 60
maternal health, 212
Mauritania, 68, 134
McNeill, Desmond, 15, 116
measles, ix, 41–42, 55, 151
measles-rubella, 42
Mectizan Donation Program, 15
Médecins sans Frontières/
   Doctors Without Borders
   (MSF), 119, 125–26, 131,
   180
membership policies
   due vs/ voluntary
      contributions, 87–88
   and the Global Fund, 133–40
   membership standards for
      multilaterals, 121–22
   for multilateral institutions,
      121–22
   and nonstate actors, *136–39*
   and the World Bank, 126
   and the World Health
      Organization, 122–26
meningitis A, 42
Merck, 133
Merson, Michael, 12
Mexico, 95–96

miasma theory, 24
microcephaly, 2, 144.
   See also Zika virus
Middle East Respiratory
   Syndrome (MERS), 1
Millennium Development
   Goals (MDGs)
   and annual disbursements
      over time, *104*
   and background of global
      health cooperation, 10–11
   and changing WHO
      priorities, 35
   and consequences of new
      institutional models, 166
   and DAH funding, *84,*
      88–89
   and development assistance
      for health funding, *29*
   and funding shifts, *33*
   and influence of the Gates
      Foundation, 76,
      78, 81
   and World Bank funding,
      105
Millennium Development
   Summit, 78
mosquito-borne illnesses, 2,
   134, 215–16
Mozambique, 151
Multilateral Investment
   Guarantee Agency
   (MIGA) (World Bank
   program), 38, *99,* 193
multilateral organizations
   and alignment of global
      health objectives, 59–61,
      63
   bilateral vs. multilateral aid,
      27, 28
   and changing accountability
      standards, 119–20
   and consequences of new
      institutional models,
      161–63
   and Gavi funding, 117
   and Global Fund's impact
      on aid landscape, 174–75,
      177
   and the Global Fund's
      mission, 44, 46
   and growth of public-private
      partnerships, 15–16

impact of new vertical
    initiatives, 161–65
and incentive structures, 64,
    68
and information
    asymmetries, 69
and legitimacy of
    public-private
    partnerships, 17
and mechanics of
    international
    cooperation, 26–27
and monitoring of global
    agencies, 72–75
and noncommunicable
    disease efforts, 207, 209
and pandemic preparedness,
    214
principal-agent perspective
    on, 29–30
and revolutionizing global
    aid, 18
and rise of public-private
    partnerships, 13
and shifts in governance
    structures, 49, 51, 53
and source vs. channel
    funding, 86
and transparency, 141,
    145–47, 153–54
and trend toward vertical
    initiatives, 56
and WHO governance, 125
and World Bank funding,
    101
See also specific organizations
multiple principal model, 30–31
Murray, Chris, 203
Musgrove, Philip, 199

Nakajima, Hiroshi, 12
Nature, 153
Netherlands, 51, 102, 109, 114, 115
new actors. See Global Alliance
    for Vaccines and
    Immunization (Gavi);
    Global Fund to Fight
    AIDS, Tuberculosis and
    Malaria
Nigeria, 53
noncommunicable diseases
    (NCDs), 3, 94,
    204–9, 215

nongovernmental
    organizations (NGOs)
and alignment of global
    health objectives, 61–62
and changing accountability
    standards, 119–20
and composition of
    governing boards, 58
and consequences of new
    institutional models, 165
cooperation with "new"
    institutions, 129
and critiques of the WHO,
    37
and fraud in Global Fund
    grants, 175
and Gates Foundation aid,
    28, 203
and Gavi's mission, 43
and Global Fund funding,
    54, 111
and Global Fund
    governance, 134–35
and Global Fund's Board
    composition, 45
and global institution
    governance structures,
    136–38
and growth of public-
    private partnerships, 15
and membership standards
    for multilaterals, 121
and monitoring of global
    agencies, 74–75
and noncommunicable
    disease efforts, 207
and pandemic preparedness,
    212–13
and polio eradication
    efforts, 215–16
and revolutionizing global
    aid, 18
and rise of public-private
    partnerships, 12–13
and shifts in governance
    structures, 50, 51
and source vs. channel
    funding, 86–87
and transparency, 140–41,
    147
and universal health
    coverage efforts, 210, 212
and WHO funding, 89

and WHO governance,
    122–25
and WHO reforms, 179–82,
    186, 188
and World Bank
    governance, 126–29
and World Bank reforms,
    189, 195
and World Bank's
    comparative advantage,
    197
See also Civil Society
    Organizations (CSOs);
    nonstate actors
nonstate actors
and case study
    methods, 46
and changing accountability
    standards, 119–21
cooperation with "new"
    institutions, 129
and Gavi's impact on aid
    landscape, 168
and Global Fund
    governance, 133, 135
and Global Fund's impact
    on aid landscape, 171
and global institution
    membership policies,
    136–39
and growth of public-
    private partnerships, 15
and the ILO, 40
and legitimacy of
    public-private
    partnerships, 17
and mechanics of
    international
    cooperation, 23–24, 27
principal-agent perspective
    on, 29
and purpose of study, 21
and rise of public-private
    partnerships,
    12–13
and transparency, 142, 147
and WHO governance,
    122–25
and WHO reforms, 178–82,
    186–88
and World Bank
    membership and
    governance, 126

Norway, 26–27, *51*, *95*, 96, *114*,
    115, *116*, 206
  and Global Fund funding,
    109
nutrition programs
  and background of global
    health cooperation, 6
  and composition of HNP
    commitments, *105*
  and influence of the Gates
    Foundation, 78–79
  and noncommunicable
    disease efforts, 205, 207
  principal-agent perspective
    on, 33
  and World Bank funding,
    97, 101, 103, *103*, 105
  and World Bank
    governance, 126
  and World Bank practices,
    39
  and World Bank reforms,
    190
  and World Bank's
    comparative
    advantage, 199
Nye, Joseph, 142–43, 150

Office International
    d'hygiène Publique
    (OIHP), 6–8
Office of the High
    Commissioner for
    Human Rights
    (OHCHR), 187
Official Development
    Assistance (ODA), 9,
    83–85, *85*, 113, 200
old actors. *See* World Bank;
    World Health
    Organization (WHO)
onchocerciasis (river
    blindness), 15
ONE Campaign, 110–11
Organization for Economic
    Cooperation and
    Development (OECD),
    29–30, *85*
outbreak prevention and
    response, 163. *See also*
    pandemics and pandemic
    preparedness
output legitimacy, 17

Pacini, Filippo, 5
Pan American Health
    Organization (PAHO), 5,
    6, 13
pandemics and pandemic
    preparedness, 211–14
  and alignment of global
    health objectives, 61
  and background of global
    health cooperation, 5, 11
  and changing WHO
    priorities, 35
  and critiques of the WHO,
    37
  and information
    asymmetries, 69
  and mechanics of
    international
    cooperation, 26
  and need for coalitions, 204
  and purpose of study, 22
  and rise of public-private
    partnerships, 13
  and WHO funding, 91, 93,
    96
  and WHO reforms, 182, 188
  and World Bank reforms,
    195
Parran, Thomas, 8
Partners in Health, x
pentavalent vaccine, 41–43, 131,
    151, 167, 227n53
performance-based funding
    (PBF), 166, 170–73, 176,
    253n13
pertussis, 41, 167
philanthropic organizations
  and background of global
    health cooperation, 5–6
  and consequences of
    new institutional
    models, 162
  and Gates Foundation
    influence, 203
  and Gavi funding, 116
  and Gavi governance, 130
  and global institution
    membership policies, *136*
  and growth of public-
    private partnerships, 15
  and IAVI funding, 241n97
  and influence of the Gates
    Foundation, 77

  and membership standards
    for multilaterals, 121
  and noncommunicable
    disease efforts, 207–9
  principal-agent perspective
    on, 32
  and rise of public-private
    partnerships, 14
  and shifts in governance
    structures, 50, 52
  and source vs. channel
    funding, 86
  and WHO funding, 89
  and WHO governance,
    124–25
  and WHO reforms, 178, 181,
    185
  and World Bank
    governance, 127
  and World Bank's
    comparative advantage,
    197
  *See also specific organization
    names*
Piot, Peter, 95
pneumococcal vaccine, 167
pneumonia, ix, 42
Pogge, Thomas, 17–18
polio
  eradication program, 214–16
  and Gavi grants, 55
  and Gavi's impact on aid
    landscape, 167
  and Gavi's mission, 41, 42
  and importance of
    governance, 1
  and legitimacy of
    public-private
    partnerships, 17
  and revolutionizing global
    aid, 18
  and World Bank funding,
    106
Population Services
    International (PSI), 207
Portugal, *51*
post-war institutions, 16
PricewaterhouseCoopers, 153
principal-agent theory
  and alignment of global
    health objectives, 59–60
  and changing accountability
    standards, 121

described, 29–33
and Gavi funding, 42
and Gavi governance, 132
and Global Fund funding,
    108, 113
and information
    asymmetries, 69
and monitoring of global
    agencies, 72–73
and new funding and
    governance patterns, 59
and purpose of study, 20–21,
    21–22
and shifts in governance
    structures, 48
and shirking, 32
and slippage, 32
and WHO governance, 125
and World Bank funding,
    102, 107
principal recipients (PRs) of
    Global Fund grants
and Global Fund
    governance, 134, 138
and Global Fund grants, 54
and Global Fund's impact
    on aid landscape, 172,
    174, 176
and the Global Fund's
    mission, 44–45
and monitoring of global
    agencies, 73
and noncommunicable
    disease efforts, 207
and transparency, 153
Programme to Eliminate
    Lymphatic Filariasis, 36
Project Concept Note, 191
Project Implementation
    Plan, 192
Public Health Emergency of
    International Concern
    (PHEIC), 2, 144–45,
    147, 155
public-private partnership
    (PPP)
and legitimacy of
    public-private
    partnerships, 16–18
and noncommunicable
    disease efforts, 206, 208
and polio eradication
    efforts, 215–16

and purpose of study, 21
and rise of public-private
    partnerships, 12–14
and source vs. channel
    funding, 86
and WHO reforms, 177
See also specific PPP names

(Red) program, 53, 68, 108–10,
    112, 138, 171
reform efforts
and financing functions,
    184–86
and the Gates Foundation,
    178, 181, 184
and Gavi, 166–70
and the Global Fund,
    170–77
and inclusion of nonstate
    actors, 178–82
and oversight, 183–84
and transparency,
    performance, and
    accountability, 182–83
and the WHO, 177–78,
    178–82, 182–83, 183–84,
    184–86, 186–88, 187, 188
and the World Bank,
    188–89, 189–90, 189–93,
    193–94, 194–96, 196–200
refugee health, 7–8
Reinicke, Wolfgang, 13
replenishment mechanisms
and dues vs. voluntary
    contributions, 88
and Gavi funding, 43–44,
    113
and Gavi governance, 132
and Global Fund funding,
    108, 111
and Global Fund's impact
    on aid landscape, 177
and IDA funding, 38, 100,
    102
and incentive structures,
    66–68
and shifts in governance
    structures, 53
and World Bank funding,
    99–101
and World Bank Group
    structure, 99
and World Bank reforms, 189

respiratory infections, 212
Rockefeller Foundation, 6, 77,
    166–67
Roll Back Malaria, 15, 37, 51,
    123, 136
Rotary International, 123, 214,
    215
rotavirus, 42
rule-making powers, 186
Russia, 5, 115, 116, 193, 194,
    228n9
Rwanda, 212

Sandberg, Kristin, 116
Sarbib, Jean-Louis, 195
Saudi Arabia, 193
Save the Children, x, 15, 17
Second Italian War, 5
selective primary care, 10
short message service (SMS),
    216
Sierra Leone, 198
smallpox eradication, 8, 215
Snidal, Duncan, 16, 25
South Africa, 16, 53, 87, 115,
    169, 189
Soviet Union, 8
Spain, 51, 95–96, 102, 109, 115
Sridhar, Devi, 59, 162
Strategic Investment Plan
    (SIP), 191, 260n100
sub-Saharan Africa, 14
Supari, Siti Fadillah, 164–65
Sustainable Development Goals
    (SDGs), 35, 209, 214
Sweden, 51, 95, 96, 102, 109,
    115, 206
Switzerland, 50, 206

Tanzania, 19
technical assistance
and changing role of
    nonstate actors, 119
and Gavi governance, 131
and Global Fund's impact
    on aid landscape, 173,
    176–77
and the Global Fund's
    mission, 44
and growth of public-
    private partnerships, 15
and "old" institutions, 108
and transparency, 146–47

technical assistance (*continued*)
  and WHO reforms, 188
  and World Bank funding,
    101
  and World Bank reforms,
    192
tetanus, 41, 167
text messaging, 216
Thailand, 53, 206
tobacco industry, 207
Trade-Related Aspects of
  Intellectual Property
  Rights (TRIPs), 16
traffic accidents, 3
transparency, 140–59, *155*,
  182–83
tuberculosis, 19, 20, 205
  and background of global
    health cooperation, 8, 11
  and changing WHO
    priorities, 35
  and critiques of "old
    actors," 40–41
  and the Global Fund,
    45–46, 53–54, 110
  and importance of
    governance, 3
  and information
    asymmetries, 70
  and transparency, 153
  and World Bank funding,
    106
  See also Global Fund to
    Fight AIDS, Tuberculosis
    and Malaria
2011 Report on Multilateral Aid
  (OECD), 29–30
typhus, 5

Uganda, 151, 206
UN Children's Emergency
  Fund (UNICEF)
  and background of global
    health cooperation, 9
  and Gavi governance, 131, *139*
  and Gavi grants, 55
  and Gavi's impact on aid
    landscape, 166–69
  and Gavi's mission, 41–43
  and the Global Fund's
    mission, 44–45
  and growth of public-private
    partnerships, 14–15

and incentive structures, 65
and influence of the Gates
  Foundation, 76
and mechanics of
  international
  cooperation, 26
and polio eradication
  efforts, 214–15
and shifts in governance
  structures, 51, *52*
and source vs. channel
  funding, 86–87
and transparency, 145
and WHO funding, 92
and WHO reforms, 178
UN Development Programme
  (UNDP), 15, 26, 54, 93,
  117, 166, 207
UN Educational, Scientific
  and Cultural
  Organization
  (UNESCO), 26
UN Food Programme (WFP),
  26, 92
UN General Assembly, 90
UN Human Settlements
  Programme (UN-
  HABITAT), 64–65
UN Industrial Development
  Organization (UNIDO),
  64
UN Interagency Working
  Group on Child
  Mortality Estimation
  (UN-IGME), 167–68
UN International Strategy for
  Disaster Risk Reduction
  (UNISDR), 64–65
United Kingdom (UK)
  and alignment of global
    health objectives,
    62–63
  bilateral vs. multilateral aid,
    27, *28*
  and consolidation of
    influence, 203
  and DAH funding, 84
  Department for
    International
    Development (DFID),
    13, 63, 65, 72, 75
  and development assistance
    for health funding, *29*

and dues vs. voluntary
  contributions, 87
and Gavi funding, *114*, 115,
  116
and Global Fund funding,
  109, 112
and IDA funding, *101*, *102*
and incentive structures,
  64–66
and mechanics of
  international
  cooperation, 23
and monitoring of global
  agencies, 72, 75
and noncommunicable
  disease efforts, 206
scope of global health aid, 28
and shifts in governance
  structures, 51
and transparency, 145, 149
UK Multilateral Aid
  Review, 64, 145
and WHO funding, *95*
and World Bank reforms, 193
United Nations (UN), 90, 186
United Nations Charter, 186
United States
  and alignment of global
    health objectives, 62
  and background of global
    health cooperation, 5–6,
    8–10
  bilateral vs. multilateral aid,
    27, *28*
  and changing accountability
    standards, 119
  and consequences of new
    institutional models, 163
  and consolidation of
    influence, 203
  and corporate sector
    funding, 247n69
  and development assistance
    for health funding, *29*
  and dues vs. voluntary
    contributions, 87
  and Gavi funding, *114*
  and Gavi's impact on aid
    landscape, 169
  and Global Fund funding,
    108, *109*, 112–13
  and Global Fund
    governance, 133, 135, 140

and Global Fund's impact
on aid landscape, 171,
173–74, 177
and the Global Fund's
mission, 44–45
and IDA funding, *101*
and incentive structures, 64,
66–68
and influence of the Gates
Foundation, 76–78
and mechanics of
international
cooperation, 23,
26–28
and monitoring of global
agencies, 72–74
and noncommunicable
disease efforts, 206
and pandemic preparedness,
213
scope of global health
aid, 28
and shifts in governance
structures, *51*
and source vs. channel
funding, 86–87
and transparency, 147, 159
and universal health
coverage efforts, 209
US Treasury, 86
voting power of, *194*
and WHO funding, 89,
90–91, 94–95, *95*
and WHO reforms, 187
and World Bank funding,
98–99, 100
and World Bank reforms,
193–94
Universal Declaration of
Human Rights, 186
universal health coverage, 22,
36, 195, 198–99, 204,
209–11
UN Office for the
Coordination of
Humanitarian Affairs
(OCHA) @@, 26
UN Office on Drugs and
Crime (UNODC), 26
UN Population Fund
(UNFPA), 14, 26, 76, 92
UN Programme on HIV/
AIDS (UNAIDS)

and alignment of global
health objectives, 61
and background of global
health cooperation, 11–12
and consequences of new
institutional models, 162
and Global Fund grants, 54
and Global Fund's Board
composition, 45
and Global Fund's impact
on aid landscape, 173–74
and growth of public-
private partnerships, 14
and influence of the Gates
Foundation, 76
and mechanics of
international
cooperation, 25–26
and rise of public-private
partnerships, 13
and shifts in governance
structures, 50, *51*
and WHO funding, 95
and WHO reforms, 178
UN Refugee Agency
(UNHCR), 26, 117
UN Resolution 1308, 211
USAID, 14, 172
US Centers for Disease
Control (CDC), 117, 163,
214, 215
US Congress, 19, 61, 67, 87, 90
US Government
Accountability Office
(GAO), 72
US Presidential Emergency
Plan For AIDS Relief
(PEPFAR)
and alignment of global
health objectives, 62
and data sources, 228n64
and Gavi's impact on aid
landscape, 168
and Global Fund's impact
on aid landscape, 170–71
and Global Fund's mission,
45–46
and legitimacy of
public-private
partnerships, 17
and mechanics of
international
cooperation, 26

and purpose of study, 20
and universal health
coverage efforts, 211
and World Bank's
comparative advantage,
197
Uzbekistan, 149

vaccines
DPT$_3$ vaccine, 41–42
and the Gates Foundation,
78, 79
pentavalent vaccine, 41–43,
131, 151, 167, 227n53
pneumococcal vaccine, 167
vaccination rates, ix, 41, 167
vaccine gap, 16, 28, 40, 41
vaccine paradigm, 166
See also Global Alliance for
Vaccines and
Immunization (Gavi)
Vaubel, Roland, 30
vertical approach to
health-care challenges
and background of global
health cooperation, 8–12
and consequences of new
institutional models,
161–62
and DAH funding, 84
and Gavi governance, 131–32
and importance of
governance, 4
and influence of the Gates
Foundation, 77–79, 81
and pandemic preparedness,
212–13
and shifts in governance
structures, 52
trend toward vertical
initiatives, *55*, 56
and universal health
coverage efforts, 210
vertical trust funds, 213
and World Bank funding,
104
and World Bank practices,
39
and World Bank's
comparative advantage,
196–98
See also horizontal approach
to health-care challenges

Vietnam, 147
voluntary contributions
and alignment of global
health objectives, 60
and background of global
health cooperation, 12
and consequences of new
institutional models, 162
and Global Fund funding,
108, 111
and incentive structures, 65,
67
and influence of the Gates
Foundation, 76, 81
and shifts in governance
structures, 53
vs. membership dues, 87–88
and WHO funding, 89–90,
92, 94–97, 95, 96
and WHO governance,
122–23
and WHO reforms, 185–86
and World Bank funding,
99

Wall Street Journal, 175
Walt, Gill, 13
West Africa, 211
WHO Framework
Convention on Tobacco
Control, 162–63, 187, 207
Widdus, Roy, 14
William H. Gates Foundation,
76
Woods, Ngaire, xi, 59, 162, 192
World Bank
advantage as economic
institution, 196–200
and alignment of global
health objectives,
61–63
and background of global
health cooperation, 10
Bangladesh Integrated
Nutrition Project, 190–91
and the case for good
governance, 202–4
and case study methods,
38–39, 46
challenges and reform
proposals, 188–200
and changing accountability
standards, 120–21

Civil Society Policy Forum,
126, 127–29
commitments and
disbursements over
time, 103
composition of governing
board, 57
and composition of
governing boards, 59
and composition of HNP
commitments, 105
and consequences of new
institutional models,
161–63, 165
cooperation with civil
society, 126–29
and critiques of the WHO,
35–37
and DAH funding, 86
and dues vs. voluntary
contributions, 87
funding for global health
efforts, 97–107, 98
and funding for global
health initiatives, 97–107
and funding shifts, 33
and Gavi funding, 113
and Gavi governance, 130,
139
and Gavi's impact on aid
landscape, 166, 168–69
and Gavi's mission, 41–43
Global Fund contrasted
with, 107–10
and Global Fund's impact
on aid landscape, 170, 173
and Global Fund's mission,
45
and global HIV/AIDS
battle, 25
governance structure of, 137
and growth of public-
private partnerships,
14–15
Health, Nutrition, and
Population Sector
Programme, 191
Health, Nutrition and
Population Global
Practice, 198
and IDA funding, 101, 102
and incentive structures,
64–67

Independent Inspection
Panel, 67, 74
influence of donor
countries, 40
and influence of the Gates
Foundation, 76, 81
and information
asymmetries, 69, 71
knowledge bank role,
194–96
and legitimacy of
public-private
partnerships, 17
loan approval process,
189–93
and loan approval process,
189–93
Matrix Programme Cycle,
191
and mechanics of
international
cooperation, 23
and membership standards
for multilaterals, 122
and monitoring of global
agencies, 74
Multi-Country HIV/AIDS
Program (MAP), 25, 39, 62
and noncommunicable
disease efforts,
206–7
Open Contracting, 148
and pandemic preparedness,
212–13
Pandemic Preparedness
Financing Facility,
212–13
policy lending, 196
and polio eradication
efforts, 215
Pre-Appraisal Mission,
191–92
Preparation Mission, 191
principal-agent perspective
on, 30, 32–33
Project Appraisal, 192
project lending, 196
and purpose of study, 20,
21–22
Quality Assurance Group
(QAG), 192
Quality Enhancement
Review (QER), 191–92

and revolutionizing global
aid, 18–19
and shifts in governance
structures, 48–50, 51, 52,
53–55
and stakeholder
engagement, 159–60
and transparency, 141–42,
144, 145–46, 147–50,
150–52, 156, 159, 193–94
and trend toward vertical
initiatives, 55
voting power of member
countries, 194
and WHO funding, 97
and WHO reforms, 178, 183
and World Bank Group
structure, 99
and World Bank reforms, 195
World Bank Strategy, 104
See also International Bank
for Reconstruction and
Development (IBRD)
World Bank Group, 38, 49–50,
98, 99, 106, 127, 137
World Bank Independent
Evaluation Group, 170
World Cancer Report, 36
World Development Report,
10
World Development Report:
Investing in Health, 104
World Health Assembly
and composition of
governing board, 56
and critiques of the WHO,
34–37
and incentive structures, 65
and monitoring of global
agencies, 73
and polio eradication
efforts, 214
and shifts in governance
structures, 49
and transparency, 144, 155
and universal health
coverage efforts, 209
and WHO funding, 90–91,
92–94, 95, 96, 97
and WHO governance,
122–24, 123, 136
and WHO reforms, 179,
183, 185

and World Bank
governance, 127
World Health Organization
(WHO)
and alignment of global
health objectives, 59–61
annual disbursements over
time, 104
and background of global
health cooperation, 6, 8–12
and the case for good
governance, 202–4
and case study methods,
34–38, 46
and changing accountability
standards, 119–21
Commission on
Macroeconomics and
Health, 105
and composition of WHA
governing board, 56
conflict of interest, 180, 182
and consequences of new
institutional models, 162–65
and DAH funding, 86, 88–89
Department of
Immunization, Vaccines,
and Biologicals, 43
and dues vs. voluntary
contributions, 87–88
Emergency Committee, 144
Expanded Program on
Immunization, 41
extrabudgetary funding, 93
funding for, 89–97
and funding of global health
initiatives, 89–97
and Gates Foundation aid,
28
and Gavi funding, 116–18
and Gavi governance,
130–31, 139
and Gavi's impact on aid
landscape, 166–69
and Gavi's mission, 41–43
Global AIDS Programme, 60
Global Fund contrasted
with, 107–11
and Global Fund's impact
on aid landscape, 171,
174, 177
and Global Fund's mission,
44–45

Global Health Observatory
(GHO), 147
and growth of public-
private partnerships,
14–15, 16
and importance of
governance, 2, 4
and incentive structures,
63–65
influence of donor
countries, 40
and influence of the Gates
Foundation, 76–77, 81
and information
asymmetries, 69–71
Intensified Malaria
Eradication
Programme, 92
Intensified Smallpox
Eradication
Programme, 92
law-making powers, 187
and mechanics of
international
cooperation, 23, 25–26
membership and
governance of, 122–26
membership policy, 136
and monitoring of global
agencies, 73–75
and noncommunicable
disease efforts, 205–7
and ODA trends, 200
Onchocerciasis Control
Programme, 17, 106, 200
Pandemic Influenza
Preparedness
Framework, 188
and pandemic preparedness,
212–14
and polio eradication
efforts, 214–15
principal-agent perspective
on, 30, 32–33
and purpose of study, 20,
21–22
Regional Committees, 73
and revolutionizing global
aid, 18–19
and rise of public-private
partnerships, 13
and shifts in disbursements,
33

World Health Organization
   (WHO) (*continued*)
   and shifts in governance
      structures, 48–56, *51*, *52*
   and stakeholder
      engagement, 159–60
   and transparency, 141–42,
      143–47, 150–52, 154,
      155, 159
   and trend toward vertical
      initiatives, *55*
   and universal health
      coverage efforts, 209

voluntary contributions, *96*
WHO Centre for
   Emergency Preparedness
   and Response, 213
and WHO reforms,
   178–88
and World Bank funding,
   97–100, 105, 107
and World Bank
   governance, 126–27,
   129
and World Bank practices,
   38–39

World Health Organization
   Constitution,
   186
World War II, 8

yellow fever, 5, 6, 42
Yip, 2

Zacher, Mark, 17
Zambia, 68, 151
Zika virus, 1–2, 144, 200, 202,
   215–16
Zoellick, Bob, 190